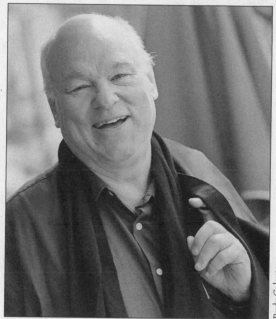

Rudy Gelenter

about the author

JOHN BAXTER is an acclaimed film critic and biographer whose subjects have included Woody Allen, Steven Spielberg, Stanley Kubrick, and Robert De Niro. The co-director of the Paris Writers' Workshop, he also is the author of *Immoveable Feast: A Paris Christmas*, *We'll Always Have Paris*, and *A Pound of Paper: Confessions of a Book Addict* and the translator of Harper Perennial's Naughty French Novels series. Mr. Baxter lives in Paris.

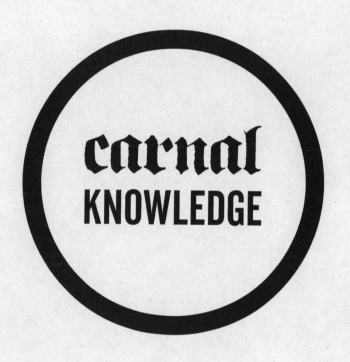

Also by John Baxter

Immoveable Feast

We'll Always Have Paris

A Pound of Paper

Science Fiction in the Cinema

The Cinema of Josef Von Sternberg

Luis Buñuel

Fellini

Stanley Kubrick

Steven Spielberg

Woody Allen

George Lucas

Robert De Niro

Baxter's Concise Encyclopedia of Modern Sex

John Baxter

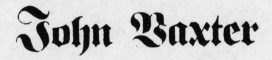

HARPER ⬤ PERENNIAL

NEW YORK • LONDON • TORONTO • SYDNEY • NEW DELHI • AUCKLAND

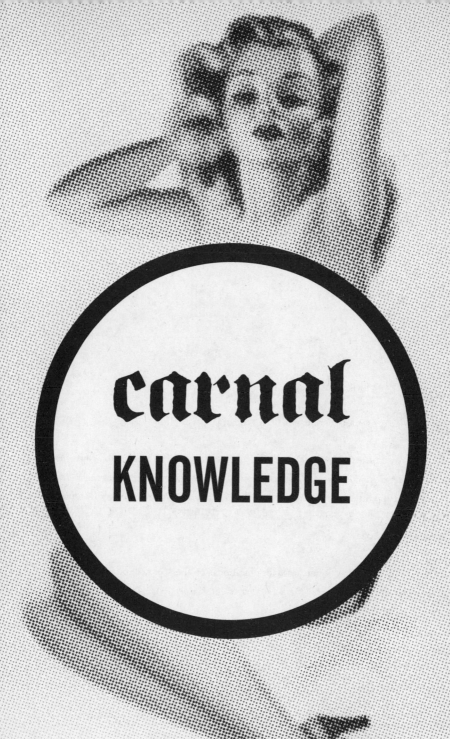

HARPER ● PERENNIAL

HarperCollins books may be purchased for educational, business, or sales promotional use. For information please write: Special Markets Department, HarperCollins Publishers, 10 East 53rd Street, New York, NY 10022.

FIRST EDITION

Designed by Justin Dodd

Library of Congress Cataloging-in-Publication Data is available upon request.

ISBN 978-0-06-087434-6

09 10 11 12 13   OV/RRD   10 9 8 7 6 5 4 3 2 1

Preface

If there's nothing new under the sun, one would think there's even less new between the sheets. A kiss is still a kiss, a sigh still a sigh, whether a generation goes by or a millennium. So what can have happened in human sexuality during the last hundred years that makes it worth writing a book about?

In one sense, the skeptic would be right. Many of our sexual habits and customs are traceable back not just a hundred years but thousands. "Peeping Tom," the archetypal voyeur, lived—if he lived at all—about 1050. We still speak of teenage lovers in terms of Romeo and Juliet, when the real couple first emerged on the page in the thirteenth century. Blinded Oedipus still stalks the world of incest as he did centuries before Christ, and modern lesbians have kept Sappho alive as an entity and a symbol well after most of her poems have been lost.

A pimp is still, as he was in the time of Elizabeth I, a pimp, and a bordello—whether or not Shakespeare called it a "nunnery"—is still a bordello. The function of a modern vibrator would be readily recognizable to Boccacio, author of *The Decameron,* as it would to Vatsyayana, who compiled the *Kama Sutra.* Nor, for all the talk of "sex workers," are we unaware of what Thomas Ryder meant when, in 1715, he wrote, "I was very warm with drinking wine and had a mighty inclination to fill a whore's commodity."

Some things don't change—but many do. And this book is about those things in the world of sexual sensation that the years since 1900 have transformed, rediscovered, or renewed.

The twentieth century brought us plastics and the movies, electronics and aircraft, cheap printing, the Internet, refrigeration, and automobiles—all of which had their impact on that universe of the mind and body we call "sex."

Far more influential, however, than the technical advances of the last hundred years were those in the areas of society. The twentieth century, rightly called "the century of the common man," didn't so much introduce new modes of sensual satisfaction as make available to everyone those pleasures that for centuries the rich had reserved for themselves.

If this compilation has one lesson to teach, it is that while sex has changed in matters of detail and degree, in its essentials it has remained very much the same. The song was right. The fundamental things apply as time goes by.

Author's Note

Entries in all capital letters indicate a separate entry devoted to that person or topic.

AC/DC (American slang, 1960s-present). Bisexual.

A pun on the common term for the two types of electricity, alternating current and direct current.

ADLER, Pearl "Polly" (1900-1962). U.S. brothel owner.

Adler emigrated from Russia as a teenager. By her early twenties, she was leasing Manhattan apartments and stocking them with girls, good liquor, and even books. Clients didn't come just for sex, but also to talk, drink, play backgammon or cards, or join Adler's all-night parties. Horny playwright George S. Kaufman ran a tab. Robert Benchley sometimes went there to write his reviews, and drink with Dorothy Parker. Both comic MILTON BERLE and actor JOHN GARFIELD were clients. "The world knew Polly as a madam," said Berle, "but her friends knew her as an intelligent woman, fun to be with, and a good cook."

During the 1929 stock market crash, ruined brokers visited Adler's establishment for a last fling before jumping out of their windows. In 1930, Adler refused to inform on her many mobster friends to the Seabury Commission on police and judicial corruption, and was put out of business. She retired to Los Angeles in 1943, earned a college degree, and in 1953 published a bestselling memoir, *A House Is Not a Home*. Shelley Winters played her in a dismal 1964 film version.

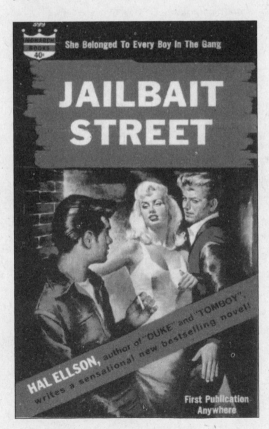

She Belonged To Every Boy In The Gang

JAILBAIT STREET

HAL ELLSON, author of "DUKE" and "TOMBOY" writes a sensational new bestselling novel

First Publication Anywhere

AGE OF CONSENT. The age at which a person can legally consent to sex.

The age of consent varies between countries. Some nations forbid sex completely outside marriage. Many Anglo-Saxon countries choose sixteen, though there are variations— sometimes, as in Australia, between individual states. In certain countries, different ages apply for men and women, for gay sex, and for anal and vaginal intercourse, while Finland requires only that "there is no great difference in the ages or the mental and physical maturity of the persons involved." Norway also demands that the couple be "about equal in age and development." Germany allows sex at age fourteen, provided the older partner is under eighteen and not "exploiting a coercive situation" or paying. In Japan, the age of consent is technically thirteen, but individual prefectures often ignore this, preferring eighteen.

Songs and jokes of the 1920s and 1930s often turned on the attractions of very young women, frequently from rural societies—hence stories involving a FARMER'S DAUGHTER, and the popularity of books such as Erskine Caldwell's *God's Little Acre*, about child brides in the Deep South. Since anyone having sex with a minor risked a charge of "statutory rape," a nubile underage woman became known as "jailbait." One song celebrated "The sweetest l'il gal to come from a cotton field / Rather make love than eat a decent meal / She's jailbait . . ."

While it was far from unknown for older women to pleasure themselves with young men, such situations turned up far less in Anglo-Saxon literature than in more cosmopolitan France, where they became in particular a specialty of Colette, author of the *Cheri* series, about a middle-aged woman and her TOY BOY, and of *Le Blé en Herbe*, in which a worldly mondaine on a summer holiday initiates a local sixteen-year-old.

ALSO
AGE OF CONSENT (1938). Australian novel by Norman Lindsay.

On a rural painting expedition, a middle-aged artist meets an adolescent girl who becomes his model and lover. The book was published in Britain, but banned in Australia until 1962.

AGE OF CONSENT (1969). Australian/UK film. Directed by Michael Powell. James Mason played the painter, and Helen Mirren, then a mature twenty-four, his model. See also *LOLITA;* LORDS, Traci.

AIDS. Acquired immune deficiency syndrome. Health condition caused by the human immunodeficiency virus, or HIV, which lowers the body's capacity to resist infection.

First officially recognized in 1981, AIDS has been traced back to the 1950s. Though its source is still contested, the virus may have migrated from certain West African primates. Responsibility may even lie with SERGE VORONOFF, who experimented in 1920s Paris with transplanting organs between monkeys and humans.

AIDS is most readily transmitted during anal sex, making the male gay community uniquely vulnerable. For some time before the virus was isolated, its existence fostered rumors of a "gay plague." Subsequently, it became clear that all members of society were at risk. In January 2006, the Joint United Nations Programme on HIV/AIDS and the World Health Organization estimated that AIDS has killed more than 25 million people. The impact is greatest in Africa, where the disease was initially spread along the main trade routes by truck drivers and the prostitutes they patronized. It has since become epidemic among the general population, exacerbated by the common disinclination to use CONDOMS, the absence of effective and consistent medication, the proliferation of quack remedies, and the publicly expressed skepticism of certain African leaders that AIDS and HIV are connected.

In developed countries, AIDS induced fundamental changes in sexual practice that favored MASTURBATION, VOYEURISM, BONDAGE, and other forms of nonpenetrative intercourse. In particular, it hastened the rise of INTERNET PORNOGRAPHY and PHONE SEX.

Most art dealing with or inspired by AIDS has concentrated on the gay community or emanated from it. It includes *Angels in America: A Gay Fantasia on National Themes* (1990), by Tony Kushner, comprising two plays, *Millennium Approaches* and *Perestroika*, which were conflated and filmed by Mike Nichols in 2003; *Philadelphia* (1993), directed by Jonathan Demme, in which Tom Hanks plays an AIDS-afflicted lawyer successfully fighting his wrongful dismissal; the AIDS Memorial Quilt, begun in 1987 and now comprising forty thousand panels, each memorializing a victim; and *And the Band Played On: Politics, People,and the AIDS Epidemic*, a 1987 book by Randy Shilts excoriating the sluggish social, medical, and political response to the disease. See VORONOFF, Serge Abrahamovitch.

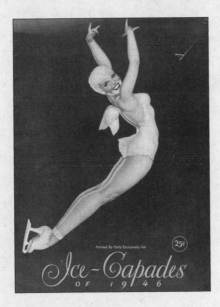

FRANK PETTY AIRBRUSHED PINUP

AIRBRUSH. Illustrator's tool that uses a compressor to distribute a fine mist of paint over precise areas.

Before computer programs such as Photoshop, the airbrush was an essential tool of illustrators and picture retouchers. It expunged pubic hair and genitalia from nude photographs, eradicated blemishes, and peeled fat from waists and chins. Artists such as Emilio Vargas and Frank Petty also used it to create original work, since its smooth fields of color and subtle gradations were ideal for PINUPS.

AIRCRAFT.

"The wish to fly," wrote SIGMUND FREUD in 1910, "is a longing to be capable of sexual performance." As soon as aircraft had room for passengers, aviators explored the machines' sexual potential. The first authenticated case of sex in powered flight dates from November 1916. New York socialite Mrs. Waldo Polk was enjoying a "flying lesson" with handsome aviator Lawrence Sperry when she spasmodically bumped the controls, and the Curtiss floatplane plunged five hundred feet into South Bay. Though neither passenger was harmed, duck hunters who dragged Polk and Sperry from the wreck found them naked. Undeterred, Mrs. Polk continued lessons, and won her license. Sperry, before his early death at thirty-one, invented that crucial aid to airborne sex, the automatic pilot.

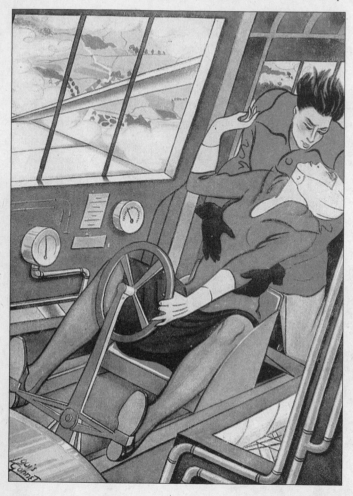

FRENCH CARTOON OF THE 1920s ILLUSTRATING THE AMOROUS TEMPTATIONS OF AVIATION

Post–World War I, ex-fighter pilots bought war surplus fighters and "barnstormed" across the United States, giving shows by day and sheltering themselves and their planes in barns by night. Heroic figures to the girls who staggered away, weak-kneed, from their first aptly named "joy ride," these men coaxed some into becoming "wing walkers," climbing out on to the wings in flight to do gymnastics or even play musical instruments. The 1933 musical *Flying Down to Rio* culminates in an aerial leg show, with chorus girls dancing on wings and having their costumes whipped off by the slipstream.

The reality is shown more graphically in *The Great Waldo Pepper* (1975), where a girl trying a similar stunt loses her clothes and her life.

World War II offered few opportunities for airborne fornication, though in Steven Spielberg's *1941* (1979), Nancy Allen plays a girl who finds flight an aphrodisiac, a fact exploited by Tim Matheson as a horny captain. That sex was frequently on the minds of fliers, however, was evident from the PINUPS painted on the noses of USAF bombers. A widespread and false rumor suggested that a sexy image of actress Rita Hayworth decorated the nose of the *Enola Gay*, which dropped the first nuclear bomb on Hiroshima, or even the bomb itself. However, a photograph of Hayworth was in fact pasted to the first postwar bomb to be exploded at Bikini Atoll in 1946.

The golden age of airborne sex arrived in the mid-1950s, with CinemaScope. In 1963, *Come Fly with Me* showed most of the clichés already in place: horny or larcenous passengers date complaisant stewardesses eager for sex or marriage. In 1965, publicist Mary Wells, revamping struggling Braniff International, dressed its stewardesses in outfits by Emilio Pucci. "When a tired businessman gets on an airplane," Wells explained, "we think he ought to be allowed to look at a pretty girl." Overnight, women who'd been dismissed as little more than airborne waitresses were transformed into the figures of sexual legend celebrated in Trudy Baker and Rachel Jones's 1967 book *Coffee, Tea or Me?* Braniff depicted one murmuring, "I'm Mandy. Fly me." In the early 1970s, Southwest put their stewardesses into HOT PANTS and white go-go boots, and adopted the motto "Sex Sells Seats."

Soon, passengers no longer had to delay sexual satisfaction until landing. In 1974, SYLVIA KRISTEL enjoyed two lascivious interludes en route to Bangkok in *EMMANUELLE*—parodied in the porn feature *THE OPENING OF MISTY BEETHOVEN*, where passengers are offered a choice between "First Class with Sex" and "First Class Non-Sex." In Bob Fosse's 1979 *All That Jazz*, Roy Scheider's pill-popping choreographer, creating a musical number about flight, drives his dancers into a frenzy of aerial erotica, making an aircraft resemble a flying brothel.

Flight crews weren't slow to realize that the option of cruise boat staff to have "a girl in every port" now extended to them as well. The comic possibilities were thoroughly explored in Marc Camoletti's play *Boeing Boeing*, about a Paris bachelor juggling three flying "fiancées." In 1963's *Sunday in New York*, pilot Cliff Robertson and his stewardess mistress chase each other around the country, never both in any city at the same time. Steven Spielberg's *Catch Me If You Can* shows con man Leonardo DeCaprio impersonating a pilot and exploiting the sexual opportunities of the position. However, the most poignant evocation of the emotional aridity of modern aviation remains Steven Sondheim's song "Barcelona," for his musical *Company*, where a man coaxes his stewardess one-night-stand to skip her flight to the Spanish city and stay in his bed. See also MILE-HIGH CLUB.

ALBERT. Metal chain with a crosspiece at one end, used to secure a pocket watch to a Victorian gentleman's waistcoat.

Named for Prince Albert, husband of Queen Victoria, who would Not Be Amused to find the Albert latterly popular with PIERCING enthusiasts, who threaded similar chains through a pierced penis. See AMPALLANG; PIERCING.

ALCOHOL.

"Candy is dandy / But liquor is quicker," wrote U.S. poet Ogden Nash. (He might have continued, "Though a pill or joint / Does not disappoint.") The twentieth century did not discover alcohol's erotic effects; it only saw the invention of new and more potent mixtures to disguise, delay, or accelerate them. Alcoholic oblivion was widely exploited to excuse sexual lapses, both of performance and of control. Matt Crowley's 1968 play *The Boys in the Band* attacked closeted gays who indulged their homoerotic inclinations and then protested, "I was *so* drunk last night."

Despite claims as early as 1903 that "ABSINTHE Makes the Heart Grow Fonder," the liquor most often associated with decadence was actually—like its fashionable companion OPIUM—a sexual suppressant. Still, many seducers swore by the nose-tickling effects of champagne, and the British comedy duo of Michael Flanders and Donald Swann persuasively celebrated the aphrodisiac value of sweet dessert wines in their song *Have Some Madeira, M'dear,* but the preferred "LEG OPENER" was, and remains, gin. See BREWER'S DROOP.

ALLBRITTON, Cynthia. See "CYNTHIA PLASTER CASTER."

ALLEN, Woody (né Allan Stewart Konigsberg) (1935–). U.S. writer, film director, and performer.

For years, Allen was credited with joking that if he were to be reincarnated, he'd like it to be as the fingertips of Warren Beatty. While he denied having said this ("although I could have"), Allen had much in common with arch-seducer Beatty—including Diane Keaton, a sometime mistress of both men. Vicky Tiel, the costume designer whom Allen failed to seduce during production in Paris of *What's New Pussy-*

cat, remarked, "The girls that would go with Woody are the same that would go with Warren, because they were interested in being with men that are successful. But with Warren they would fall in love with him because he would dominate them sexually, and Woody couldn't."

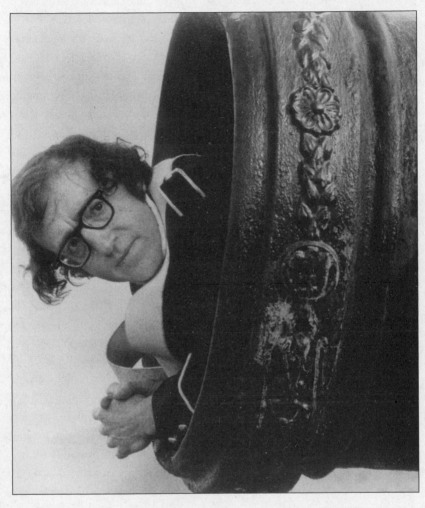

WOODY ALLEN ABOUT TO BE BLOWN OUT OF A CANNON IN HIS NAPOLEONIC COMEDY *LOVE AND DEATH*

Audiences habitually confused the real actor-director with the "Woody" character of his films, a weedy, aging social and sexual failure, chronically self-aware, who succeeds by playing on the appeal of his timidity. The real Allen was reflected more accurately by *Manhattan*, in which his scruffy New York TV writer is harried by a bisexual ex-wife as he pursues the mistress of his best friend and shares the bed of a beautiful high school girl—the latter based on Stacey Nelkin, the teenager with whom he was at that time having an affair. Allen even used the film to advertise the sexual appeal of men like him. When he and Keaton encounter the latter's ex-husband, described by her as a dynamic eroticist who "opened her up" to sex, it amused Allen to choose for the part the tubby, balding but effortlessly articulate Wallace Shawn.

Allen met his equal in self-absorption when he took Mia Farrow as a mistress in 1980. He was unprepared to deal with her complex sexual history and her eccentric activities as a "gatherer" of orphan children. The revelation of his affair with the oldest of these, Soon-Yi Previn, via a set of pornographic POLAROIDS, led to a public brawl, with unsupported allegations from Farrow of child abuse and resulting damage to Allen's public persona.

These bruising experiences confirmed Allen as the preeminent chronicler of mid-century Manhattan's sexual habits. His fascination with infidelity among the chattering classes (particularly affairs between wised-up middle-aged intellectuals and manipulative young women) and his preoccupation with call girls and prostitutes underscore a lubricious, if often weary, acceptance of sex as one of the few pleasures that matter. In the words of his character in *Stardust Memories*, "Sex without love is an empty experience—but as empty experiences go, it's one of the best."

AMPALLANG.

Barbell-shaped metal rod inserted horizontally through a hole pierced in the penis, usually transecting the glans, or head, but sometimes the shaft itself. A vertical piercing through the penis is known as an *apadravya*. See PIERCING.

AMPUTATION.

Whether elective amputation for sexual reasons represents a genuinely erotic impulse or a psychotic one is still debated. There is anecdotal evidence of masochists having themselves castrated as the extremity of satisfaction, and some S&M groups routinely mime the act, using a hot or cold knife to mimic the effect of a cut.

Elective amputation of other body parts is more common. Victims of the condition known as body dysmorphia (also known as body integrity identity disorder) become convinced that a limb—usually a leg below the knee—"no longer belongs" to them. Surgeons are sometimes persuaded to amputate, and in a few cases, subjects have attempted the surgery themselves. The ultimate amputation fantasy is Bernard Wolfe's 1952 novel *Limbo*, about a future in which voluntary amputees, or "vol-amps," have all their limbs replaced by computerized prosthetics. See AUTO-FELLATIO.

ANAL PENETRATION.

The practice of forcing foreign objects into the rectum, always popular as an adjunct to masturbation, increased in popularity as the industrial revolution offered items machined to a tempting smoothness. United States emergency rooms have extracted at various times a bottle of Mrs. Butterworth's syrup, an ax handle, a 9-inch zucchini, countless dildoes and vibrators, including one 14-inch model complete with two D-cell batteries, a plastic spatula, a 9 1/2-inch water bottle, a deodorant bottle, a Coke bottle, a 3 1/2-inch Japanese glass float ball, an 11-inch carrot, an antenna rod, a 150-watt light bulb, a 100-watt frosted bulb, a cucumber, a screwdriver, four rubber balls, 72 jeweller's saws, a paperweight, an apple, an onion, a plastic toothbrush package, two bananas, a frozen pig's tail (it got stuck when it thawed), a 10-inch length of broomstick, an 18-inch umbrella handle and central rod, a plantain encased in a condom, two Vaseline jars, a whisky bottle with a cord attached, a teacup, an oil can, a 6-by-5-inch tool case weighing 22 ounces, a 6-inch stone weighing two pounds (in the latter two cases, the patients died due to intestinal obstruction), a baby powder can, a test tube, a ball-point pen, a peanut butter jar, candles, baseballs, a sand-filled bicycle inner tube, sewing needles, a flashlight, a half-filled tobacco pouch, a turnip, a pair of eyeglasses, a hard-boiled egg, a carborundum grindstone (with handle), a suitcase key, a syringe, a file, tumblers and glasses, a polyethylene waste trap from the U-bend of a sink, and much, much more. In 1955, one man who confessed to "feeling depressed" inserted the paper tube from a roll of kitchen paper into his rectum, dropped in a lighted firecracker, and blew a hole in his anterior rectal wall. See also GERBILS; FISTING.

ANDERS ALS DIE ANDERN (Not Like the Others). German film (1919). Directed by Richard Oswald.

The earliest film to deal with homosexuality, which was criminalized at the time in Germany under Paragraph 175 of the country's Criminal Code. In one sequence, famous homosexuals from history parade past a banner reading "Paragraph 175," each one shrinking from it.

In a plot almost identical to VICTIM, set in Britain half a century later, a concert violinist becomes the lover of a young student, and is blackmailed by another gay man. Rather than pay, the musician publicly reveals his homosexuality and, with his career ruined, kills himself.

ANDERS ALS DIE ANDERN was co-written by the director and sexologist MAGNUS HIRSCHFELD (who also appears in an epilogue). Its many references to CROSS-DRESSING reflect Hirschfeld's theory that homosexuals were simply heterosexuals handicapped by an excess of female hormones. The film's blackmailer frequents a DRAG club, and there are documentary sequences on transvestism, a word coined by Hirschfeld, illustrated by items from the latter's Berlin sexology institute. Bisexual dancer ANITA BERBER also has a small role.

"The great film star sat apart at his own table, impeccable in evening tails. He watched the dancing benevolently through his monocle as he sipped champagne and smoked a cigarette in a long holder. He seemed a supernatural figure, the guardian god of these festivities, who was graciously manifesting himself to his devotees."

—CHRISTOPHER ISHERWOOD ON CONRAD VEIDT AT BERLIN'S ANNUAL CHRISTMAS DRAG BALL

To evade censorship, Oswald made forty copies of ANDERS ALS DIE ANDERN, shipping them simultaneously all over Germany. The authorities quickly restricted access to the film to physicians and court-appointed lawyers. Subsequently, the Nazis destroyed most prints, and no complete copy survives. See HIRSCHFELD, Magnus; BERBER, Anita.

ANGER, Kenneth (1927–). U.S. filmmaker and author.

Through his grandmother, a movie costume mistress, Anger was cast as the changeling boy in Max Reinhardt's 1935 *A Midsummer Night's Dream*. However, despite actorish good looks, he preferred directing to performing, claiming to have made his first movie at nine. He also discovered occultism, via Aleister Crowley, and while living in San Francisco, Paris, London, and Egypt, created a sporadic series of obscure but inspired short films, all displaying strong CAMP and mystical elements. They include *Fireworks* (1947), hailed by JEAN COCTEAU as issuing "from that beautiful night from which emerge all true works"; *Scorpio Rising* (1964); *Kustom Kar Kommandos* (1965); *Inauguration of the Pleasure Dome* (1969); *Invocation of My Demon Brother* (1969); and *Lucifer Rising* (1972). Anger also began a version of *HISTOIRE D'O*, but filmed only a few scenes. He is best known, however, as author-compiler of the book *HOLLYWOOD BABYLON*.

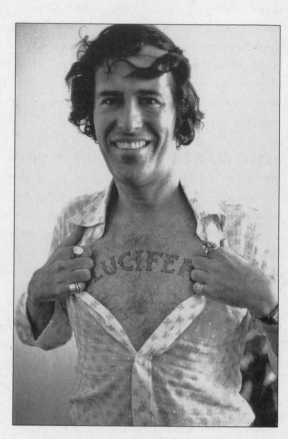

ANIME. Japanese animated films, often sado-erotic in nature.

ANSONIA HOTEL. See CONTINENTAL BATHS.

APACHE DANCING (pronounced "Apash") (1890s–1930s). Style of exhibition dancing, based on the French *java*, in which the male, dressed as a French street crook or *apache*, throws his sullen but adoring girlfriend around the floor.

APOLLINAIRE, Guillaume (Guillaume Albert Vladimir Apollinaire de Kostrowitzky) (1880–1918). French author.

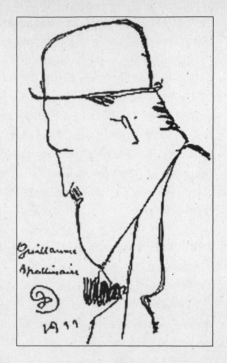

The illegitimate son of an Italian nobleman, Apollinaire kept his mother's name when he moved from Rome to Paris and launched himself as poet, playwright, art critic, champion of the avant garde, and both scholar and writer of pornography.

Plump, with a slightly comic moustache and a pipe usually clamped between his teeth, Apollinaire, despite his placid exterior, was fascinated with the outrageous and forbidden. In 1917, he would label his play *Les Mamelles de Tirésias* "surrealist," a term adopted by André Breton and his followers.

"Artists," Apollinaire wrote, "are, above all, men who want to become inhuman." His first pornographic novel, *Mirely, ou le petit trou pas cher* (*Mirely, or the Inexpensive Little Hole*), is lost. In 1907 he published two, *Les Exploits d'un jeune Don Juan* (aka *Amorous Exploits of a Young Rakehell*) and *Les Onze mille verges* (aka *The Debauched Hospodar*).

Rakehell, despite its flamboyant title, recounts a gently traditional story, probably autobiographical, of a boy's sexual initiation in the family chateau, starting with erections in the bath, but graduating to sex with his sister and aunt. By contrast, *Hospodar* has been called "a brilliant fantasy in which all the demons of some insane Sadeian hell are unleashed." The hero, Mony Vibescu, is a horny Rumanian "Hospodar," or prince, who fights and fornicates his way from Bucharest to Paris and finally Port Arthur, in China, where, in 1904, he continues between battles in the Russo-Japanese War. Few sexual activities are left undescribed. Many are morbid: a Russian general sodomizes a Chinese boy, and a medical orderly fellates a dying soldier whose legs and arms have been blown off.

Volunteering for the French Army, Apollinaire sustained a head wound in 1916, and never fully recovered. He supported himself with journalism, and by writing introductions, compiling bibliographies, and sometimes discreetly expurgating the reprints of porn classics. He died of influenza in 1918. In 1953, the OLYMPIA PRESS published a vigorous translation of *Verges* that skillfully showcased its comic violence. Credited to "Oscar Mole," it was actually by the Scots Beat poet Alexander Trocchi.

APPLEGATE, Colleen (aka Shauna Grant, Callie Aimes) (1963–1984).
U.S. actress.

Cheerleader Applegate ran away with her boyfriend from Farmington, Minnesota to Los Angeles in 1982. She appeared over the next two years in thirty porn films, as "Callie Aimes" in *The Young Like It Hot* and *Feels Like Silk*, then as "Shauna Grant" in, among others, *Summer Camp Girls, Valley Vixen, Suzie Superstar,* and *Virginia,* her last film. She earned, she claimed, $100,000 in her two-year career. Most of it, however, went toward cocaine. When her lover was arrested in March 1984, Colleen, then living with her mother in Palm Springs, killed herself from a shotgun blast to the head. She was twenty. Her story was told in the films *Death of a Porn Queen; Shauna Grant, Superstar;* and *Shattered Innocence.*

ARBUCKLE, Roscoe "Fatty" (aka William Goodrich) (1897–1933). U.S. actor/director.

Despite weighing three hundred pounds, Roscoe Arbuckle was an inspired physical comedian who turned his improbable athleticism into a $1 million-a-year movie career. On September 5, 1921, he drove with friends to San Francisco for Labor Day weekend. The group checked into the St. Francis Hotel, where Arbuckle's friend Bambina Maude Delmont provided alcohol and put out a call for PARTY GIRLS. Those who responded included Virginia Rappe, a minor actress who'd worked with Arbuckle in Hollywood but who'd blighted her career by spreading a sexual disease through the studio.

Hours later, with everyone drunk and partly undressed—Arbuckle wore pajamas and a robe—Rappe fled the party. She subsequently died of peritonitis from a ruptured bladder, probably related to her infection. Delmont, who had convictions for blackmail and extortion, saw the possibility of profit and proposed to Arbuckle's lawyers that she hush up the story in return for a bribe. They refused, since the coroner who autopsied Rappe was emphatic that he found "no marks of violence on the body . . . no evidence of a criminal assault, no signs that the girl had been attacked in any way."

Delmont then offered to invent a crime if the price was right. District Attorney Matthew Brady, planning to run for governor, saw the news value of such a high-profile case, and paid up. Testifying before the grand jury, Delmont claimed that Arbuckle spent an hour alone with Rappe, who then fled, screaming of rape. Quickly leaked, the lie started new rumors that Arbuckle, too drunk to get an erection, had raped Rappe with a Coca Cola bottle—or maybe a champagne bottle—or perhaps a piece of ice. Alternatively, his penis was so big that he did the damage himself. None were true, but on September 17, Brady arraigned Arbuckle on rape and murder charges.

Though studio head Adolph Zukor paid for the best defense, newspaper publisher William Randolph Hearst, who backed Brady's ambitions, pilloried Arbuckle in his rags. Hearst later boasted that the case "sold more newspapers than any event since the sinking of the *Lusitania.*"

Arbuckle endured three trials before being acquitted of all charges. However, the public preferred to believe that the funny fat man had raped the poor starlet, and refused to watch Arbuckle again onscreen. He found work as a comedy director under the name William Goodrich, and was set to make a comeback when he died of a heart attack at age forty-six.

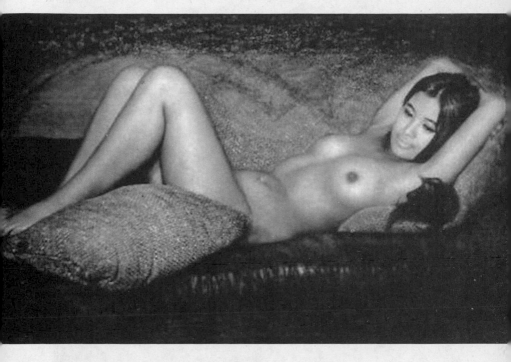

EMMANUELLE ARSAN PHOTOGRAPHED BY PIERRE MOLINIER

ARSAN, Emmanuelle (aka ROLLET-ANDRIANE, Maryat, aka BIBIDH, Maryat) (193?–).

Every French literary season brings its sexual page-turner, but few had the impact of a pale green paperback issued by Éric Losfeld in the spring of 1959, and called simply *Emmanuelle*. The novel was supposedly the fictionalized memoirs of Emmanuelle Arsan, a twenty-year-old innocent who followed Jean, her older and more sexually experienced diplomat husband, to Bangkok, where she plunged into a life of group sex and lesbianism.

Even more exciting to readers than its echoes of France's lost colonial empire was the revelation, carefully leaked by Losfeld, that a real French diplomatic wife wrote *Emmanuelle*. De Gaulle's government banned the book as yet another slur on a foreign service already battered by the gay confessions of Roger Peyrefitte in *Les Ambassades*. Although Grove Press's U.S. edition made it an international bestseller, the novel remained illegal in France until 1992.

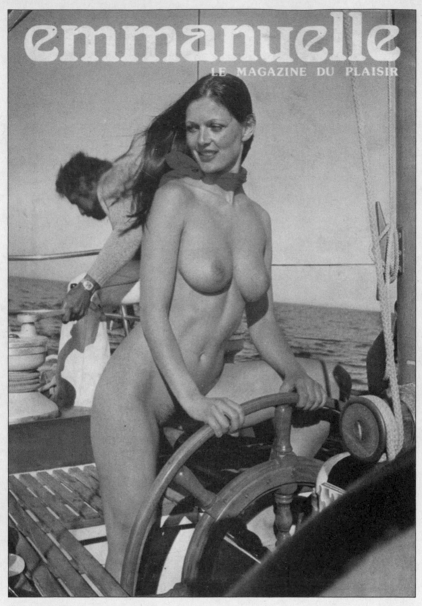

emmanuelle
LE MAGAZINE DU PLAISIR

MAGAZINE NAMED FOR THE ARSAN CHARACTER

Losfeld let the public visualize Arsan as a pale white ingenue as embodied in the 1974 film by Dutch model SYLVIA KRISTEL. Yet the real Emmanuelle was neither white nor European but the daughter of a Thai politician and diplomat. Married to Louis Andriane, a Bangkok-based official of the Southeast Asia Treaty Organization, Arsan had a brief movie career as "Maryet Andriane," playing the Chinese slave-prostitute Mally opposite Richard Attenborough and Steve McQueen in Robert Wise's 1966 *The Sand Pebbles*.

Once Arsan was "outed," no exhibition of erotic art was complete without her patronage, and no new piece of up-market porn lacked her introduction, or at least a cover quote. She published five volumes of essays on sexual subjects and went into film production, after which she and her husband retired to rural France. In her absence, the name Emmanuelle lived on, adopted by a French magazine of soft-core erotica, and attached to numerous films, many with no connection to the original. See MOLINIER, Pierre; *EMMANUELLE*.

ARSE ANTLERS (Australian slang, present). Wide symmetrical tattoos on the small of the back, just above the crease of the buttocks.

ASHES HAULED, TO HAVE ONE'S (U.S. slang, 1930s–1970s). Unlovely simile for intercourse, which equates the satisfaction of sexual need with removing garbage. Equivalent terms include "to get laid" and the Australian "to get the dirty water off your chest."

AUDEN, W(ystan). H(ugh). (1907–1973). UK poet.

The reading of *Funeral Blues* by John Hannah at the memorial service for his lover in the 1994 film *Four Weddings and a Funeral* decisively confirmed the austere Auden as laureate of the gay community. Yet during his lifetime, his sexual preference remained, to a large extent, "the love that dare not speak its name." He was embarrassed enough about some of his homoerotic poems to change their "he" to "He," suggesting that Christ, and not some lover, had inspired them, and he never acknowledged authorship of "The Platonic Blow," a graphic 1948 evocation of a sexual encounter with one of the young working-class boys he favored.

> Well-hung, slung from the fork of the muscular legs,
> The firm vase of his sperm like a bulging pear,
> Cradling its handsome glands, two herculean eggs,
> Swung as he came towards me, shameless, bare.
> We aligned mouths. We entwined. All act was clutch,
> All fact, contact, the attack and the interlock
> Of tongues, the charms of arms. I shook at the touch
> Of his fresh flesh. I rocked at the shock of his cock.
> —FROM "THE PLATONIC BLOW," ATTRIBUTED TO W. H. AUDEN

AU PAIR (1950s–present). French for, literally, "equal to." Arrangement under which a person, usually a girl from another country, exchanges domestic services for room, board, and pocket money.

French, Swedish, and German students frequently took au pair places in Britain during the 1960s, feeding a rich mythology in which British reserve and sexual naïveté encountered continental liberalism. See SWEDEN.

AUTOEROTIC ASPHYXIATION. Dangerous sexual variation exploiting the fact that strangulation can trigger orgasm.

Devotees, known as "gaspers," tighten a ligature around their throat during masturbation, encourage lovers to strangle them, or place plastic bags over their heads. Death by heart failure is common. Celebrity victims include actor Albert Dekker, novelist Jerzy Kosinski, rock star Michael Hutchence, illustrator Vaughn Bodé, and British politicians Stephen Milligan and Kristian Etchells. The practice has been used for dramatic purposes in *The Ruling Class* (film and play), *Rising Sun* (book and film), and the films *Ken Park, Hannibal, An Unsuitable Job for a Woman,* and *In the Realm of the Senses.*

William Burroughs frequently refers to the fact that hanged men ejaculate spontaneously at the moment of death. In the 1920s, German Expressionist dancer ANITA BERBER and her husband Sebastian Droste created *The Depraved Woman and the Hanged One,* in which Berber, having murdered her lover, arranged herself under his corpse so as to catch the sperm ejaculated in his last moments.

AUTO-FELLATIO. Ability of some men to suck their own penises.

French surrealist and cross-dresser PIERRE MOLINIER practiced this fetish, documenting it in some of his photographs. American actor Ron Turner can claim the honor of first displaying the skill on film, followed shortly by RON JEREMY, in *Inside Seka, BEHIND THE GREEN DOOR: THE SEQUEL,* and other films. By then, he had rivals, including gay performer "Doctor Infinity," who performed the feat in the 1977 film *The Double Exposure of Holly,* and Philadelphia artist Albo Jeavons, aka Al Eingang, who, relates an admiring Jeremy, "devoted his entire career to the art of sucking his own penis, putting out films such as *Blown Alone* and *The Young Man From Nantucket.*"

There was a young man from Nantucket
Whose dick was so long he could suck it.
While wiping his chin,
He said with a grin,
"If my ear were a cunt, I could fuck it."

—TRADITIONAL LIMERICK

Latterly, some men, in an innovative adaptation of sexual AMPUTATION, have had their lower ribs surgically removed to facilitate the practice.

AUTOMOBILES.

Sex in motor cars has a book to itself in *Crash,* the 1973 novel by J. G. Ballard, in which a cult derives erotic satisfaction from watching and experiencing car crashes, and re-creating those involving celebrities such as James Dean and Jayne Mansfield. (David Cronenberg filmed the book in 2002.) Ballard himself never disguised his interest in the sexuality of the automobile. He famously organized an exhibition of crashed cars at

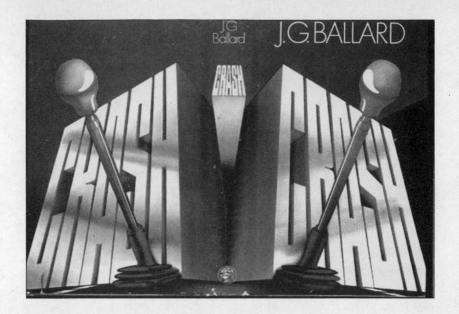

the Institute of Contemporary Arts in London, the opening of which degenerated into a drunken riot during which a scantily clad hostess was nearly raped in the backseat of a mangled Studebaker.

In the JAMES BOND novels, Ian Fleming insists that driving a girl at high speed turns her weak at the knees and unable to resist. Neither the Dean nor Mansfield accident took place during sex, but there have been fatalities under such circumstances. Legend holds that in 1931, German film director F. W. Murnau died in a California car crash while fellating his chauffeur. In John Irving's *World According to Garp*, one car rear-ending another causes the woman fellating her lover to bite off his penis.

Backseats predominate in automobile erotica, their anthem being "Seven Little Girls Sitting in the Back Seat (Huggin' and a-kissin' with Fred)," a 1959 hit for Paul

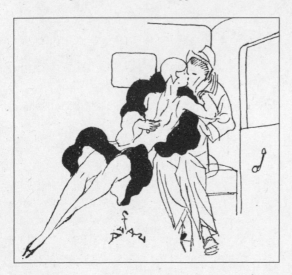

Evans and the Curls, in which seven girls prefer the backseat with Fred to the front seat with the car-proud narrator. When cars were simpler, the backseat "squab" could be removed entirely to make an al fresco bed. A *New Yorker* cartoon of 1932 shows a couple carrying such a seat and reporting to a smirking policeman, "Someone stole our car."

Among the most potent images of backseat sex is the photograph by Larry Kent, generally called "Teenage Lust," of two Tulsa teenagers curled naked in their car. Front seats, however, have their adherents, despite the hazards of the gear shift and other potential disasters—exploited in *Only Two Can Play*, the film adaptation of *That Uncertain Feeling*, by Kingsley Amis, in which Peter Sellers and Mai Zetterling become entangled with brake lever, radio, and windshield wipers. The front seat received a celebrity endorsement when actor Hugh Grant was arrested in 1995 while being fellated in his car by a Los Angeles prostitute.

AV (Japanese slang; 1990s-present). "Adult Video"—shorthand for videos with hardcore porn content.

AXILLISM. Using the armpit for sex. Evoked by Luis Buñuel in *Un Chien Andalou*, where armpit hair is compared with pubic hair.

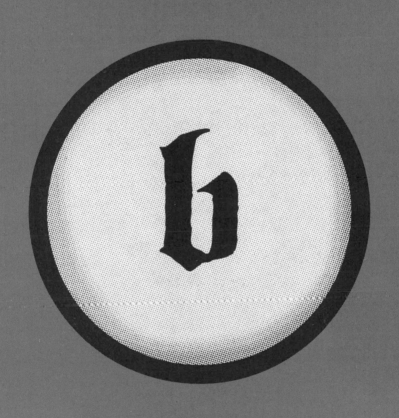

BABB, Howard W. "Kroger" (1906-1980). American film and TV producer, and distributor.

The archetypal exploitation film distributor, Babb is mainly remembered for the sex education movie *MOM AND DAD*.

Renting small-town cinemas for the day, he wasted no money on advertising, but barraged local newspapers with fake letters protesting the film, and distributed hand-outs designed to stir up controversy. So effective was this technique that, according to *Time* magazine, it "left only the livestock unaware of the chance to learn the facts of life."

During intermission, "Fearless Hygiene Commentator Elliot Forbes," a role played by various performers, made a standard speech from the stage. (In the South, African American Olympic gold medal athlete Jesse Owens sometimes substituted.) "Forbes" urged the purchase of two booklets, *Man and Boy* and *Woman and Girl*, which yielded Babb his real profit. Written by his wife and sold in the theater by "nurses," who were often local strippers or prostitutes hired for the day, the pamphlets cost eight cents each to print but were sold for a dollar. Estimates of Babb's total profit on the film vary from $40 million to $100 million.

After selling the rights to *Mom and Dad* worldwide, Babb applied his methods to films sensationalizing marijuana and African tribal life. On the strength of a brief nude bathing scene, he also acquired the American rights to Ingmar Bergman's *Sommaren med Monika (Summer with Monika)*, cut about a third of it, and released it successfully as *Monika: The Story of a Bad Girl*.

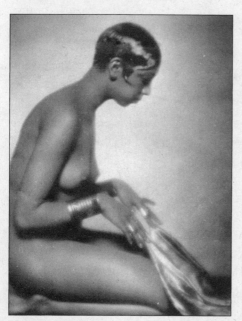

BAKER, Josephine (née Frida Josephine McDonald) (1906-1975). U.S. entertainer.

Daughter of a white or mixed-race father and an African American laundress in St. Louis, Missouri, Josephine left school at twelve, was dancing in the chorus at fifteen, and married twice before she was seventeen, the second time to Pullman porter Willie Baker, whose name she retained.

Baker's gangling movements and goofy grin won her spots in the chorus at Harlem's Plantation Club, the Cotton Club's 1924 show *Choco-late Dandies*, the Broadway revue *Shuffle Along*, and, in October 1925, a featured role in the *Revue Nègre* when it opened at Paris's Théâtre des Champs-Élysées. Her entrance, naked but for a skirt of feathers, slung over the shoulder of a brawny colleague, electrified the audience. Ernest Hemingway called her "the most sensational woman anyone ever saw." *New Yorker* columnist Janet Flanner, a lesbian, acknowledged that she, too, was sexually stirred by Baker. "Her magnificent dark body, a new model to the French, proved for the first time that black was beautiful."

When the rest of the troupe moved to Germany, Baker stayed in Paris, where the Folies Bergère starred her in their revues, dressed in what became her trademark skirt of phallic stuffed bananas (designed by couturier Paul Poiret). Not everyone loved her. Critics disparaged her dances, which were little more than comic variations on the Charleston and the Camel Walk. She was scorned by French "racial purists," who preferred their Africans primitive and submissive. But the majority of Parisians, accustomed to simple tribal people from the French African colonies, were enchanted by a wised-up black woman whose acrobatic seminude dances made a joke of sex yet were intensely provocative.

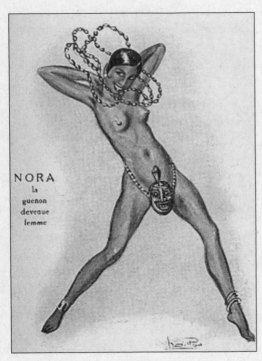

A CARICATURE OF JOSEPHINE BAKER

Although Baker took numerous lovers—among them the writer Georges Simenon, and Paul Colin, who designed her exaggerated art deco posters—she married her manager, Sicilian ex-stone mason but self-styled "count" Giuseppe "Pepito" Abatino. He orchestrated her career, attaching her name to ghosted "memoirs" and "confessions," and even to a novel. She also improved her thin voice sufficiently to record six songs, including "J'ai deux amours" ("I have two loves," went the lyrics, "My country and Paris"), which became a hit, and her lifelong signature tune.

Films such as *Zouzou* (1934) and *Princesse Tamtam* (1935) widened her fame still further, though she lacked the discipline to develop as an actress. She habitually arrived on the set after a sleepless night and accompanied by some of her private menagerie. This included a chimp, a piglet, a goat, a snake, multiple parakeets, fish, three cats, seven dogs, and a cheetah named Chiquita, which wore a diamond collar and sometimes escaped, causing panic among the crew.

Smarting from racial discrimination and hostile reviews during a U.S. tour, Baker became a French citizen in 1936. Remaining in Europe during World War II, she was active as a courier in the Resistance. The French government recognized this with various awards, culminating in 1961 with the Legion d'Honneur. See ZOOPHILIA.

BARA, Theda (Theodosia Burr Goodman) (1885–1955). U.S. actress.

According to S. J. Perelman, Bara "immortalized the VAMP just as LITTLE EGYPT at the World's Fair of 1893 had the HOOCHIE-COOCHIE." Hollywood producer William Fox created Bara to compete with slinky European stars. For publicity photographs, she squatted amid snakes and skeletons, while the studio credited her with occult powers. Her name, they pointed out helpfully, was an anagram of "Arab Death."

Though Fox claimed Bara was the Saharan-born child of a French painter and an Egyptian princess, she actually came from Cincinnati, Ohio, where her father was a tailor. After a brief Broadway career as Theodosia de Coppett, the blond Goodman dyed her hair black and plastered her face with makeup to star in Frank Powell's *A Fool There Was* (1915), as a seductress who could transfix men with her murmured invitation "Kiss me, my fool." Though *Cleopatra, Camille* (both 1917), and *Salome* (1918) followed, Bara lost ground to more skilled temptresses such as Jetta Goudal and Nita Naldi. She effectively retired in 1921.

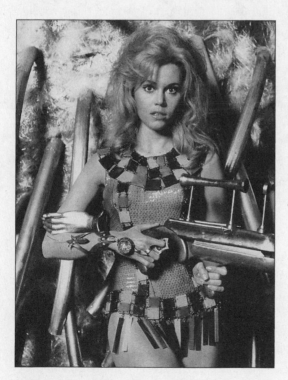

JANE FONDA IN ROGER VADIM'S FILM OF *BARBARELLA*

BARBARELLA. French comic strip.

In 1962, the French science fiction magazine *V* proposed an erotic strip about Tarzela, a female Tarzan. Artist Jean-Claude Forest (1930–1998), countersuggested *Barbarella*, featuring a voluptuous but innocent space girl. Based in looks on BRIGITTE BARDOT, Barbarella ricochets from one fantastic society to the next, most of which exploit her sexually. Her lovers include Diktor, a robot, Dildano, a revolutionary who introduces her to old-fashioned face-to-face fornication, and Pygar, a blinded angel. The villain Duran Duran tortures her by inducing extremes of pleasure with his Excessive Machine. *Barbarella*, though his most durable creation, backfired on Forest. "For two years, I couldn't find any work," he said. "I was considered a distinguished erotomaniac by the comics industry! They thought, 'If it's Forest, there will be sex in it and we'll be in trouble!'"

ALSO
BARBARELLA (1968). French film. Directed by ROGER VADIM.

Vadim envisaged "a kind of sexual *Alice in Wonderland* of the future," starring thenwife Jane Fonda, who, frugally dressed in fiberglass and vinyl, cruises the universe in a fur-lined spaceship. ANDY WARHOL called this his favorite film, in part because the Excessive Machine represented his ideal of sex without physical contact. See SEX MACHINES.

BARDOT, Brigitte (1934–). French actress.

Film history dates the *nouvelle vague* from 1960 and the films of Alain Resnais, Jean-Luc Godard, and Francois Truffaut, but credit for tapping the new young audience eager to see performers of their own age rightly belongs to Brigitte Bardot

Bardot was twenty-one when her husband ROGER VADIM starred her in *Et Dieu… Créa La Femme*. She'd already made seventeen mediocre films, but this romance, set in the then-sleepy fishing village of St. Tropez, showed her in a new light. Trashy, pouting, half-naked, she strutted around town, tossing her mane of golden hair and switching her rump while the matrons tut-tutted and her male co-stars, Curd Jürgens, Jean-Louis Trintignant, and Christian Marquand, panted in her wake.

French film heroines had traditionally been either young and innocent or mature and knowing. This "sex kitten"—who, even though barely out of her teens, knew what she wanted and exploited her sexuality to get it—was something new, and the kids flocked to see her. "In her role of confused female, of homeless little slut," wrote one critic, "BB seems to be available to everyone." By 1962, she'd become the darling of the French intelligentsia. As Simone de Beauvoir wrote in her essay "Brigitte Bardot and the Lolita Syndrome," "paradoxically, she is intimidating. . . . [T]here is something stubborn in her sulky face, in her sturdy body. . . .There is nothing coarse about her. She has a kind of spontaneous dignity . . ."

Almost overnight, "BB" became the face of the new France. She posed for the bust of Marianne, the symbol of France that occupies a place of honor in every town hall, divorced Vadim to have affairs with a succession of handsome young men, recorded a few songs in her frail little-girl voice, and made the occasional foray into serious cinema with roles as murderess and prostitute. Through it all, however, she remained the archetypal tease, at her most effective when she could toss her head, pout, and wiggle. Once she became too old for such gestures, she retired, devoting her energies to political causes, in particular animal rights.

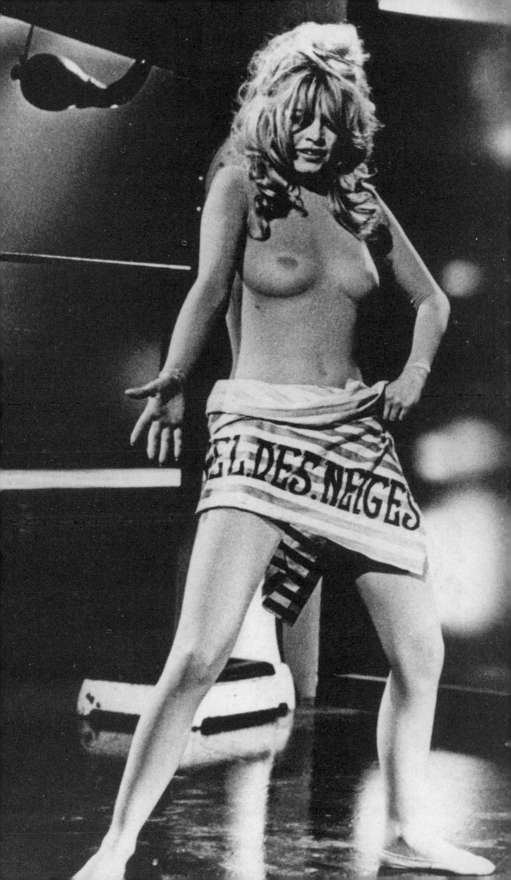

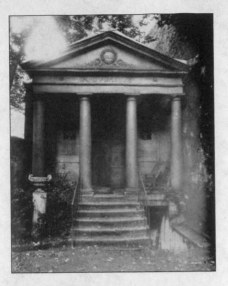

BARNEY, Nathalie Clifford (1876–1972). Hostess and writer.

Wealthy Boston dilettante Barney turned up in Paris dressed as a boy and seduced one of the most famous *grandes horizontales* of her day, Liane de Pougy. Subsequently she became the doyenne of Paris lesbian society between the wars. "I invented lesbianism," she announced. Her home at 20 Rue Jacob served as salon and court, where she and her companion, painter Romaine Brooks, entertained a succession of literary and artistic lesbians, including Gertrude Stein and Alice B. Toklas, Djuna Barnes, Janet Flanner, Dolly Wilde, and RADCLYFFE HALL, as well as "honorary" Sapphists such as Truman Capote,

THE TEMPLE TO FRIENDSHIP BUILT BY NATHALIE CLIFFORD BARNEY ON THE GROUNDS OF HER PARIS HOME

Noël Coward, and Raymond Duncan, eccentric brother of the more famous Isadora. Barney's garden contained a Greek-style "Temple of Friendship," where she conducted genteel celebrations of Sappho, complete with Hellenic robes and dances. She inspired the character of Valérie Seymour in Radclyffe Hall's novel *THE WELL OF LONELINESS*, and was parodied by Djuna Barnes in her comic fantasy *The Ladies' Almanack*.

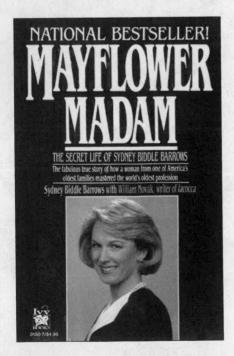

BARROWS, Sydney Biddle (1952–). Socialite and brothel keeper.

Dubbed the "Mayflower Madam" because of her Social Register roots, Barrows, an out-of-work Manhattan fashion buyer, spotted the need in the newly affluent 1970s for an up-market CALL-GIRL service. Cachet (pron. "Cash-AY"—French for a distinctive mark or style) opened in 1979. Barrows's girls initially cost $125 an hour, half of the fee going to the house. Cachet boasted of employing only students and professional girls, supposedly earning a little on the side to keep themselves solvent in the Big Apple. Barrows fired one girl after discovering she'd appeared in porn films. "We couldn't risk anyone finding out that we weren't as sterling and as pure as we promised, and as we wanted to be." Police closed her down in 1984, but the articulate and unrepentant Barrows wrote a bestselling autobiography, *Mayflower Madam*, filmed in 1987 with Candice Bergen as Barrows.

BDSM (1960s-present). Imprecise term encompassing a range of sexual behaviors, e.g., BONDAGE, SADOMASOCHISM, dominance, submission, and role-playing.

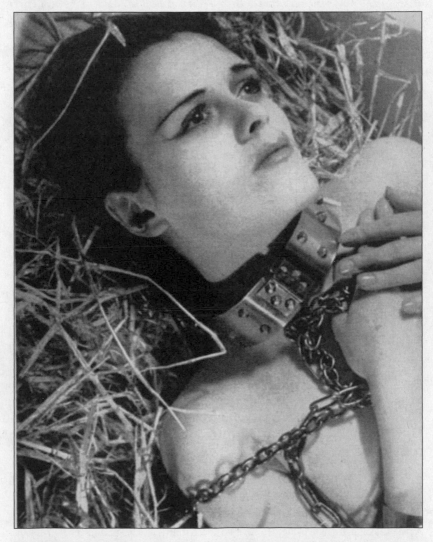

BEACH INSPECTORS (Australian, 1920s-1980s). Municipal employees who prowled the beaches of Australia, ejecting women whose costumes they regarded as too brief. See BIKINI.

BEACH PARTY FILMS (1963-1966). Cycle of low-budget Hollywood films in which fun-loving teenagers—played mostly by Frankie Avalon, Annette Funicello, and friends—are harried by unsympathetic oldsters, whom they eventually discourage, convert, or humiliate.

Beach Party (1963) was followed by Muscle Beach Party (1964), The Horror of Party Beach (1964), Dr. Goldfoot and the Bikini Machine (1965), Beach Blanket Bingo (1965), How to Stuff a Wild Bikini (1965), and The Ghost in the Invisible Bikini (1966). Made mostly by horror/action specialists American International Pictures, the films exploited the teenage drive-in audience and the surfing craze. Well-filled bikinis featured prominently. Asked who'd played opposite him in Dr. Goldfoot and the Bikini Machine, Vincent Price said wearily, "Every high-breasted woman in Hollywood."

BEARD (U.S. slang, 1960s). A person who accompanies a couple to public events to camouflage their interest in one another.

Typified by stock gay actor Franklin Pangborn in Stage Door (1937), in which he's hired to sit at a nightclub table with Adolphe Menjou and pretend to be the escort of his mistress, Gail Patrick. In Sweet Smell of Success, ruthless columnist J. J. Hunsecker (Burt Lancaster) attacks a senator for being seen in public with a mistress while his publicist acts as a transparent beard. Further anatomized by Paul Schrader in his 2007 film The Walker, with Woody Harrelson as an elegant gay in Washington, D.C., whose duties as companion to its wealthy matrons involve him in murder. See MERKIN; GIGOLO; WALKER; ESCORT.

BEAVER. U.S. slang for female pubic hair. Adapted from a 1920s slang term for a beard.

BEEFCAKE (U.S. slang, 1950s-present). Male glamour, represented in photography or film.

CHEESECAKE was one of the cornerstones on which Hollywood built its international popularity, but beefcake wasn't far behind. The popularity of early stars such as RUDOLPH VALENTINO and Douglas Fairbanks Sr. can be traced in part to the appeal to the female audience of a naked male torso.

Even the most pigeon-chested stars stripped down. Ben Lyon, ordered to try out for the starring role in the 1925 Ben-Hur, had to have muscles painted on before he looked halfway credible. Ramon Navarro, who finally played the role, was, though gay, marginally more athletic, a fact emphasized by photo layouts showing him in running shorts.

After Clark Gable removed his shirt to show a bare chest in the 1934 film It Happened One Night, sales of undershirts plunged, further demonstrating the value of sturdy pecs. Throughout the 1930s, Hollywood put under contract every personable new male athlete in sight. All were immediately featured in photo shoots showing them in swimming trunks or less. The same went for actors such as Steve Reeves and ARNOLD SCHWARZENEGGER,

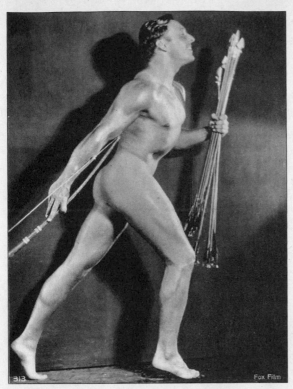

recruited in the 1960s from the ranks of body-builders.

BEHIND THE GREEN DOOR (1972). U.S. film. Directed by James and Artie, the MITCHELL BROTHERS.

Needing product for their San Francisco cinema, the Mitchells, prolific producers of LOOPS, turned to an anonymous pornographic booklet that circulated among American soldiers during World War II. Their title came from *The Green Door*, a number one *Billboard* hit in 1956,

ACTOR GEORGE O'BRIEN IN A CLASSIC "BEEFCAKE" POSE OF THE LATE 1920s

in which the sleepless Jim Lowe frets about the wild party going on behind the green door of a nearby house. Impatient with scripts, the Mitchells improvised the action and dialogue, frequently consulting the original text, a few age-yellowed sheets of paper.

In a diner, a truckdriver (George MacDonald), asked by the cook and a fellow driver to explain about "the green door," describes a sex coven that preys on young girls. Gloria (MARILYN CHAMBERS) is abducted from a hotel. After being "calmed" by lesbian caresses, she's paraded before an audience wearing masks and evening dress. Though silent throughout, she submits enthusiastically to sex with African American Johnny Keyes, a trio on trapezes, and members of the audience. These include the truckdriver, who, at the climax of the orgy, runs onstage, snatches her up, and flees from the club. The film ends with an extended sex sequence between MacDonald and Chambers that uses psychedelic color effects, including a COME SHOT with giant gouts of SEMEN leaping in multicolor slow motion.

This sequence, inspired by the work of San Francisco experimental filmmakers such as Jordan Belson, indicates the film's hippie heritage. So does the casting of lesser roles, which run the gamut of physical variety. The orgy, soon to become a Mitchell trademark, includes a FELLINI-esque cast of midgets and cross-dressers, middle-aged baldies, and a few tattooed people, as well as the gargantuan V. VENUS.

The Mitchells opened *Green Door* in New York City, and, with typical chutzpah, advertised in the trade press recommending the film to Academy members for consideration for the 1973 Oscars.

"We got up at 6am, and went down to the bad part of town, to a sound studio called Stage 8. It was the size of a 747 hangar. It was a big shoot. My forty-seventh film and Marilyn's first. We had full body make-up; that had never been done before. We got to stand around on a cold concrete floor, naked, till ten, when the lights were set up and we were ready to go. Then they moved us over to a three-quarter-inch plywood platform covered with black photo paper so the shot could be run through an optical printer. . . . We've got full body make-up on black photo paper, so we can't move. Under full direction, the first scene took two hours. When they said "Stop", not only did you have to think about keeping it up, but, with fourteen technicians, they could afford to have a make-up girl come over and touch up your testicles."

—GEORGE MACDONALD ON SHOOTING *Behind the Green Door.*

BELLOCQ, E. J. (né John Ernest Joseph Bellocq) (1873–1949). U.S. photographer.

In between bland commercial work in New Orleans, Bellocq secretly documented the underside of the city, in particular its OPIUM dens and the brothels of the STORYVILLE district.
His work remained unknown until 1958, when another photographer, Lee Friedlander, discovered a cache of Bellocq's glass plates. They were published as *Storyville Portraits* and provided the basis for the film *Pretty Baby*.

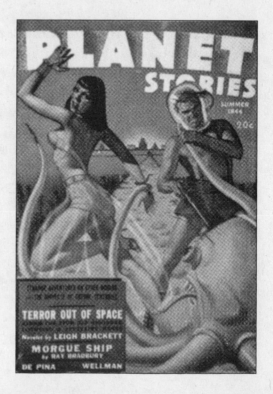

BEM, BUM, BEAUTY (U.S. slang, 1930s–40s). Short-hand recipe for successful cover art on science fiction pulp magazines of the 1930s and 1940s, i.e., a BEM (bug-eyed monster) battling a bum, or spaceman, for the virtue of a voluptuous beauty, usually depicted in a spacesuit made of cellophane.

BERBER, Anita (1899–1928). German dancer and choreographer.

An alcoholic and cocaine addict, Berber frequently performed naked, which even BERLIN in the Weimar era found scandalous. She once urinated in the drink of a customer who'd annoyed her, and would habitually calm a riotous crowd by promising to fuck every spectator. Her favorite snack was a single rose dipped in chloroform and ether.

In 1919 she married the artist Eberhard von Nathusius, but soon became the lover of lesbian club owner Susi Wanowsky. Rumors circulated that she was the sex slave of Wanowsky and her fifteen-year-old daughter. She had small roles in more than twenty movies, including Fritz Lang's *Dr. Mabuse, Der Spieler* (1922), and the 1919 *ANDERS ALS DES ANDERN*. Meanwhile, she developed her Expressionist dance performances, choreographing pieces to Debussy and Richard Strauss.

Over the years, her material grew increasingly macabre, in keeping with her extravagant bisexual lifestyle and drug use. In 1922, she married Sebastian Droste, a gay writer and dancer, with whom she created dance works with titles such as *Morphium, Suicide, Insane Asylum,* and *The Corpse on the Dissecting Table.* They published a book of poetry, photographs, and drawings called *Die Tänze des Lasters, des Grauens, und der Ekstase (Dances of Vice, Horror, and Ecstasy)*, based on their performance of the same name. For their most startling ballet, *The Depraved Woman and the Hanged One*, Berber crouched under the hanged Droste to catch the sperm ejaculated in his last moments.

The couple divorced in 1923 and Berber married American dancer Henri Chatin-Hoffman, also gay. At the end of their European tour, which left a swathe of scandal, Berber collapsed, and was cared for by sex researcher MAGNUS HIRSCHFELD. In 1928, during a Middle Eastern tour, she contracted pulmonary tuberculosis, untreatable and fatal. Friends arranged for her to be brought back to Berlin, where she died on November 10, 1928, aged twenty-nine. According to one report of her funeral, "prominent film directors marched beside the whores of Friedrichstrasse, young male hookers with hermaphrodites from the El Dorado [nightclub], famous artists next to barmen, men in top hats beside the most famous transvestites of Berlin." Berber is best remembered in the portrait by Otto Dix showing a sepulchrally pale woman in a draped crimson gown. See AUTOEROTIC ASPHYXIATION.

BERLE, Milton (né Milton Berlinger) (1908–2002). U.S. comedian.

"Mr. Television," and the first TV comedy star, Berle possessed a penis of legendary size. When a drunk challenged him to a barroom comparison, a friend, aware of Berle's superiority, advised him, "Go on, Miltie, just take out enough to win." Compulsively horny even in his adolescent vaudeville days, Berle, rather than waste time and energy on seduction, let his stagestruck mother find him girls. Celebrity partners included evangelist Aimee Semple Macpherson, whom he shared with Anthony Quinn, and silent movie vamp THEDA BARA. He pleasured Betty Hutton, Lucille Ball, and even a young MARILYN MONROE when they appeared together in *Ladies of the Chorus*

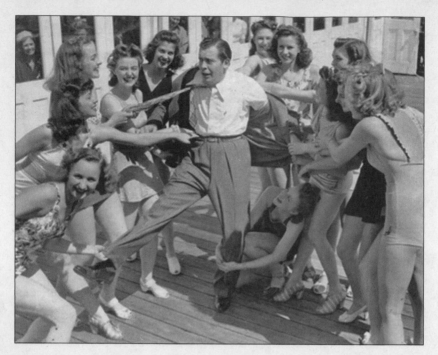

MILTON BERLE

in 1948. He was also a regular client of the brothels of POLLY ADLER. Age slowed him
little. Berle's wife of forty-five years once confided wearily that "she couldn't wait for
Miltie to get old." In the end, he outlived her and, in his eighties, married an attractive
blonde half his age.

BERLIN.

"For Christopher," wrote gay novelist Christopher Isherwood of his life in pre–
World War II Europe, "Berlin meant boys." When both he and W. H. AUDEN moved
there in the 1930s, male homosexuality, though technically illegal, flourished. It was
even the subject of academic study at the Institut fur Sexualwissenschaft (Institute for
Sexual Research) of MAGNUS HIRSCHFELD.

Although Isherwood's stay would inspire *Cabaret,* the most popular celebration of
1930s Berlin's everything-for-sale culture, the Kander/Ebb musical barely skimmed the
surface. Bankrupted by the reparations demanded by the victors of the First World War,
even bourgeois and aristocratic Germans were forced to sell everything simply to survive. Families collectively prostituted themselves in their own homes, with wives, husbands, and children offering themselves for sex. Child prostitution services were listed
in the phone book as *apoteken* (pharmacies). If you phoned for aspirin, they'd ask how
long you'd had the headache. Depending on whether you said "nine hours" or "fifteen
minutes," a cab would deliver a nine- or fifteen-year-old to your hotel. At actual pharmacies, any drug was readily available, in particular cocaine.

In cabarets, stars such as ANITA BERBER performed nude, while prostitutes of all ages, sexes, and types roamed streets designated for their particular specialty. On Munzistrasse, only pregnant women offered themselves. Another thoroughfare drew *Heuschreken* (grasshoppers), women with physical deformities: hunchbacks, club feet, or faces slashed by razors or burned by acid. Elsewhere, dominatrices strolled in high leather boots, the color and pattern of the laces indicating their particular expertise.

Ostensibly moralistic, the Nazis attacked Berlin's vice industry while covertly, particularly in the case of Ernst Rohm's SA Brownshirts, enjoying a homoerotic culture, celebrated in the opening of Leni Reifenstahl's *Berlin Olympiade,* with nude bodies of both sexes leaping and twining in an ecstasy of sensuality. Luchino Visconti, himself bisexual, highlighted this double standard in his film *The Damned.* He staged the confrontation of June 1934, when Hitler liquidated his rival in the so-called Night of the Long Knives, as a slaughter at an idyllic lakeside resort, with his SS Blackshirts descending on their victims as they sprawl naked and insensible after a gay orgy.

Having wiped out all opposition, the Nazis "cleaned up" Berlin, looting and burning Hirschfeld's institute, and driving him into exile, along with numerous other "decadent" artists, from MARLENE DIETRICH and Kurt Weill to Max Reinhardt and Arnold Schoenberg. Many more creators died in the war, or in concentration camps. Proof that the spirit of Berlin could not, however, be extinguished came in 1948, when director Billy Wilder returned to make *A Foreign Affair,* with Dietrich as a cabaret star who consorts with both her old Nazi lover and a new American admirer. See HIRSCHFELD, Magnus; DIETRICH, Marlene; BERBER, Anita.

BESTIALITY. See ZOOPHILIA.

***BEST LITTLE WHOREHOUSE IN TEXAS, THE* (1978).** U.S. stage and film musical. Written and composed by Larry L. King and Carol Hall.

News reports of the Chicken Ranch brothel outside La Grange, Texas, inspired this story of a reporter who campaigns to close a bordello that's been operating discreetly for more than a century. This throws the local sheriff into conflict with his friend and sometime lover, the bordello's madam.

The original starred little-known Carlin Glynn and Henderson Forsythe, but was so successful that Ann-Margret headed the touring company. (An unsuccessful 1994 sequel, *The Best Little Whorehouse Goes Public,* ran briefly on Broadway.) This use of the word *whorehouse* and the show's acknowledgment that brothels operated openly and often legally in some states marked a significant advance in American COMMUNITY VALUES.

ALSO

BEST LITTLE WHOREHOUSE IN TEXAS, THE (1982). U.S. film. Directed by Colin Higgins. Dolly Parton played the madam and Burt Reynolds the sheriff in this fairly faithful film version.

BETTAKU (JAPANESE). LITERALLY "SECOND HOUSE." A residence where one or more Japanese men keeps a mistress. Customarily in foreign countries a small apartment complex. A *bettaku* in Los Angeles provides a setting for scenes in Michael Crichton's novel *Rising Sun* and Phil Kaufman's film version.

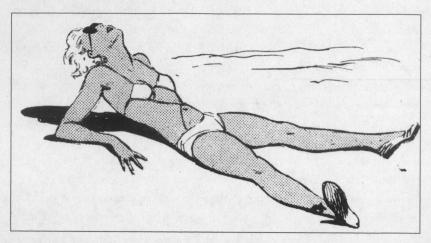

AN EARLY VERSION OF THE BIKINI AS IMAGINED BY RENE GIFFEY IN 1931.

BIKINI (1946–present). Two-piece swimsuit.

Two-piece suits had been around for years, but it took the July 1946 U.S. test of an atomic bomb at Bikini Atoll to explode them into public consciousness. In May 1946, Jacques Heim, a Paris couturier, had shown a two-piece suit called L'Atome, and hired a plane to skywrite "The Atom—World's Smallest Swimsuit" above the city.

However, he was trumped by the more flamboyant Louis Réard, a swimsuit shop owner, who, four days after the Bikini test, held a parade of two-piece suits at the Piscine Molitor, a large public swimming pool. Réard's suits used only thirty square inches of fabric, and were little more than handkerchiefs taped at the hips and across the breasts; he claimed they could fit in a matchbox, and were "brief enough to pass through a wedding ring." Professional models refused to wear them, so Réard hired Micheline Bernardini, a Casino de Paris showgirl (and wife of CRAZY HORSE SALOON owner Alain Bernardin). Punning on the concept of "splitting the atom," he called the outfits bikinis, and had a plane skywrite "Bikini—Smaller Than the World's Smallest Swimsuit" over Paris. On July 18 he officially registered the name and design. See MONOKINI.

BIMBO (U.S. slang, 1919–present). A pretty but dumb woman. From *bimbo*, Italian for "little child."

BINIBONG (Japanese, 1990s). Porn magazines so extreme that they are sold wrapped in plastic. See also BROWN-WRAPPED and TOP-SHELF.

BIRDBATHING. Sex act in which the recipient takes not only the penis and testicles into the mouth but also a good portion of the male ass, containing him much in the way a birdbath would if he sat in one. See also TOSSING SALAD.

BITE (pronounced "beet") (French slang, traditional). Erect penis. See also FOUFOUNE.

BLACK VELVET (1900s-present). Omnibus term for a taste for sex with African women. Regarded as an occupational hazard in the tropics, where it was usual for colonial administrators to take local mistresses.

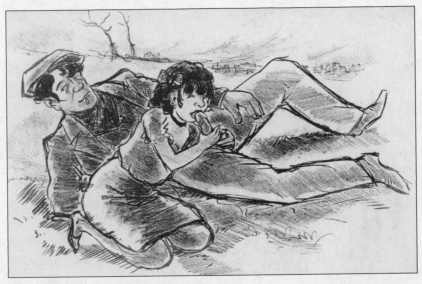

BLOW JOB (U.S. slang, 1920s-present). Fellatio. Initially in widest use among gays, particularly in the navy and army, *blow job* quickly replaced the euphemism *French*. Christopher Hitchens suggests the phrase is "possibly derived from the jazz scene and its oral instrumentation," but it's more likely a corruption of Victorian brothel slang "below job," the suffix *job* also implying that it began as part of a whore's repertoire; compare, for instance, *hand job*.

BLUE (1700s-present). Adjective implying a sexually suggestive element, e.g., BLUE MOVIE, BLUE JOKES.

"BLUE FILM, THE" (1954). Short story by Graham Greene.

A middle-aged couple holidaying in Thailand attend a pornographic movie show during which the man recognizes himself as the performer in one of the films, made during his student days. The experience inspires the couple to share their first sex for some time, but while the woman is excited, the man is nostalgic for the forgotten girl in the film. A detailed description in the story of the well-known French pornographic film *Massages* indicates Greene's real-life familiarity with STAG FILMS.

BLUE LAWS (1781–present). Legislation, usually local, promulgated to impose a moral agenda, e.g., to ban markets or public entertainment on Sundays.

BLUE LIGHT CLINICS (1914–1960s). Before penicillin, silver salts constituted the main treatment for sexually transmitted diseases. British and Australian army personnel exposed to infection were required to report to clinics, signified by a blue light, where they were treated crudely with argynol, potassium permanganate, and Calomel salve. Soldiers going on weekend leave were issued with "Blue Lights," prophylactic packs of the same chemicals, for self-medication.

BLUE MOVIE. Any pornographic film. Title was also used for a number of feature films.

ALSO
BLUE MOVIE (1970). U.S. novel, by Terry Southern, and aborted Stanley Kubrick film project.

During the 1963 production of *Dr. Strangelove, or How I Learned to Stop Worrying and Love the Bomb*, a guest brought a porn film to the London home of the film's reclusive director, Stanley Kubrick. Later, Kubrick remarked to screenwriter Terry Southern, "It would be great if someone made a movie like that under studio conditions." This inspired Southern's *Blue Movie*, a novel about the production of Hollywood's first big-budget porn film. "I thought Kubrick would be the ideal person to direct such a movie," says Southern, who based the character of the director, Boris Adrian, on Kubrick. "I would send him pieces [from the novel] from time to time. I still have a great telegram from him saying, 'You have written the definitive blow job!' in the scene with the Jeanne Moreau–type, Arabella." Once *Blue Movie* was published in 1970, however, Kubrick, to whom it's dedicated, backed out. "It turned out he has an ultra-conservative attitude to things sexual," said Southern.

The project circulated until, around 1974–75, John Calley, then president of Warner Brothers, decided to produce it, and persuaded his companion, Julie Andrews, to play Angela Stirling, the squeaky-clean star who agrees to appear in the film. On this basis, Mike Nichols, whose eyes had been opened to the possibilities of porn by three visits to *DEEP THROAT*, agreed to direct.

All seemed set, until Warners tried to reacquire the rights to Southern's book and script from Ringo Starr, who then held the option. But Starr's lawyer vetoed any such deal without payment. In 1981, Blake Edwards, Julie Andrews's then-husband, fictionalized the incident in his comedy *S.O.B.*, in which a director with a flop on his hands decides to rescue it by adding sex scenes. Andrews appears demurely but defiantly bare-breasted. The film is a pale shadow of what *Blue Movie* might have been.

BOARDING SCHOOL. Residential school, usually for adolescent boys.

The mythology of boarding schools invariably involves bullying, corporal punishment, and homosexuality. Mr. Wackford Squeers's Dotheboys Hall, in Charles Dickens's *Nicholas Nickleby*, established the benchmark, rivaled by Thomas Hughes's 1857 *Tom Brown's Schooldays*, set at Rugby School, where the eponymous hero is victimized by the villainous Flashman, whose later exploits on the battlefields and in the bedrooms of the British empire were dramatized by George Macdonald Fraser in a highly successful series of novels.

Homosexuality was endemic in most British boarding schools, exacerbated by the "fagging" system, in which newcomers acted as servants and, sometimes, sexual partners for older boys. The 1972 LONGFORD report on pornography described incidents in an unnamed British boarding school in which "new boys had been held down by groups of second-year boys and masturbated by them or forced to masturbate each other, or taken to the toilet for oral masturbation. A first-year boy had been held down and submitted to buggery.... [First-year boys] had been taken into the prefects' room and there shown a large scrap book full of pornographic material, both written and pictorial [containing] pictures of all variations and perversions of sexual behaviour, heterosexual, homosexual, group sex, anal, oral and sadistic sex ..."

Not all students found the experience entirely objectionable. In his 1988 novel *The Swimming Pool Library*, Alan Hollinghurst writes of clandestine meetings at the select school of Winchester with like-minded boys in the open-air baths. "On high summer evenings . . . three or four of us would slip away from the dorms and go with an exaggerated refinement of stealth to the pool, [where] soap, lathered in the cold, starlit water, eased the violence of cocks up young bums. Fox-eyed, silent but for our breathing and the thrilling gross little rhythms of sex—which made us gulp and grope for more—we learnt our stuff."

Films and books about boarding school life are mostly autobiographical, and represent the experience of those who survived and prevailed. The best contain a healthy element of revolt, in particular Lindsay Anderson's *If...*, where a radical not only survives the hierarchical social structure and brutal beatings but turns a machine gun on his tormentors. In *Another Country* (1984), from Julian Mitchell's play, the homophobia of his school sets the young Guy Burgess on the path to becoming a Soviet spy.

BOB (U.S. slang, 2000s). Acronym for "Bend Over, Boyfriend," coded reference for the practice of PEGGING, in which a male lover is penetrated anally by a female wearing a STRAP-ON.

BOBBITT, John Wayne (1967–). U.S. adult film actor.

An ex-Marine and nightclub bouncer whose penis, severed by his vengeful wife in 1993, was thrown from a speeding car, but then retrieved and reattached in a nine-hour operation. (Wife Lorena, supposedly suffering from stress following an abortion three years earlier, was acquitted.) Bobbitt, described as "good-looking and well-built, but inarticulate and slow-witted, with no discernable talents," tried to raise money for the medical bills by forming a rock group, the Severed Parts. He also had a brief, inglorious career in porn films directed by RON JEREMY. Following his appearance in *John Wayne Bobbitt Uncut* (1994) and further surgery to enlarge his penis, Bobbitt appeared in *Frankenpenis* (1997), playing a creature made up of spare parts whose penis becomes detached, and who, given a new and enormous organ, is pursued by a voracious "Bride of Frankenpenis." He subsequently relocated to Nevada, where he worked as both construction worker and minister of religion, and experienced numerous brushes with the law.

> Two women are driving at night. A dismembered penis smacks into their windshield and just as quickly disappears.
>
> **Woman 1:** Was that a fly?
> **Woman 2:** If it was, it had the biggest penis I've ever seen.
>
> Opening scene from first-draft screenplay for *John Wayne Bobbitt Uncut.*

BODICE RIPPER. Romance novel, usually with period setting, described as "five parts sex to one part history."

The genre is typified by *FOREVER AMBER*, in which the heroine experiences violent but satisfying sex, usually involving torn clothing. The genre was not defined in print until December 1980, when *The New York Times* noted "Women too have their pornography: Harlequin romances, novels of 'sweet savagery'—bodice-rippers." The first modern "bodice ripper" (a term despised by the romance industry) is generally agreed to be the 1972 novel *The Flame and the Flower*, by Kathleen Woodiwiss.

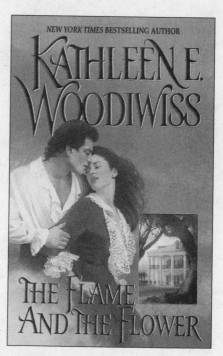

BODY DOUBLE. Actor who replaces another for nude shots.

Few actors and actresses are sufficiently confident about their bodies to appear naked. Britt Ekland showed her breasts in 1973's *The Wicker Man* but demanded a double for her buttocks on the grounds that she "had a butt like a ski slope." In the film *Notting Hill* (1999), Julia Roberts, playing a movie star, elucidates for Hugh Grant the contractual prohibitions on nudity, and the concept of a "stunt bottom" and "ass work."

ALSO
BODY DOUBLE (1984). U.S. film. Directed by Brian DePalma.

Actor Craig Wasson, house-sitting a luxury Los Angeles home, spies on a beautiful young woman through her bedroom window—until he sees her murdered there. Or does he? Trying to find the truth leads him into the porn film world and the orbit of sex star Holly Body. Trapped in a Hitchcockian murder plot, Wasson tracks down Holly by impersonating a STUNT COCK, but is quickly exposed as an amateur. "He didn't even know what a CUM SHOT was," sneers Holly.

Body Double was inspired by the opening scenes of DePalma's 1980 film *Dressed to Kill*, during the shooting of which Angie Dickinson, playing a middle-aged wife enjoying masturbatory rape fantasies in the shower, was replaced in close-ups by someone younger and more voluptuous. (*Body Double* ends with Wasson playing a similar shower scene—opposite a body double.) DePalma wanted real-life porn star ANNETTE HAVEN to play Holly, but despite intensive grooming and training, she was rejected by the studio in favor of Melanie Griffith. See HAVEN, Annette.

BODY PAINTING. Painting designs or images on the nude body, usually female.

Body painting extends back to tribal societies, but flourished most vigorously after the arrival of chemically safe paints in the 1920s. Models at the QUATZ'ARTS BALL in Paris would appear nude as living statues, coated all over in paint. During World War II, women short on stockings painted their legs, even drawing false seams down their calves. The sixties ushered in a more decorative use of paint, with bodies covered in swirling psychedelic patterns. French artist Yves Klein took it to the extreme; his nude models rolled in blue paint, then pressed their torsos to virgin canvases. Most recently, covers on *Vanity Fair* magazine featured movie stars, including Demi Moore, who appeared to be fully clothed but were actually nude, in painted garments. See BOND, James.

BOND, James. Fictional secret agent created by Ian Fleming.

"The name's Bond; James Bond." The moment in 1951 when forty-three-year-old Ian Lancaster Fleming typed these words in a Jamaican villa deserves to be commemorated as a significant cultural event.

Fleming visualized a truly *secret* secret agent, a soft-spoken Royal Navy commander who lived alone in a small London flat and was fussy about his coffee and boiled eggs. If someone did play Bond on-screen, Fleming imagined actor-songwriter Hoagy Carmichael or Humphrey Bogart. However, the role went to an unknown, one-time swimwear model and milkman Sean Connery. Harry Saltzman and Albert "Cubby" Broccoli, pro-

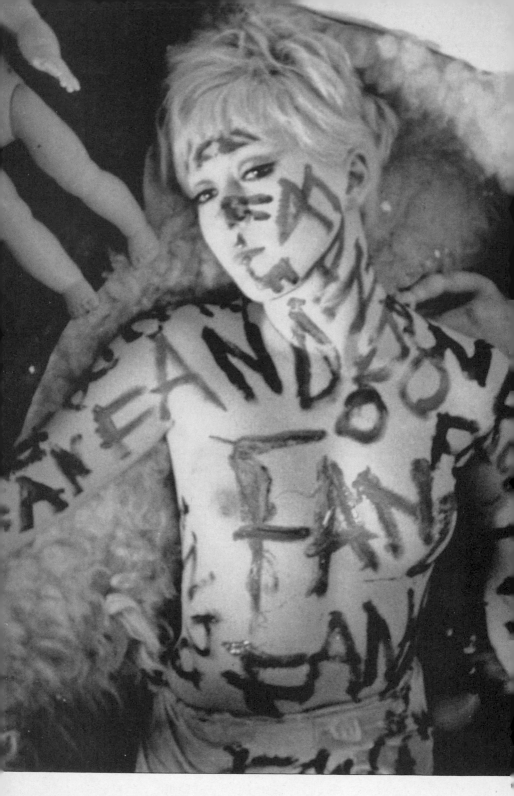

DIANA MARISCAL IN ALEXANDER JODOROWSKY'S *FANDO AND LIS* (1968)

ducers of the 1962 *Dr. No*, watched Connery cross the street after the interview and decided that he moved "like an animal."

Connery was impatient with Bond. "He has no mother. He has no father. He doesn't come from anywhere and he hadn't been anywhere when he became 007." Why so popular, then? "He likes to eat. Likes to drink. Likes his girls. He is rather cruel, sadistic. That takes in a big percentage of the fantasies of lots of people."

Sex and sadism were central to the success of the Bond books and films, in each of which the secret agent has repeated erotic encounters, but is also tortured, usually sexually. In *Casino*

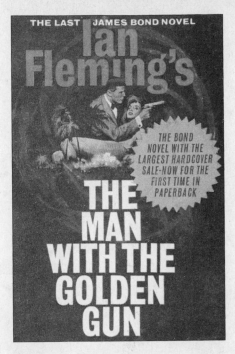

Royale, his testicles are battered with a carpet beater, and in the film of *Goldfinger*, the villain spreadeagles him on a table with a laser beam inching toward his crotch.

In almost every case, however, he is freed by a woman who begins as an enemy yet becomes another conquest, only to sacrifice her life to save his. Filmmakers followed Fleming's lead and gave these characters comic-erotic names—Pussy Galore, Plenty O'Toole, Holly Goodhead, Mary Goodnight, Kissy Suzuki. Of the actresses who played

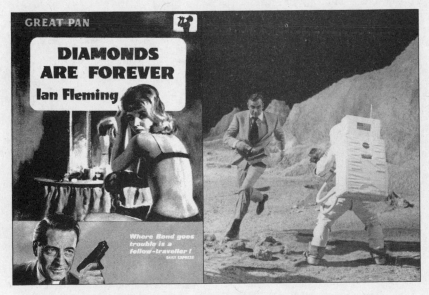

COVER OF *DIAMONDS ARE FOREVER* WITH A SOBER EARLY VERSION OF JAMES BOND, AND SEAN CONNERY AS HE APPEARED IN THE MORE FANTASTIC MOVIE

them, best remembered is Shirley Eaton, who's BODY-PAINTED to death with gold paint in *Goldfinger*. Her gilded seminude body was so distinctive in the cinema that nobody much cared that such a demise was a medical impossibility.

"I don't think you can take it too seriously [being called] the Sexiest Man Alive. There are very few sexy dead ones."
—Sean Connery

Fleming eventually wearied of Bond, calling the character "a cardboard booby." He disliked the movies, and just about endured Connery. The author died in 1966, so never saw Roger Moore, Timothy Dalton, Pierce Brosnan, or Daniel Craig in the role—which is just as well. Asked to distinguish between his performances as Bond and Simon Templar, "The Saint," Moore purred, "For one, I wear a black dinner jacket, for the other a white one."

BONDAGE. General term to describe forms of sexual satisfaction achieved with the use of restraints: ropes, handcuffs, chains, straps, etc.

Among the formerly clandestine sexual practices to increase most in popularity since 1900, bondage is a leader. Its complex rituals and degrees of involvement, and the intricate hardware and flattering costumes of rubber and LEATHER, appealed to a culture preoccupied with externals.

Following the success of the 1955 novel *HISTOIRE D'O*, bondage entered the mainstream. Numerous shops sold costumes and equipment. In music videos, the S&M sensorium was exploited by such stars as MADONNA, and by Billy Idol, whose video for "Eyes Without a Face" (1984) features the singer in black leather, including a spiked wristband and single black glove. FIST FUCKING is evoked in repeated shots of hands beating rhythm on leather-clad buttocks, a palm sliding into a back pocket, and a fist thrust into the camera.

Australian star Kylie Minogue and her lover Michael Hutchence, of the group INXS, were often associated in the popular press with bondage. Hutchence boasted of having a seventeen-year-old sex slave whom he led around on a dog collar and chain. During her relationship with Hutchence, Minogue was stopped by London Customs for carrying handcuffs—which she claimed were only the "fun" handles of her handbag. (In 2005, a line of "Cuffz" handbags was launched by Linz, with handles that incorporated a single cuff—supposed to secure it to the wrist.) In 1997, after their relationship ended, Hutchence was found strangled in a Sydney hotel in what was believed to be a case of AUTOEROTIC ASPHYXIATION. See *MAITRESSE*.

BOOGIE NIGHTS (1997). U.S. film. Directed by Paul Thomas Anderson.

Film à clef of the Hollywood porn scene at the end of the 1970s and early 1980s. Burt Reynolds plays producer Jack Horner and Julianne Moore his mistress and star Amber Waves. They discover Eddie Adams, a WELL-HUNG but naïve busboy, agree to his new name Dirk Diggler, and star him in movies with Horner's stock company of equally dim performers and technicians. Horner and Diggler, both ambitious for acceptance by the mainstream cinema, resist the arrival of video and amateur performers, but in vain.

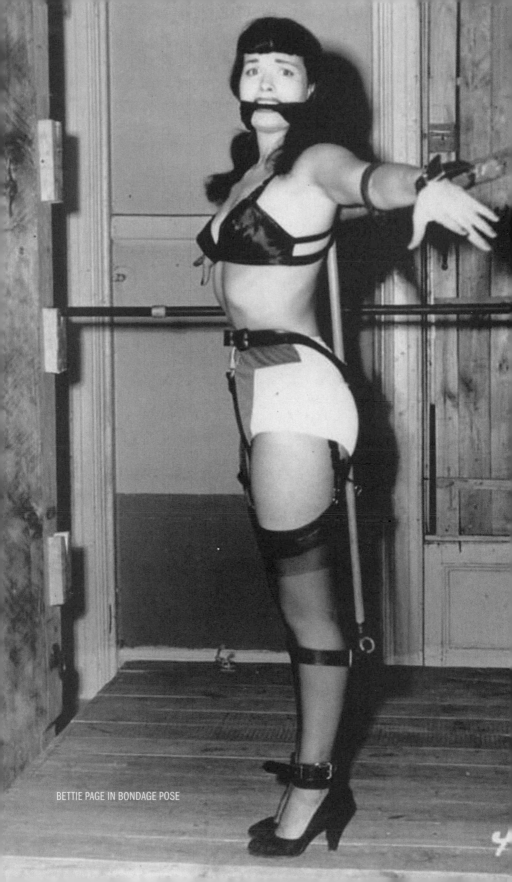

BETTIE PAGE IN BONDAGE POSE

One by one, the group's members, helped by cocaine and jealousy, destroy themselves or each other. Real-life porn diva NINA HARTLEY, the inspiration for Amber Waves, plays the NYMPHOMANIAC wife of director William H. Macy. Mark Wahlberg's Eddie has elements of JOHN C. HOLMES, while Horner has been compared to, among others, RADLEY METZGER.

BOOTY (U.S. slang, 1990s–present). Buttocks.

Like *ass*, *booty* came to mean not only buttocks but sex. Cf, BOOTY CALL, an invitation to a HOT DATE.

BREASTS.

The shift of emphasis from the waist and hips to the breasts is one of the defining characteristics of modern erotica. The medium-breasted wide-hipped ideal represented by the Venus de Milo gave way to the hourglass figure, and then, in the second half of the twentieth century, to a scaled-down version represented by the classic dimensions (in inches) 36-24-36.

Later in the century, this changed even more as the ability to bear children became less pressing. A narrow waist, long legs, and average breasts came to be preferred, as typified by the exaggerated proportions of the Barbie doll. To achieve her dimensions, a woman would have needed to possess thirty- to thirty-six-inch hips, an eighteen- to twenty-three-inch waist, a thirty-eight- to forty-eight-inch bust, and be seven feet tall.

Despite the folk wisdom that "anything over a mouthful was wasted," many Western men remain fixated on breasts, making icons of the grotesquely disproportioned ANITA EKBERG, Jayne Mansfield, and CHESTY MORGAN. With the arrival of silicone injections and implants in the 1960s, such breasts soon became available to every woman. Show business was quick to take advantage. In *A Chorus Line*, a showgirl sings "Dance: 10, Looks: 3" (aka "Tits and Ass"), explaining how plastic surgery gave her a body commensurate with her dancing talent.

Among the first to exploit the trend was STRIPTEASER Carol Doda, whose 1964 silicone injections had ballooned her bra cup size from 34B to 44D. In June of that year, wearing a TOPLESS swimsuit designed by RUDI GERNREICH, she debuted at the Condor Club in San Francisco's North Beach, descending on a grand piano lowered from the ceiling. Journalist Tom Wolfe, mesmerized, wrote of "two incredible mammiform protrusions, no mere pliable mass of feminine tissues and fats there but living arterial sculpture—visceral spigot—great blown-up aureate morning-glories." The record for the largest breasts was held by Italian porn star LOLO FERRARI.

"For STAR WARS, they had me tape down my breasts, because there are no breasts in space. I have some. I have two".

—CARRIE FISHER

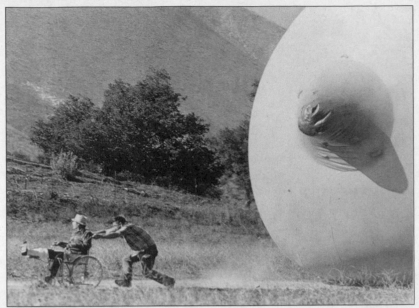

PURSUED BY A GIANT BREAST IN "ARE THE FINDINGS OF DOCTORS AND CLINICS WHO DO SEXUAL RESEARCH ACCURATE?"—AN EPISODE FROM WOODY ALLEN'S *EVERYTHING YOU ALWAYS WANTED TO KNOW ABOUT SEX* *BUT WERE AFRAID TO ASK*

BREATH THRILL (UK slang, 1890s–1920s). Arousing a woman to orgasm with a combination of licking and blowing on her vagina.

BREEN OFFICE. See PRODUCTION CODE.

BREWER'S DROOP (British and Australian slang, 1940s–present). Impotence caused by alcohol.

BROTHEL. House of prostitution. (Also bordello, whorehouse, cathouse, callhouse, *maison close*, bawdy house, house of ill-fame, etc.)

Though *brothel* is often a derogatory term, indicating chaos and untidiness, there's little evidence to suggest brothels are more prone to this than any other establishment. On the contrary, brothels in capitals such as Paris, London, and Berlin have traditionally catered to a wealthy clientele by offering discreet sex in the atmosphere of an exclusive private club, with bar, restaurant, and theatrical entertainment.

Numerous books, films, and plays have dramatized brothel life, including Guy de Maupassant's *Le Maison Tellier*; the play *SEX*, by MAE WEST; *A Walk on the Wild Side*, by Nelson Algren; *Pretty Baby*, Louis Malle's film based on the photographs of E. J. BELLOCQ; *A House Is Not a Home*, the memoirs of POLLY ADLER; and FEDERICO FELLINI's *Fellini Roma*. Early in the twentieth century, some brothels catered to cultural or racial minorities, e.g., the Chinese brothels of San Francisco

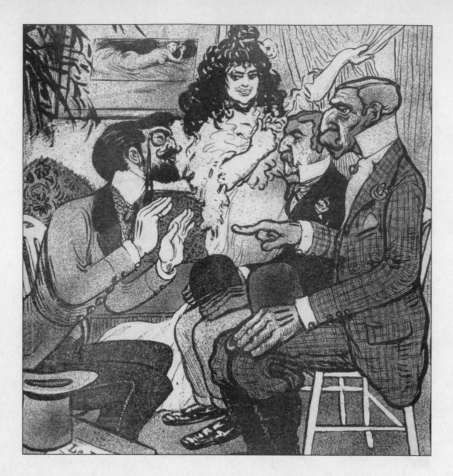

FRENCH AND ENGLISH CLIENTS IN A PARIS BROTHEL DISCUSS WHO'S TO GO FIRST, 1910s

and the Jewish brothels of New York, described in Jonathan Demme's film *Last Embrace*. Others have offered sexual specialties, e.g., Edwardian London's Verbena Lodge, for flagellants; 1940s Hollywood's LEE FRANCIS, for movie-star lookalikes, as featured in the book and film *L.A. Confidential*. See RICHARD, Marthe; LE CHABANAIS ; LE SPHINX.

Madame,

You will have me taken up to the flagellation room. You will see I am given 5 strokes by the ladies of the house, each in her turn. Then I shall crawl down the main staircase, right down to the ground floor, on my knees the whole time, viewed by as many of your young ladies as possible. After that, I wish to lie down in the selection salon and to have ten of your ladies urinate on me.

I remain, Madame, yours most sincerely . . .

—LETTER SENT BY A CLIENT TO THE PROPRIETOR OF "LE 122" BROTHEL AT 122 RUE DE PROVENCE, PARIS

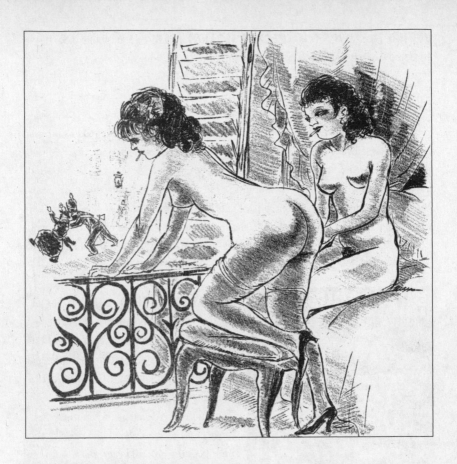

BROWN-WRAPPED (UK, 1960s–present). Pornography so extreme it is sold in a brown-paper wrapper. See TOP SHELF; BINIBONG.

BUFFET FLATS (U.S., 1910s–1940s). Sometimes "good-time flats."

Until the mid-twentieth century, African American travelers, particularly richly tipped Pullman servants, who were barred from white clubs and bars, patronized Buffet Flats—the *t* hard, as in *butter*. These illicit composites of speakeasy, hotel, brothel, and casino offered whores, sex shows, porn films, high-stakes poker, booze, drugs—and anonymity. (Blues diva Bessie Smith used one in Detroit for her lesbian trysts.) "It was nothing but faggots and bulldykers, a real open house," testified a patron. "Everything went on in that house—tongue baths, you name it. They called them 'buffet flats' because 'buffet' means everything, everything that was in The Life."

BUKKAKE (Japanese, 1990s–present). Pornography in which groups of men ejaculate on the face and body of a woman, who is normally bound. Supposedly inspired by a traditional Japanese punishment for unfaithful wives, who were displayed in the public square, tightly bound, and forced to endure every man in town ejaculating on them. See SEMEN; FACIAL.

BURIED TREASURE (also **PECKER ISLAND**) (1925). Anonymous U.S. animated film, attributed to Walter Lantz.

A proficient pornographic animated film—probably the first ever produced. Part of a series called "Climax Fables," though no other titles appear to have survived. Its hero, "big-hearted" Eveready Harton, is a small moustachioed figure with gigantic and near-autonomous genitals. Stranded on an island where birds, dogs, and snakes all boast large penises, Harton glimpses a naked girl masturbating on a rock and, carrying his giant dick before him on a small trolley, offers to satisfy her. She squirts him with milk from her breast while her vagina, exhibiting a life of its own, sucks greedily at his penis. Trying to enter her, he encounters bits of debris, then a huge crab, which pinches him so painfully that his genitals detach themselves and run away. He coaxes them back, treating them like a nervous puppy. Generally attributed to Walter Lantz, creator of the popular "Woody Woodpecker" cartoons.

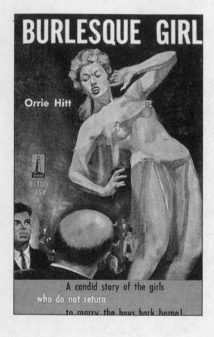

"Take Ten Terrific Girls (But Only Nine Costumes)"

—SONG TITLE FROM *THE NIGHT THEY RAIDED MINSKY'S*, LYRICS BY CHARLES STROUSE

BURLESQUE (1840–1960s). Sexual stage revue. Sometimes mispronounced—intentionally—"Berly-cue." From *burle* (Italian), a padded stick used in the *commedia dell'arte* to slap players for comic effect; the origin of "slapstick" comedy.

Burlesque developed when music halls dropped the sentimental and novelty acts but kept the girls and gags, the latter often BLUE and frequently racist. Charlie Chaplin played burlesque in Chicago in 1910, and remembered "a coterie of rough-and-tumble comedians supported by twenty or more chorus girls. Some were pretty, others shopworn. Some of the comedians were funny, most of the shows were smutty harem comedies—coarse and cynical affairs."

Talking pictures destroyed burlesque, while also, paradoxically, providing work for its performers, such as George Burns, MILTON BERLE, W. C. Fields, Bob Hope, and Red Skelton, who trained in its hard school and mastered its snappy, aggressive humor. Top theaters such as MINSKY'S responded to the shrinking audience with more lavish and bawdy shows, but in 1942, Mayor Fiorello LaGuardia, branding it "commercialized vice" and "entertainment for morons and perverts," closed every burlesque house in New York. Some lingered in other states, until TV administered the coup de grace. The last to close was the Folly in Kansas City, supplanted in 1969 by an adult cinema.

BUTTERFLY KISS. Brushing the cheeks or lips of a lover with the eyelashes only. Claimed as her invention by ELINOR GLYN.

BUTT PLUG. Dildo designed for rectal use.

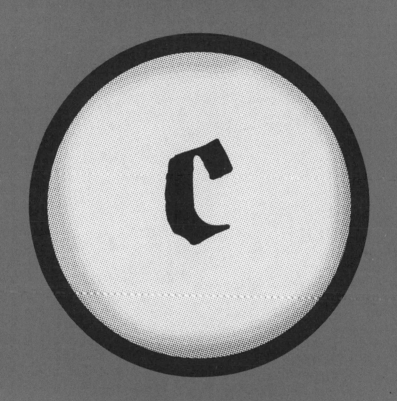

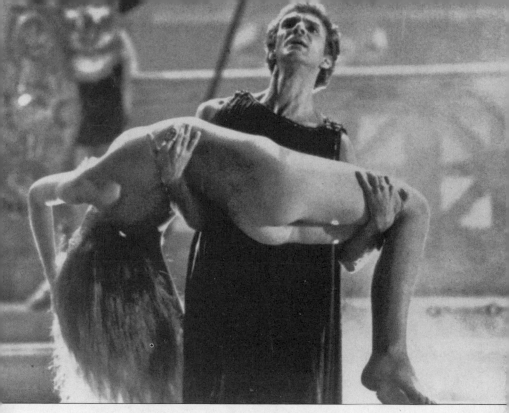

MALCOLM McDOWELL IN *CALIGULA*

***CALIGULA.* (1979)**. Italian film. Directed by Tinto Brass and (uncredited) Robert Guccione.

Ill-fated attempt to created an X-rated epic, bankrolled by Bob Guccione of *PENT-HOUSE* magazine, with Malcolm McDowell as the deranged emperor and some distinguished character actors (e.g., Peter O'Toole, John Gielgud, Helen Mirren) as courtiers and victims.

Gore Vidal's screenplay shows Caligula obsessed to madness with lust for his sister, Julia Drusilla. He appoints a horse to the Senate, forces Roman matrons to become whores, and stages bloody spectacles in which intricately sadistic machines torture and execute his enemies.

Guccione rejected Brass's cut, and inserted lesbian porn sequences with anonymous performers. Brass disowned the result, and Vidal sued to have his name removed. When every major distributor shunned *Caligula*, Guccione leased cinemas in world capitals, and in time saw a profit on his $17 million investment. Numerous versions exist, ranging from a TV cut of 90 minutes to the Imperial version of 160 minutes, containing all the new hardcore material.

CALL GIRL. (U.S. slang, 1950s–present). Prostitute, usually independent, who visits the client in his own home or at a hotel. Presumably so-called because one made the arrangement by telephone.

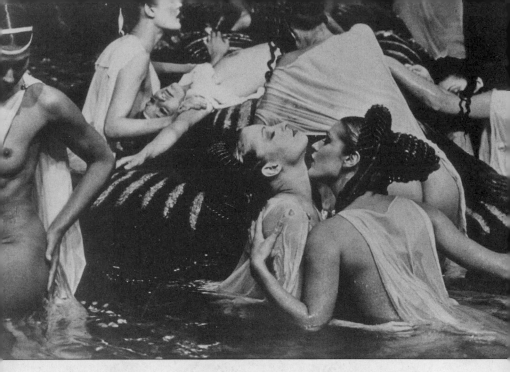

ONE OF THE ADDITIONAL PORN SEQUENCES ADDED TO *CALIGULA* BY PRODUCER BOB GUCCIONE

CAMEL TOE. (U.S. slang, 1990s-present). Pulling trousers tight over the female pubic area divides the vaginal lips, creating the impression of a camel's toe.

In the Chinese province of Guangzhou (formerly Canton), women engage in camel toe competitions, showing off degrees of labial separation for the benefit of tourists and TV camera crews.

CAMP (gay slang, U.S., 1900s-present). To behave in an exaggerated and effeminate manner. Also to **camp up; high camp.**

As early as 1909, the *Oxford English Dictionary* defined *camp* as connoting anything "ostentatious, exaggerated, affected, theatrical; effeminate or homosexual; pertaining to or characteristic of homosexuals." The *OED* called its origin "etymologically obscure." It's been variously attributed to the police acronym KAMP, for "Known as Male Prostitute," or to the practice of prostitutes becoming "camp followers" by migrating in the tracks of military units.

In her 1964 essay "Notes on Camp," Susan Sontag cited examples of camp as varied as the *Flash Gordon* serials, Bellini's operas, *King Kong*, Ronald Firbank, Noël Coward, and the performances of Carmen Miranda. Camp, she asserted, should be relished, not derided. Thus a film scorned by both public and critics, such as John Huston's 1954 *Moulin Rouge*, could be relished for the "campness" of its gaudy color photography, Zsa Zsa Gabor's exaggerated Jane Avril, and Jose Ferrer tottering about on his knees and, in the phrase of S. J. Perelman "polluting the memory of Toulouse Lautrec." In *High Camp*, the exaggeration and adulation reach delirious proportions, as in the stage performances of MARLENE DIETRICH and Judy Garland.

CANDY, as in "arm candy," "eye candy" (U.S. slang, 1980s–present). Woman whose primary appeal is as an ornament for her male escort.

ALSO

CANDY (1964). U.S. novel, by "Maxwell Kenton" (Terry Southern and Mason Hoffenberg).

"If homosexuals have an enemy, it is age. And [Judy] Garland is youth, perennially, over the rainbow.... Homosexuals tend to identify with suffering. They are a persecuted minority group, and they understand suffering. And so does Garland. She's been through the fire and lived."

—WILLIAM GOLDMAN, SCREENWRITER, *THE SEASON*

Written for MAURICE GIRODIAS's OLYMPIA PRESS, *Candy* was a parody of Voltaire's satire *Candide*. Candy Christian, the ultimate innocent, is exploited for her sexuality by a succession of charlatans and swindlers.

CANDY (1968). French film. Directed by Christian Marquand.

Despite a script by the talented Buck Henry, the film traduces the Southern/Hoffenberg original, with lamentable performances by the unknown Uwe Aulin as Candy, Marlon Brando as a guru, and Richard Burton as a Dylan Thomas–like poet.

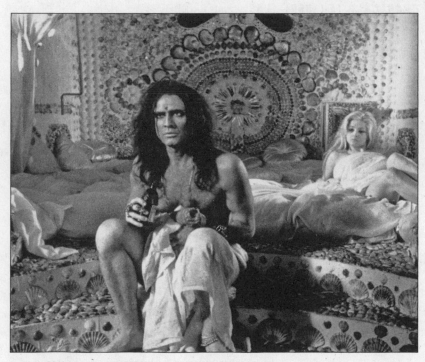

MARLON BRANDO AND UWE AULIN IN THE FILM VERSION OF *CANDY*

CARTE DE FRANCE (French slang, ?-present). Literally "map of France"—slang for the stain left on sheets by dried semen.

CASANOVA CLIP. Sexual technique, sometimes called the "Shanghai Squeeze," in which the woman constricts her vaginal entrance around the base of the penis. This acts like a COCK RING, conserving the blood supply and maintaining the male erection. See SIMPSON, Wallis.

CASTING COUCH (U.S. slang, 1920s-1960s). The practice, common in Hollywood, of trading sexual favors for professional success. A STAG FILM of the 1920s called *The Casting Couch* stars what appears to be the young Joan Crawford. See *PROMOTION CANAPÉ.*

CAT FIGHT. Scratching/wrestling match between two women, often nude or partially clothed.

Cat fights appealed particularly to U.S. STAG FILM audiences, and a number were produced by IRVING KLAW. The KEFAUVER COMMITTEE of 1955 concluded "presumably there is some special sexual bang that results from the sight of a dumb blonde, with her breasts flopping, clawing aimlessly at another dumb blonde with her breasts flopping. The acting is ludicrously poor. The girls are not attractive; their appeal is nudity alone."

CHABANAIS, LE (1880s-1946). Paris BRÔTHEL.

Le Chabanais was the most distinguished of Paris WHOREHOUSES, catering to crowned heads, including the future British king Edward VII and important figures of literature and art. Situated at 12 rue Chabanais, it was within easy walking distance of both the Stock Exchange and the National Library.

Any fantasy could be realized there—for a price. Its wardrobe contained costumes for nuns, brides, eighteenth-century courtesans, and harem girls (or boys). Retired provincial administrators nostalgic for France's African colonies often requested the Moorish room, which boasted tropical plants and a swimming pool. For even greater authenticity, a canvas panorama of desert scenes could be unrolled in the background—the same one that provided a moving landscape outside the window of the simulated Orient Express sleeping car.

Visiting this *bordel de luxe* was less like having sex than attending a reception at one of the best houses in Paris. Certainly the furnishings were no less elaborate. Ten years after a member of the exclusive Jockey Club opened Le Chabanais, he acquired the Japanese chamber that won first prize at the 1896 Universal Exposition. He added a suite in the style of Louis XVI, with porcelain medallions painted with plump pink nudes à la François Boucher.

In an unheard-of refinement, water from the house's taps was filtered, to remove impurities that might give clients anything less than the smoothest ride. For Prince

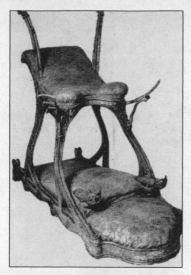

Edward, the house provided a gold-plated bath, decorated at both ends by large-breasted sphinxes. The future king liked to fill it with champagne, watch his favorite whore bathe in it, then sit around the tub with his friends and drink the "bathwater." Also for the benefit of the corpulent prince, the management created an art nouveau chair on which his companion would arrange herself, legs spread, while England's future king stood or kneeled between them.

Salvador Dalí, arriving in Paris for the first time, directed the cab driver to take him to a brothel. Delivered to Le Chabanais, he demanded an instant sexual education. Sensing his voyeur tastes, the madame placed him in the room fitted with peepholes. Dalí confessed that he left "with enough to last me for the rest of my life in the way of accessories to furnish, in less than a minute, no matter what erotic reverie, even the most exacting."

Like all French brothels, Le Chabanais was closed in 1946 on the instigation of MARTHE RICHARD. The owner enjoyed revenge of a sort by publicly auctioning its furniture and fittings, including the Prince of Wales's chair and bath.

CHAMBERS, Marilyn (née Marilyn Ann Briggs) (1952-).
U.S. actress.

New York actress and advertising model Chambers was working in a San Francisco TOPLESS bar when the MITCHELL BROTHERS began auditions for their first feature, *BEHIND THE GREEN DOOR*. They looked through her portfolio, noticed a packet shot she'd done for Ivory Soap, cuddling a baby next to the slogan "99 and 44/100% Pure," and said, "You're just what we're looking for—the girl next door."

Chambers's relish for sex went beyond simple performance. WILLIAM ROTSLER watched her with Johnnie Keyes on the set of *The Resurrection of Eve* (1973). "Keyes was laying sprawled on a couch and she was kneeling between his legs. What was remarkable about this is that, as she came up on him, her whole body was *sinuous*. It was like she was sucking him *to her toes!* It was the most physically beautiful act of that nature I'd ever seen, and I just stared at this. It was just *gorgeous*."

Chambers pioneered shaving her PUBIC HAIR and wearing a LABIAL RING— including one of platinum and diamonds, a gift of SAMMY DAVIS, JR. Like many porn stars, she aspired to enter the mainstream. However, her appearance in David Cronen-

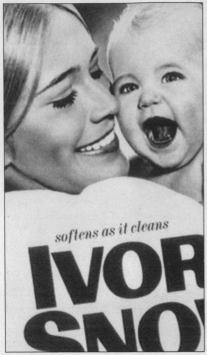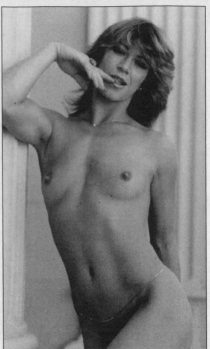

MARILYN CHAMBERS, BEFORE AND AFTER

berg's horror film *Rabid* (1977) produced few serious offers. Nor did a stage play, *The Sex Surrogate*, or a Las Vegas cabaret show.

Her frustration shows in her films of the 1970s. Mostly made for the Mitchells, they are edgy, plotless, violent. In *Beyond De Sade* (1979), she performs masochistically at the O'Farrell Theater's Kopenhagen Lounge to an audience of masked men, all of whom wield large phallic flashlights. *Never a Tender Moment* (1979) is a compilation of LOOPS, including *Southern Belles*, in which a mixed-race cast of ladies in Civil War costumes pleasure one another with dildoes; and *Hot Nazis*, an S&M fantasy set to German martial music, in which Chambers does a nude dance focusing on her labial ring.

Approaching forty, Chambers found her niche at last with *Insatiable* (1980) and *Insatiable II* (1981), playing Sandra Chase, a wealthy retired model who flits around the world—an excuse for a travelogue drive around London and sex in the pool of a stately home. In both films, she's joined by actresses of her own age, a calculated appeal to the emerging MILF market.

In 1985 Chambers returned to the O'Farrell as a stripper. High on cocaine, on which she later confessed a dependency, she courted arrest by allowing members of the audience to fondle her. Duly detained by the vice squad, she made a celebrity appearance in court, allowing herself to be photographed with the dozens of cops who flocked to be seen with the porn legend.

CHEESECAKE (1934–present). Erotic but unpornographic photographs or drawings of women.

Defined by generative anthropologist Eric Gans as "innocent erotic art [which] represents the desirable without directly arousing desire," the term dates from 1934, though the comparison between women and cake or pie is older, perhaps inspired by a fancied resemblance between the conventional wedge-shaped slice of cake and the pubic area; hence the English slang description of cunnilingus as "eating a slice of hearth rug pie." See also BEEFCAKE; GLAMOUR; PINUP.

CHICKEN HAWK. Pedophile with a preference for young boys.

CHICKEN RANCH (sometimes TEXAS CHICKEN RANCH). Brothel in La Grange, Texas, that was the inspiration for *THE BEST LITTLE WHOREHOUSE IN TEXAS.*

CHICKENS. "Eroticism is using a feather—perversion, the whole chicken" (folk wisdom). In the 1977 Italian film *Padre Padrone,* Sardinian farmboys, caught up in the fury of spring, are shown having sex with chickens, suggesting that in rural areas at least, the practice was common. Closer to home, *Hustler* publisher LARRY FLYNT confessed that his first sexual experience was with a chicken, which he killed afterward but, showing a good taste not always demonstrated in his later life, didn't eat.

CHIKAN DENSHA (Japanese). Literally "pervert train" or "molester train."

Themed sexual encounter in a replicated train compartment, where clients can act out fantasies with girls dressed as office workers, schoolgirls, etc. See TRAINS.

CHIPPENDALES (1980–present). U.S. "male revue."

Bare-chested, dressed in pants of spandex or leather, with bow ties, white cuffs, and sometimes bowler hats, Chippendales project an image of "flirty fun," which belies their seedy beginnings in 1979 in a Los Angeles club called Destiny II, owned by Somen "Steve" Bannerjee and Paul Snider, the latter the murderer of *PLAYBOY* Playmate and sometime movie star Dorothy Stratten.

After failing with female mud wrestling, Bannerjee hired Emmy Award–winning choreographer Nick DeNoia to create a show that combined male dance, striptease, and sexual fantasy. The Chippendales were an instant success, but in 1987 Bannerjee and DeNoia fell out over touring rights to the group. DeNoia was later found murdered in what many charged was a "hit" arranged by Bannerjee, who was also suspected of torching rival clubs. When three dancers broke away to form their own team, Bannerjee tried to have them killed also. Exposed by an FBI informant in 1993, he admitted to arson, racketeering, and murder for hire. He hanged himself in his cell before sentencing.

The Chippendales, much imitated, went on to become a major franchise, merchandising clothes and other products, and offering Broadway-style shows worldwide. In 1997, the film *The Full Monty* showed unemployed British factory workers teaming up to present a Chippendales-style show, but with the added appeal of total nudity. A 2002 Broadway stage musical of *The Full Monty* ran for 770 performances.

CHONG, Annabel (née Grace Quek) (1972–). Singapore-born actress who specialized in films of sex with multiple partners, e.g., *Sgt. Pecker's Lonely Hearts Club Gangbang, I Can't Believe I Did the Whole Team*, and culminating in *The World's Greatest Gang Bang* (1995), in which she performed 251 sex acts with an estimated 70 men over a ten-hour period, setting a world record. The event and Chong herself, who has since retired, became the subject of a documentary, *Sex: The Annabel Chong Story* (dir. Gough Lewis, 1999).

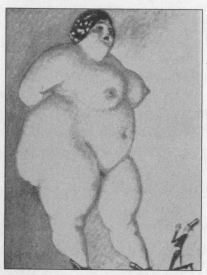

CHUBBY CHASER. Person attracted to overweight sexual partners.

CINQ À SEPT, LE (French). Literally "the five-to-seven." The French tradition whereby businessmen relax with their mistresses or visit a brothel in the two hours after leaving the office and before going home to their families.

CIRCLE JERK. Group male masturbation. Sometimes, by extension, any vanity project carried out collectively by a male group.

CLEVELAND STEAMER. Form of COPROPHILIA where participants defecate on each other's chests, then smear or play with the feces in an erotic manner.

In WOODY ALLEN's *Crimes and Misdemeanors*, his character's sister, after having been tied up by a casual sex partner, is the unwilling recipient of a Cleveland Steamer.

CLINTON, William Jefferson (1946-). U.S. politician and forty-second president of the United States.

Many U.S. presidents, notably Warren Harding and JOHN KENNEDY, have enjoyed illicit sex as one of the perquisites of power, but Clinton was the first to have his liaisons exposed while in office, and to be impeached for lying about them. If Joe Klein's 1998 roman à clef *Primary Colors* is to be believed, Clinton's philandering, even while he was governor of Arkansas, was an open secret among his family and staff. During and after his presidency, a number of women, including Gennifer Flowers, Elizabeth Ward Gracen, Sally Perdue, and Dolly Kyle Browning, alleged earlier adulterous relationships with him.

While Warren Harding confined himself to a single mistress and John F. Kennedy, for the most part, to movie stars such as MARLENE DIETRICH. Angie Dickinson, and MARILYN MONROE, Clinton's tastes ran to menials. The very insignificance of White House intern Monica Lewinsky may explain her appeal to him. Performing the role of the sex toy that every man of power secretly desires, she licked, sucked, posed, and exposed herself, and allowed him to slide a cigar tube into her vagina and ejaculate over her dress (which she fortuitously neglected to have dry-cleaned).

The playful, even adolescent nature of these acts allowed Clinton and his lawyers to argue, tortuously, that they didn't constitute *real* sex, just as smoking marijuana wasn't drug use if you didn't inhale. The American public liked Clinton sufficiently to accept this ridiculous argument, and the Republican Party emerged from the resulting scandal appearing mean-spirited and vindictive, while Clinton's approval rating rose to 65 percent. Ms. Lewinsky passed into history as little more than a footnote, although *Lewinsky* has become a synonym for fellatio.

C.O. Clothes Optional. Used by resorts to indicate areas where public nudity is acceptable.

COCK RING. Ring, traditionally of ivory or bone, but more recently of plastic, that fits around the base of the penis. As blood engorges the organ, the ring constricts it, conserving the erection and increasing its size.

COCKSUCKER. Beginning as the most extreme insult, and the only one that invariably got a sportsman sent off the field if directed at an umpire, *cocksucker* became ubiquitous and, along with *fucker*, simply a mildly hostile synonym for "man." In the Western TV series *Deadwood*, Chinese character Mister Wu (Keone Young) uses *cocksucker* to refer to all white men.

COCTEAU, Jean Maurice Eugène Clément (1998–1963). French poet, dramatist, film director, novelist, and occasional actor.

Despite his occasional affairs with women and his public scorn of homosexuality,

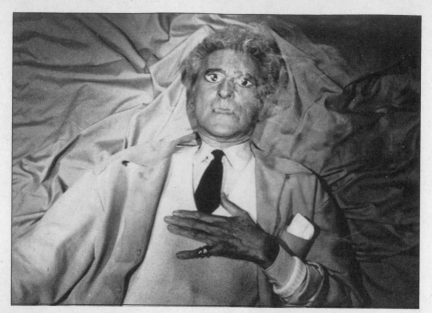

COCTEAU IN *TESTAMENT OF ORPHEUS*

Cocteau embodied better than any other twentieth-century personality the character of the gay exquisite.

Though active sexually—as a young man, he was said to have been able to achieve orgasm simply by the power of imagination—he always implied that his interest in the homo-erotic was more aesthetic than physical. As lovers, he chose only the most beautiful and talented of young men, including novelist Raymond Radiguet and the actor Jean Marais. He was also part of the group who loitered in the wings of the Ballets Russes, competing to be among those chosen to wash down the dancer Nijinsky when he left the stage. Even Cocteau's drawings of half-nude young sailors, awesomely WELL HUNG, never descend to the broad parody of TOM OF FINLAND.

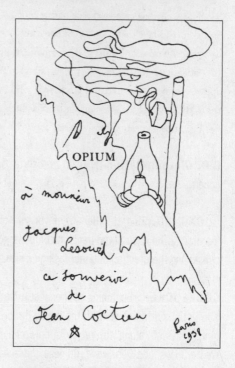

DRAWING OF MAN SMOKING OPIUM, BY JEAN COCTEAU

Cocteau knew everyone, and was admired by most of them, even those who regarded him as trivial and affected. There was no activity—from the novel to ballet to film to, briefly, boxing management—to which he did not turn his hand, and in which he did not succeed superbly. Even OPIUM, which sapped the creativity of many, could not muffle his imagination. He wrote brilliantly while an addict, and even turned the diary of one spell in a detox clinic into one of his most successful books.

COME (sometimes CUM). See SEMEN.

COMFORT, Alexander (1930–2000). British author, biochemist, anarchist, novelist, and poet.

Alex Comfort led a life of minor celebrity and modest creativity in science, literature, and politics until 1972, when, at the request of a publisher friend, he wrote—in two weeks, he claimed—a *cordon bleu* guide to fornication, THE JOY OF SEX. With the $3 million it earned him, he was able to spend most of his remaining life comfortably in California, teaching at various universities and relaxing at the SANDSTONE RANCH, which he praised so extravagantly in *More Joy of Sex* that it became his second home. According to Gay Talese, "Often the nude biologist Dr. Alex Comfort, brandishing a cigar, traipsed through the room between the prone bodies with the professional air of a lepidopterist strolling through the fields with a butterfly net. With the least encouragement—after he had deposited the cigar in a safe place—he would join a friendly clutch of bodies, and contribute to the merriment."

COMMUNISM.

That Soviet contraceptives, thick and rugged, used to be called "galoshes" hints at the state of the erotic arts under communism. Although *The Communist Manifesto* decreed "an openly legalized system of free love," the principle struggled in Soviet Russia, numbed by a hostile climate and centuries of authoritarian rule. When ex-collective farm administrator Nikita Khrushchev visited the United States in 1959 and was invited on the set of the Frank Sinatra musical *Cole Porter's Can-Can*, he was scandalized by the sight of Shirley MacLaine flourishing frilly knickers. Not that everyone shared his distaste. In the years before glasnost, Westerners disposing of their possessions before returning home from Moscow were besieged by girls trying to buy their unwanted lingerie.

Under communism, sex for visitors to Eastern Europe was difficult, even hazardous. Vigilant women, square and stern as refrigerators, guarded every floor of its hotels. A real risk existed that evidence of any escapades would end up in KGB files. Foreign Service employees were routinely the target of HONEY TRAPS. Bucharest's Intercontinental Hotel had three floors wired for sound and video, while surveillance in the German Democratic Republic was omnipresent, as documented in the Oscar-winning 2007 film *The Lives of Others*.

Nevertheless, sex flourished. In satellite countries such as Yugoslavia, prostitutes loitered in the bars of the big international hotels, their prices chalked on the soles of their shoes, which they would flash to horny businessmen. When gay defector Guy Burgess complained to visiting British MP Tom Driberg that he'd been unable to find companions in Moscow, Driberg, an inveterate COTTAGER, introduced him to Moscow's busiest gay gathering place, the toilets behind the foreign-visitors-only Rossiya Hotel.

Paradoxically, glasnost exposed the former official paradigm of Soviet beauty, a jolly, apple-cheeked peasant girl, innocent of makeup, as a fabrication of the state propaganda machine. The new Russian woman was slim, tall, even stately, and often boasted the high cheekbones and slanted eyes indicative of ancestry in Siberia, Kazakhstan, and the Asian republics of the Far East. The subsequent penetration of Western standards of beauty into the countries of the old Soviet bloc released a flood of beauties who quickly made their mark in modeling (Natalia Vodianova), cinema (the enchanting Georgian Nutsa Kukhianidze), and sport (tennis star Maria Sharapova), while their less fortunate sisters plied their trade as strippers and prostitutes in Moscow's hotels and clubs.

COMMUNITY STANDARDS. The flexible measure, first established by the U.S. Supreme Court in 1957 in *ROTH VS. UNITED STATES*, by which U.S. legislators in the 1960s judged pornography.

Instead of setting rigid rules, which had finally made the law on censorship a laughingstock, judges were required to assess, community by community, if a particular work would be regarded by its citizens as obscene.

CONCEPTUAL SEX ACT. Defined by film director John Waters as an erotic activity written and spoken about but, usually because of its repellent nature or technical difficulties, seldom performed, e.g., AMPUTATION; FELCHING; ZOOPHILIA

CONDOMS. Male contraceptive sheaths.

Before Goodyear and Hancock vulcanized rubber in 1844, condoms were made from animal intestines, thin leather, or fabric. (Hence the joke, "He's a fine boy." "He should be. He was strained through a silk handkerchief.")

Ostensibly, condoms existed only to prevent the spread of sexually transmitted disease—hence the Anglophone description "prophylactic" (meaning "to guard or prevent beforehand") and, in France, *préservatifs*, i.e., preservatives of good health. Paradoxically, British soldiers serving abroad during World War I, and facing a greater risk of infection, were denied condoms, on the theory that having them would only encourage promiscuity.

In Catholic countries, including France, condom sale was illegal, though a lively black market existed. In the UK and United States, the main suppliers were barbers, who in Britain enquired discreetly after a haircut, "Something for the weekend, sir?" The buyer conventionally requested "a packet of three." Condoms were packed individually in small paper envelopes known in Anglo-Saxon countries as FRENCH LETTERS and in France as "English letters."

Condom use plunged during the heyday of THE PILL, but revived with the arrival of AIDS, when condoms' prophylactic function became paramount. Between 1985 and 1995, sales doubled. Vending machines appeared everywhere, even, controversially, in schools. Newly reliable because of technological improvements, the condom was relaunched as a glamorous product, and rebranded to make it less daunting to women.

Condoms of the 1920s boasted testosterone-drenched brand names such as The Dreadnought, Trojans, Rameses, and Sheiks (named for RUDOLPH VALENTINO's most famous role, and with the actor's profile on the pack). Novelist Nelson Algren was prescient when his novel *A Walk on the Wild Side* proposed the "Oh Daddy! The Condom of the Future," multicolored, with a feather on the end. Modern condoms emerged as textured, colored, flavored, even fluorescent—Blake Edwards's film *Skin Deep* (1989) includes a scene of two glowing penises in a darkened room. Actress Ultra Violet suggested to ANDY WARHOL a condom for gays that went "Pop!" upon ejaculation. Warhol was tempted. "I'll autograph 'Andy' across each head," he suggested. See BLUE LIGHT CLINICS.

CONEY ISLAND WHITEFISH (U.S. slang, 1920s-present).
A discarded CONDOM, as seen floating off the beach at the Brooklyn resort of Coney Island.

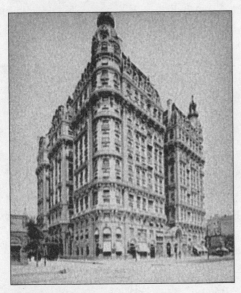

THE ANSONIA HOTEL

CONTINENTAL BATHS (1960s). Gay club, situated in the basement of the Ansonia Hotel at 2107 Broadway, in Manhattan.

The Ansonia, favorite residence of nineteenth-century opera singers visiting New York City, was in decline in the early 1960s when entrepreneur Steve Ostrow refurbished its art deco basement sports club as the Continental Baths. Courting the city's growing gay population, he restored the Olympic-size swimming pool and added a disco, cabaret, and enough steam rooms and private booths to accommodate a thousand men twenty-four hours a day. With rooms in the hotel available at eleven dollars a night, some patrons didn't leave the building for weeks on end.

Free of the risk of police harassment—a system of lights warned of imminent raids—clients of "The Tubs," as the baths became known, could indulge all but the most extreme gay tastes. (Enthusiasts for S&M patronized clubs in the meatpacking district such as THE MINE SHAFT, The Man Hole, and The Anvil.) A low-slung towel knotted round the waist was standard dress, the form of its knot indicating sexual preferences. Some clients congregated in lightless orgy rooms. Others simply lay on a bench in their booths with the door open, tacitly inviting company.

Corpulent film director John Schlesinger (MIDNIGHT COWBOY; Sunday, Bloody Sunday) was a regular at the baths. On one occasion, a young stud paused by the door to Schlesinger's booth, took one look at the director's mountainous belly, and said, "You must be joking! Never in a million years!" Without opening his eyes, Schlesinger said mildly, "A simple 'Not Interested' would suffice."

Between bouts, they could enjoy exhibitions of original art or watch cabaret shows featuring veterans such as Cab Calloway and rising talents like Manhattan Transfer or Bette Midler, accompanied by her pianist/arranger Barry Manilow. But the popularity of such shows spelled the downfall of the baths. As "straights" flooded in, the regulars, who had enjoyed their status as renegades, drifted away. Ostrow tried making the baths heterosexual, then closed them in 1975. Two years later, the Continental reopened as PLATO'S RETREAT.

The heyday of the Continental was celebrated in an amateurish 1975 feature film, *Saturday Night at the Baths*. In 1976, Richard Lester filmed Terrence McNally's play *The Ritz*, in which rotund Jack Weston, on the run from a killer, hides out in a slightly disguised version of the baths, where he's scandalized by the activities in the private booths, pestered by a cabaret singer who thinks he's a Hollywood producer, and harried by an eager CHUBBY CHASER.

COPPOLA, Francis Ford (1939–). U.S. film director.

In the 1960s, young filmmakers who a decade before would have disdained porn were seeing it as, if not their life's work, then a means to an end. At UCLA's Film School in 1961, Coppola, hungry to shoot films, was approached to make a short NUDIE in the style of *THE IMMORAL MR. TEAS*. Coppola recalls, "We shot *The Peeper*, about a little man who has reason to believe that pin-up sessions are being photographed near his house. The whole movie is the equivalent of a Tom and Jerry cartoon, with the guy trying to see what's happening. He peeks through a telescope and sees only a belly-button, or he hoists himself up with a block-and-tackle, and then falls down . . .

"Some people saw it, and offered to buy, but they themselves already had shot a vast amount of footage of a Western NUDIE, about a drunken cowboy who hits his head and sees naked girls instead of cows. They wanted me to intercut my film with theirs to leaven it, and thus make the package saleable. So they gave me money, and we devised a plot gimmick whereby both characters meet [in a Las Vegas strip club] and tell their stories, and that's how we'd unveil the two films, under the title *Tonight For Sure* (1962). Sixty to seventy percent of it was not my work, but I was so eager for recognition that I shot the credit sequence and printed 'Directed by Francis Ford Coppola' up on the screen!" Coppola also later shot twelve minutes of buxom model June Wilkinson for cutting into the German movie *Mit Eva Find Die Sunde An*, released as *The Bellboy and the Playgirls* (1962).

COPROPHAGY, or COPROPHILIA. Sexual pleasure from eating or otherwise relating to excrement. See CLEVELAND STEAMER; FARMING.

COQUILLE ET LE CLERGYMAN, LA (THE SEASHELL AND THE CLERGYMAN) (1927). French film. Directed by Germaine Dulac.

Experimental short from a screenplay by Antonin Artaud, about a clergyman whose suppressed erotic longings engender bizarre fantasies. The irrational Artaud objected to Dulac's pictorialist treatment of his idea, and persuaded the SURREALISTS to disrupt the film's premiere. The British Censor banned it, famously decreeing "this film is so obscure as to have no apparent meaning. If there is a meaning, it is doubtless objectionable."

COTTAGING (British slang, 1920s–present). Loitering in public lavatories for homosexual purposes. So called because toilet blocks, often single-story brick buildings standing alone in secluded places, resembled cottages. Sometimes called, for the same reason, tea rooms.

COUCHER DE LA MARIEE, LE (1896). French film. Directed by Eugene Pirou.

LE COUCHER DE LA MARIEE (*Bedtime for the Bride*) was the first film with sexual content. Shot in November 1896 by Eugene Pirou in Paris, less than one year after the

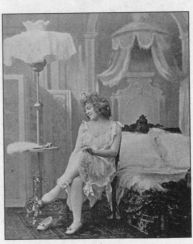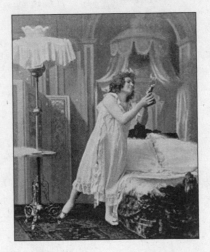

LOUISE WILLY IN *LE COUCHER DE LA MARIEE*, 1896

world's first public film screening by the Lumière brothers, it was presented with nine other short films at the Café de la Paix on December 28.

Lasting three minutes, the film recorded the STRIPTEASE that Louise Willy had already presented three hundred times at the Olympia variety theater. Her performances were especially popular since she wore no *maillot de corps* (body stocking) under her costumes.

In a bedroom setting, Willy removes a voluminous gown and a corset and chemise and, without showing much more than bare shoulders and ankles, climbs into an equally roomy nightgown. She then places the garland of flowers from her hair on the second pillow of the bed, and gets in beside it.

COUGAR (U.S. slang, 1993–present). Older woman with a sexual preference for partners young enough to be her son. Ellen Barkin plays such a character in the film *Ocean's 13* (2006).

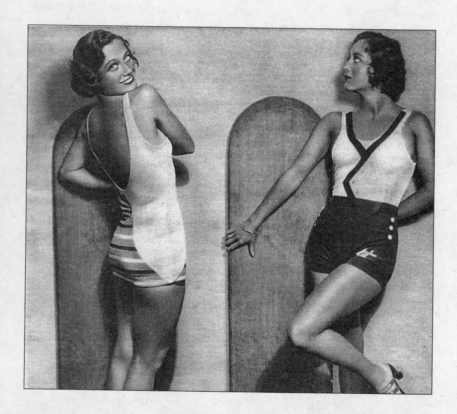

CRAWFORD, Joan (née Lucille Fay LaSueur) (1906–1977). U.S. actress.

Of the many stars reputed to have appeared in porn films, the one most confidently identified is Joan Crawford. A plump and freckled teenager dancing in burlesque in Chicago in 1924, she probably eked out her twenty-dollar-a-week wages by posing nude and appearing in STAG FILMS.

The first, made in Springfield, Missouri, in 1923, was a brief dance in the nude, made for vending machine distributor Lionel West, for viewing in Mutoscope-type single-viewer peep show machines. Once she reached Hollywood, she's said to have made *Velvet Lips*, *Coming Home*, *She Shows Him How*, and, most famous of all, *The Casting Couch*. In *The Casting Couch*, Crawford (or her lookalike) plays a starlet auditioning for a producer. He asks her to model in a bathing suit, then peeks at her through the keyhole as she changes. When he bursts in and tries to rape her, she throws him out. Her attitude changes, however, after she reads a book called *How to Become a Movie Star*. When the producer reappears, she's more than obliging; as the final title puts it, after lively exhibitions of fellatio and of sex both standing up and then recumbent on the couch of the title, "The only way to become a star is to get under a good director and work your way up."

Crawford never admitted having made these films, a line to which her biographers have staunchly clung. Arthur J. Knight, who wrote *PLAYBOY*'s history of sex movies and advised Hugh Hefner on purchases for his collection, insists that Hefner, obviously any vendor's first customer, was never offered any verifiable Crawford porn. Nor could Knight find any such film in the extensive library of the KINSEY INSTITUTE. He also dates *The Casting Couch* from around 1919, when the actress would still have been in pigtails.

CRAZY HORSE SALOON, THE (1951–present). Paris nightclub.

Alain Bernardin, founder of the Crazy Horse, was a painter and art dealer who fell for U.S. culture after World War II—not always with great discrimination. He first launched the saloon as a square dance club, complete with caller. Friends warned him the club would fail, but when it did, he redesigned it as a cabaret with strippers—one of them his then-wife Micheline.

Bernardin envisaged a show so stylish that the French president could watch without squirming, or compromising his reputation—and where, moreover, he could return the next week with his wife. There was little actual stripping at the club. Instead, singly or in groups, the dancers, dressed in a few grams of summer-weight thistledown, strolled and prowled the stage, or simply posed motionless, breathing heavily as they glowered out into the darkness. The effect on watchers ranged from hypnosis to frenzy. One tourist who, accustomed to U.S. clubs, yelled, "Get 'em off!" was shushed by disapproving neighbors. "It was like Beethoven's late quartets," the former said indignantly.

The sculptor César created routines for the dancers. Salvador Dalí saw the show often, and returned to sketch rehearsals. Bernardin added a sequence in which a dancer crawled over the famous red velvet couch designed by Dalí in the shape of MAE WEST's pouting lips.

When Abbé Pierre, France's Mother Teresa, pleaded for funds to feed the homeless during the bitter winter of 1954, Bernardin put the show at his disposal. Such gestures made it permissible, even fashionable, to be seen there. Liza Minnelli and Prince Albert of Monaco came. So did Madonna—three times. Bernardin held up the show almost an hour for SAMMY DAVIS, JR. And Jimmy Connors consoled himself there after losing the French Open to Michael Chang.

If Crazy Horse audiences weren't typical, nor were its thirty-six dancers. Well drilled, and almost identical in height and build, they were expected to conform to Bernardin's rules, which would have done credit to a high-class finishing school. Rock star Prince was one of many celebrities refused a "private meeting." "We were his girls," says one dancer of Bernardin, "almost like his daughters. He was very possessive of us."

Further to protect their incognito, Bernardin gave them fanciful stage names. An imperious Dutch dancer reemerged as Akky Masterpiece. The smallest girl in that year's cast was Tiny Semaphore. Others became Paula Flashback, Queeny Blackpool, Zia Paparazzi, and Volga Moskovskaya.

Bernardin auditioned 16,000 women over the years. He preferred British or East Europeans; French girls sulked, or arrived late. Yet it was a French girl with whom he fell in love. In 1985, to general astonishment, he married the tiny Nordic-looking blonde Marie Claude Jourdain—stage name Lova Moor—and launched her on a pop career. Her voice didn't match her looks, and the hoped-for stardom never eventuated. It was amid gossip of divorce that Bernardin shot himself in the head in his office at the theater in September 1994. See BIKINI.

In the 1965 film *What's New Pussycat*, WOODY ALLEN, playing a horny writer in Paris, tells Peter O'Toole he's found work at the Crazy Horse.

"I help the girls dress and undress," he explains. "It's twenty francs a week."

"Not much," sympathizes O'Toole.

Allen shrugs. "It's all I can afford."

CROSS-DRESSING. The practice of wearing the clothes of another sex, known in former, less politically correct, times as "transvestism."

This FETISH enjoys such widespread popularity that it has become almost totally absorbed into the culture, largely expunging earlier concepts of "male" and "female" attire. One can barely imagine that, at the turn of the nineteenth century, photographs of women who worked in trousers, such as mining coal sorters in Britain or oyster harvesters in France, were sold as pornography.

Working *en travesti* on stage or in films remains more distinct. In the twentieth century, it peaked in the European music hall of the 1920s, with the performances of the British Vesta Tilley (Matilda Powles) in male clothing and the male-to-female transformations of American acrobat Vander Clyde under his stage name, Barbette. Clyde's practice of ending his show by whipping off his wig to reveal his masculinity inspired Reinhold Schunzel's 1933 *Viktor und Viktoria*, with Renate Müller as the cross-dressing cabaret performer; the British film *First a Girl* two years later, starring Jessie Matthews; and most recently, *Victor Victoria*, starring Julie Andrews, which also transferred successfully to the stage.

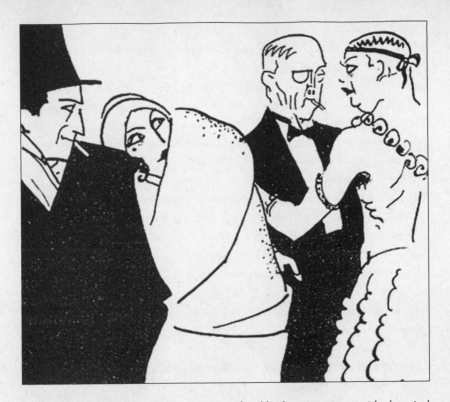

The British have always been more comfortable than Americans with theatrical cross-dressing, and plays that require it, such as Brandon Thomas's 1892 *Charley's Aunt*, are perennials. The "dame" in Christmas pantomimes is traditionally played by a man in drag, just as the "principal boy" is normally a woman. British comic Arthur Lucan made a career out of playing the drag role of Old Mother Riley in a series of low-budget films, with his pretty young wife, Kitty McShane, as his daughter.

CROTCHLESS PANTIES. A feature of erotic underwear during the 1980s and to the present, along with nipple-less bras. Not a particularly modern development, since the earliest culottes were made without crotches.

CROTCH SHOT (slang, 1980s–present). Ambiguous term, mostly interchangeable with UP SKIRT, to indicate a naked vagina glimpsed or displayed provocatively under a skirt.

Brought to prominence by Sharon Stone in the film *Basic Instinct* (1982), in which she plays a promiscuous and murderous novelist who disconcerts her police inquisitors by ostentatiously uncrossing and crossing her legs to reveal an absence of underwear.

CRUISING (gay slang, U.S., 1920s–present). Aggressively seeking sexual partners by frequenting public or semi-public locations. Certain bathhouses and parks were described as "cruisy."

ALSO

CRUISING (1980). U.S. film. Directed by William Friedkin and co-adapted by him from Gerald Walker's novel.

Al Pacino plays an undercover cop investigating serial murders in New York's gay and S&M world, who, to the dismay of girlfriend Karen Allen, is seduced by its violence and homoeroticism. The screenplay includes an arresting summary of cruising "codes," signaled by handkerchiefs of different colors. As a store clerk explains to stunned newbie Pacino, "Light blue hankie in the left back pocket means you want a blow job. Right pocket means you give one. Green one: Left side says you're a hustler; right side, a buyer. Yellow one: Left side means you give golden showers; right side, you receive."

The National Gay Task Force compared *Cruising* to the racist *Birth of a Nation* as an example of bigotry, and flyers appeared on the streets claiming "This is not a film about how we live, it's a film about why we should be killed." *Village Voice* columnist Arthur Bell predicted that it would be "the most oppressive, ugly, bigoted look at homosexuality ever presented on the screen," and advised gay activists to "give Friedkin and his production a terrible time." As a result, whistles and sirens interrupted filming, and beams of light from mirrors and reflectors ruined takes.

"CYNTHIA PLASTER CASTER" (née Cynthia Allbritton) (1947–). High-profile rock GROUPIE and sculptor.

Directed as a Chicago art student in 1966 to cast "something solid," Allbritton approached visiting rockers Paul Revere and the Raiders to make casts from their penises. Though no molds were produced that night, Cynthia did lose her virginity to lead singer Mark Lindsay, inspiring her to continue with casting as an entrée to the rock world.

Following experiments with wax and clay, she chose dentists' quick-setting alginate as the ideal medium. While a partner fellated the subject, Cynthia mixed powder and water in another room and, at a signal, entered to take the cast, after which the helper and subject continued having sex while Allbritton poured a plaster impression.

Her first success (and largest subject) was Jimi Hendrix. "He was a casting dream. When his pubes got stuck in the mold because I didn't lube them enough, he didn't freak out at all. Just very patiently fucked the mold while he waited for me to pull out one pube at a time." Subsequently cast in bronze, this model became a fetish object, much in demand at rock orgies.

Allbritton inspired the song "Plaster Caster," by the group Kiss (1977), was sponsored by Frank Zappa, and filmed by Dusan Makavajev for *W.R.: Mysteries of the Organism*, in which she's shown casting the penis of AL GOLDSTEIN, editor of *SCREW* magazine. She is also the subject of Jessica Villenes's 2001 documentary *Plaster Caster*. Having changed her name legally to "Cynthia Plaster Caster," she's recently begun casting the breasts of female performers.

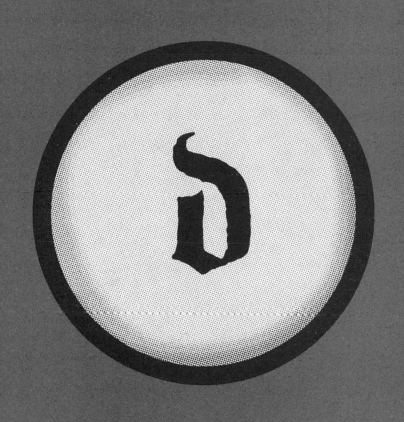

DAMIANO, Gerard (né Gerard Rocco Damiano). Aka Jerry Gerard (1928–2008). U.S. film director.

In 1967, the thirty-eight-year-old New Yorker owned two Queens hairdressing establishments. At the same time, he was learning low-budget movie-making as assistant cameraman, grip, and occasionally actor in a variety of starvation productions. When his first film as director, *Night of the Rain*, failed to gel, he added some improvised erotic scenes. Retitled *We All Go Down*, it was a modest success, and Damiano moved permanently into porn with a succession of documentaries, hard-core LOOPS, and shorter features. With this experience, he was well placed to direct DEEP THROAT when mobster LOUIE "BUTCHIE" PARAINO offered to fund the porn fiction feature.

Following *Deep Throat*, Damiano made *THE DEVIL IN MISS JONES* (1972), *The Story of Joanna*, his version of *HISTOIRE D'O*, and the chilly *MEMORIES WITHIN MISS AGGIE*, which placed him briefly in contention for an Oscar. Damiano worked mainly out of New York's Adventureland Studios and on 35mm film. He might have migrated to mainstream filmmaking, but though MGM offered him a contract, he preferred the role of renegade.

Sometimes called "Bergman-esque," Damiano's films, often violent, cynical, and suffused with what some critics identify as Catholic guilt but which is more likely simple misanthropy, stand in contrast to the yea-saying "pleasure above all" message of the porn world at large. The most joyless in sex cinema, his films certainly share some of Ingmar Bergman's despair. "In the beginning we are born. In the end we die," runs a line in his *Odyssey*. "The middle is called life."

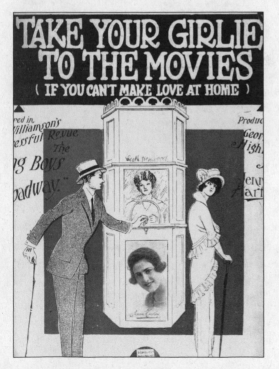

DATE MOVIE (1960s–present). Film favored by men on a date as being likely to make a partner receptive to sex later.

DEEP THROAT fulfilled this function, but escorting a woman to such outright erotica could rebound, as in the film *Taxi Driver*, where Robert De Niro scandalizes Cybill Shepherd by taking her to a porn movie. Greatest success was probably achieved with SOPHISTIQUE SOFT productions such as *EMMANUELLE*.

DAVIS, Sammy, Jr. (1925–1990). U.S. singer, dancer, and actor.

Uneducated and only semiliterate, Davis, raised on the road as a child dancer and singer, was accustomed to grabbing sex where he could, favoring tall, voluptuous blondes. After embracing Judaism to ingratiate himself with showbiz's hierarchy, he embarked on an affair with Kim Novak. Columbia studio boss Harry Cohn, whose mistress Novak had been, brought Mafia pressure to bear, and Davis hurriedly wed black chorus girl Loray White, who was paid $25,000 to acquiesce. He attempted suicide on his wedding night, then, following a speedy divorce from White, married Novak looka-like Mai Britt in 1960.

Once big-budget porn cinema arrived, Davis, an afficionado of GROUP SEX and the occult—he was inducted into the Satanic church—unashamedly pursued its stars, socially and sexually. He screened *DEEP THROAT* for Hollywood friends, and presented MARILYN CHAMBERS with a platinum LABIAL RING. LINDA LOVELACE became his house guest and sex partner. Davis briefly considered making her part of his Las Vegas act, before deciding that her only talent was sexual.

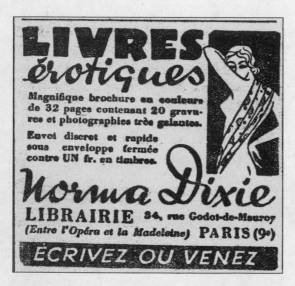

D.B. (1950s–present). Shorthand for "dirty book," a simplistic term, but surprisingly often employed, even by noted publishers such as MAURICE GIRODIAS, as perhaps preferable to the less polite "fuck book."

DEBBIE DOES DALLAS (1978). U.S. film. Directed by Jim Clark.

Inspired by a *PLAYBOY* picture story about the cheerleaders of the Dallas Cowboys football team, Clark produced this crudely made feature about two college girls who, hoping to win a place on the squad, raise money for the trip to Texas by selling sexual favors to their employers. So potent was the appeal of cheerleader sex that the film launched a franchise. *Debbie Does Dallas 2, 3, 4,* and *5* followed, then numerous rip-offs, including *Debbie Does New Orleans, Debbie Does Wall Street,* and *Debbie Does Dallas: The Musical,* which later became a successful stage show, though without explicit sex.

Debbie's success owed much to the clean-cut charm of Debra DeSanto, who, as "Bambi Woods," starred in the first three films. She had actually tried out for the Cowboys' squad, but failed to make it. Following *Debbie Does Dallas 3*, DeSanto disappeared, and has resisted attempts to locate her.

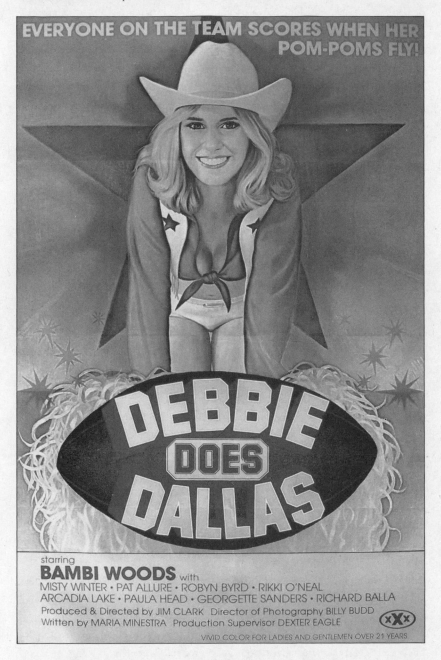

DEEP THROAT (1972). U.S. film. Directed by GERARD DAMIANO, as "Jerry Gerard."

The first feature-length hard-core pornographic film. Bachelor girl LINDA LOVE-LACE confesses to her friend Helen that sex gives her "a lot of little tingles" but no "bells ringing, dams bursting, or bombs going off." A doctor discovers that she lacks a clitoris in the normal place, but finds it deep in her throat, where it can be stimulated only by the form of fellatio in which the woman relaxes her throat to engorge the whole penis. He demonstrates by allowing Linda to fellate him, and she experiences her first orgasm.

Linda begs the doctor to marry her. Instead, she becomes a therapist in his practice, treating sexually dysfunctional patients, but returning to him frequently for total satisfaction. When he collapses, a bandaged victim of excessive sex. Linda takes up with Wilbur, a well-hung young man addicted to burglar/voyeur/rapist fantasies. His penis proves too long for her unique needs, but the doctor offers to trim it to any size Linda desires.

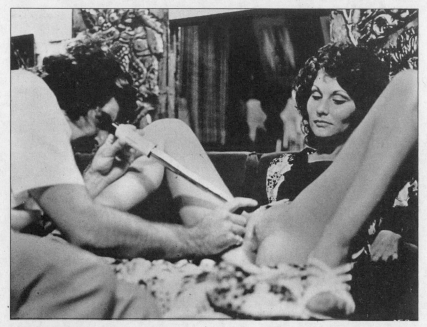

LINDA LOVELACE AND HARRY REEMS

Damiano shot *Throat* over six days in January 1972, in suburban bungalows around Miami, Fort Lauderdale, and Coral Gables, Florida, with three months of postproduction in New York. Finance came from the PARAINO Mafia family. As Lovelace's costar, Damiano sought out Harry Streicher, who, as "HARRY REEMS," a name coined by Damiano (as was "Linda Lovelace"), played the doctor in his earlier film *Doctor Love*. Dolly Sharp played Lovelace's friend Helen, and Ted Sharp the delivery boy.

Deep Throat was the standard STAG FILM writ large. Anyone familiar with porn knew these characters; the naïve heroine, eager for enlightenment; the burglar/rapist, the louche doctor and randy delivery boy. Its incidents are an anthology of popular fetishes, e.g., the MONEY SHOT, the ORGY, voyeurism, rape, even the insertion of a bottle into the vagina, here updated with a glass tube. It also includes a few not seen since the 1930s. Linda is shown shaving her PUBIC HAIR, for instance, an act elaborately parodied by portentous music and the commercial theme for Old Spice toiletries.

Though Lovelace later claimed that her husband CHUCK TRAYNOR systematically beat her throughout the filming of *Deep Throat*, forcing her participation, nobody corroborates her version of events. Given that she is nude most of the time, one would expect some sign of injury, especially on such pale skin, but aside from a small bruise on her thigh, there is none.

Throat opened in June 1972 at the World Theatre on New York's West Forty-ninth Street, just off Times Square. It took in $33,000 in its first week. Al Goldstein of *SCREW*, heading his review *"Gulp!"*, expectably hailed it as "the very best porno ever made," featuring "the greatest on-screen fellation since the birth of Christ." Journalists from *The New York Times* saw the film in its first week. In a long article, Ralph Blumenthal classified it as the latest manifestation of "porno chic." *PLAYBOY* focused on it in its issue of August 1973. Delegates to CBS's 1972 Convention abandoned a party at the home of singer Neil Diamond to queue, in some cases for hours. The entire Russian Olympic basketball team tried to see it in Albuquerque, New Mexico, but couldn't rake up the inflated ticket price.

Deep Throat became a popular DATE MOVIE, making it the first film to crack that barrier, and the last, until the SOPHISTIQUE SOFT features of the 1980s. This more than any other surprised Ned Tanen, the executive at Universal responsible for new talent. "The thing that shocked me most about *Deep Throat*," he said, "was that nobody in the audience was a dirty old man with a raincoat."

"Not to have seen it," wrote journalist and novelist Nora Ephron, "seemed somehow . . . derelict." Unlike her male colleagues, however, Ephron was alarmed by scenes such as one in which a client places a glass tube in Linda Lovelace's vagina from which they share Coca-Cola through a glass tube to a few notes from Coke's "It's the Real Thing" jingle. "All I could think about was what would happen if the glass broke," said Ephron. She was reassured when she interviewed Lovelace, who told her, as she told everyone at the time, that she was an exhibitionist who had loved doing the film, and hoped it would encourage everyone to discard their sexual inhibitions.

When a "Clean Up Times Square" campaign targeted cinemas such as the World, owner Sam Lake was arrested twice for obscenity. The judge called the film "indisputably and irredemably obscene . . . a feast of carrion and squalor [and] the nadir of decadence." In court, cinema historian Arthur Knight praised it "for expanding the audience's sexual horizons and producing healthier attitudes towards sex." Other enthusiasts included Warren Beatty, Frank Sinatra (who screened it for Vice President Spiro Agnew), and Mike Nichols, who saw it three times, and recommended it to Truman Capote. People in the trade joked that the film had "terrific word of mouth." Nevertheless, the World was closed in March 1973. Lake's derisive marquee announcement read, JUDGE CUTS THROAT: WORLD MOURNS.

By then the World had shown *Deep Throat* to 250,000 people and grossed $1 million—on one occasion $96,000 in a single week. The Pussycat Cinema in the Los Angeles beachside suburb of Santa Monica played it thirteen times a day for ten years, grossing $6.4 million. For a newly repressed New York and for foreign markets, the distributor created censored versions of both *Throat* and *THE DEVIL IN MISS JONES*. Penetration and fellation scenes were rendered legal by dividing the image diagonally (which deleted the lips and penis). Even in this form, both ran for years.

Director Damiano saw none of the film's profits, having sold his one third interest to the Paraino crime family for $25,000; almost exactly what the film had cost to make. Asked why he'd settled for so little, Damiano said, "You want me to get both my legs broken?" See REEMS, Harry; LOVELACE, Linda.

DENDROPHILIA. Sexual preoccupation with trees.

This FETISH was amusingly explored in modern times by British writers John Fortune and John Wells in their 1971 novel *A Melon for Ecstasy*, the main character of which prowls London's leafier suburbs armed with a large drill, to create orifices of appropriate size, and a tube of Germolene, to medicate against splinters. Arguably the "tree-hugging" activities of some New Age cults may disguise related tendencies.

DENMARK.

In July 1969, Knud Thaestrup, Denmark's minister of justice, announced that in line with liberalization begun in 1967, the government would lift almost all restrictions on the production, sale, and display of erotic films, books, and magazines.

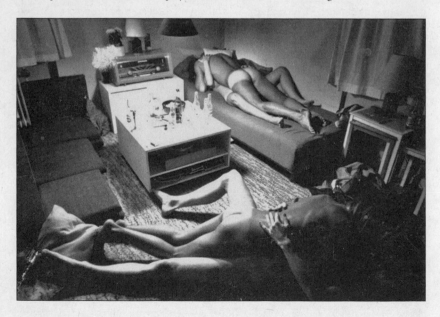

DANISH SEX FILM *KAERE IRENE* (DIRECTED BY CHRISTIAN BRAD THOMSEN, 1971)

"Why should a quiet, prosperous, introspective, Lutheran country like Denmark become the first to liberate pornography?" asked British barrister Fenton Bresler in his book *Sex and the Law*. Thaestrup's response was robust and reasoned: "Public authorities should not censor what the adult individual wants to see and to

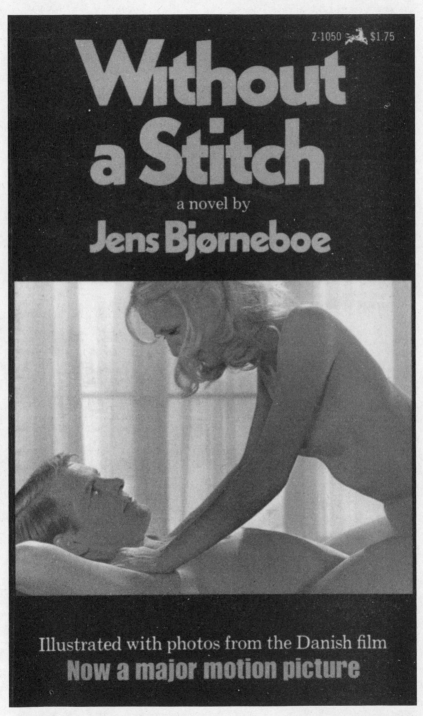

Z-1050 $1.75

Without a Stitch

a novel by

Jens Bjørneboe

Illustrated with photos from the Danish film
Now a major motion picture

read." It was an attitude that even one member of LORD LONGFORD's Committee on Pornography found persuasive. "The principle of the new law [in Copenhagen]," he wrote, "is that anything goes—providing that you don't impose it on the general public by littering the streets with it or expose it to children at any time. Seems fair enough to me."

British reformers such as Longford and MARY WHITEHOUSE imagined Denmark suffering from a national erotomania, resembling the waves of *accidie*—a sort of communal despair—that had plagued Europe in the Middle Ages. However, the Danes were anything but wild with sex. The true quality of Danish eroticism, a flaccid jollity reminiscent of English seaside POSTCARDS, is well displayed in the popular film comedies written and/or directed by JOHN HILBARD and starring Ole Soltoft. Another aspect, their rural preoccupations, is represented by the ZOOPHILIA films of BODIL JOENSON.

Behind the Danish decision to liberalize was a shrewd understanding that porn was good business. Within a year, erotica would rank second after agriculture as the country's leading export commodity. The adjective *Danish*, associated until then with bacon, bleu cheese, and modern furniture, soon acquired new connotations. In 1971, SWEDEN caught up, turning Scandinavia into the world's primary source of erotica.

Danish films such as the 1971 Hilbard-Soltoft comedy *Tandlæge på sengekanten* (*Danish Dentist on the Job*) swept Europe, where sex-starved audiences received them enthusiastically. U.S. distributors and European producers swarmed to the Danish trademark. Cinemas were bombarded with surveys of sex in Scandinavia, a form pioneered by Vilgot Sjoman's semi-documentary of one girl's exploration of the new moral climate, *I Am Curious—Yellow*, and liberated under a 1966 U.S. Supreme Court ruling that "redeeming social importance" could excuse nudity in a film.

Despite this apparent fecundity, Denmark's actual production of erotica was small. Almost all the original photographs came from Germany or France, though hardpressed publishers sometimes ranged as far as Britain for material. Nor was much sold inside Denmark. By 1979, 95 percent of all Danish pornography was being printed in other languages, notably German and English, and intended entirely for export.

By the end of the 1970s, the steam was leaking out of the Scandinavian experiment. Middle-class Swedes and Danes objected to their countries being considered as the world's sex factory, and as new liberalism in the United States and Britain reduced the market still further, production of porn in Scandinavia almost ceased.

DESCLOS, Anne, aka AURY, Dominique, and RÉAGE, Pauline (1907–1998).

Few literary reputations rest so entirely on a single work as that of Anne Desclos, who, as "Pauline Réage," clandestinely published in 1955 the sadomasochistic novel *HISTOIRE D'O* . As Dominique Aury, she made her reputation as a translator from English (e.g., Evelyn Waugh's *Loved One*) and as a journalist on the monthly *Nouvelle*

Revue Française, even compiling, with its editor (and her longtime lover) Jean Paulhan, an anthology of religious verse—of which some readers find echoes in *O*. It was to revive the flagging affair with Paulhan that she wrote her book, which she read aloud to him, episode by episode, as they drove around Paris. Published at his urging in 1955, and with a preface by him describing it as "the strangest love letter any man ever received," *O* was an immediate bestseller.

Aury maintained her incognito for decades, silent while other writers took credit, or cranked out imitations. Though posthumously "outed" as bisexual by sometime lover Edith Thomas, Aury never herself experimented with sadomasochism. "I would have enjoyed, like O, to be shared among many lovers," she confessed wistfully in old age, "but Jean would not agree. And though he was excited by whips and chains, I was not"—more evidence that the most sensitive and creative of erogenous zones remains the imagination.

DEVIL IN MISS JONES, THE (1972). U.S. film. Directed by Gerard Damiano.

Defined as "just like Sartre's *Huis Clos,* except the woman fucks a python," GERARD DAMIANO's second feature begins with a bloody suicide and subsides seventy minutes later in a cackle of laughter at the aimlessness of a life devoted to sensation.

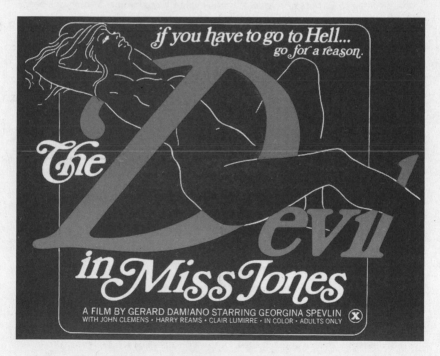

Frustrated spinster Justine Jones (Chelle Graham, aka GEORGINA SPELVIN) slashes her wrists in a bath. Waking up in a cheerless modern Hell, she's assessed by its custodian (JAMIE GILLIS), who concludes that since she's enjoyed none of the experiences for which one is normally condemned, she should return to earth for the kind of spree that might justify damnation. With the encouragement of a corporeal adviser (HARRY REEMS), she explores lesbian sex, DOUBLE PENETRATION, GROUP SEX, and ZOOPHILIA via an encounter with a python. Returning to Hell eager for more experience, she discovers that damnation is an eternity of sex without orgasm.

The bleakness of *Miss Jones* is belied by Spelvin's evident pleasure in the sex. Her lesbian pas de deux, played with her real-life lover, is believably sensual. The scene of her DOUBLE PENETRATION is remarkable for Spelvin's obligato of muttered encouragement, murmurs of pleasure, and explicit directions to her partners. Her performance becomes erotic reportage, with a corresponding voyeuristic charge.

Cinemas often double-billed *The Devil in Miss Jones* with *Deep Throat*, showing them round the clock to maximize admissions. This attracted the attention of the police, and at the height of its success, it was estimated that three quarters of the eight hundred or nine hundred legal prints of *The Devil in Miss Jones* were impounded.

DIANA, Princess of Wales (née Diana Frances Spencer) (1961–1997).

Few people could have anticipated that the blushing virgin who first entered the headlines in 1980 as the future wife of the Prince of Wales would become one of the most sensational sexual figures of the century, but little in this relationship was what it seemed. Later biographers would suggest that Diana had schemed to snare Charles ever since they met while he was dating her sister, and kept herself *virgo intacta* with this in mind. As for the prince, he never abandoned the taste, shared with his great uncle the DUKE OF WINDSOR, for older, knowing women, typified by his longtime mistress and eventual wife Camilla Parker-Bowles.

Even had Charles been the model of fidelity, Diana would never have remained dutiful. A beauty and a flirt, she bathed in her celebrity, delighting in upstaging him with slashed skirts and plunging necklines. She resisted only perfunctorily the advances of charming cads such as her riding instructor James Hewitt, revealed in his 1994 tell-all *Princess in Love*. Over the next decade, Diana watchers counted ten lovers, including football star Will Carling, art dealer Oliver Hoare, singer Bryan Adams, and Hasnar Khan, a Pakistani heart surgeon, who apparently roused Diana's greatest passion. Butler Paul Burrell described her leaving for an assignation as if in a Jackie Collins novel, wearing nothing under her mink coat except high heels and jewels.

On the rebound from Khan, she took up with his wealthy lookalike Dodi Fayed, an act eerily like the decision of the exalted, supposedly inviolate Jackie Kennedy to marry vulgar Greek shipping magnate Aristotle Onassis. Diana's shocking death in a Paris underpass, fleeing from the press, no more than fulfilled the creed of all seekers after sensation, as articulated by novelist Willard Motley in *Knock on Any Door*: "Live fast, die young and leave a good-looking corpse."

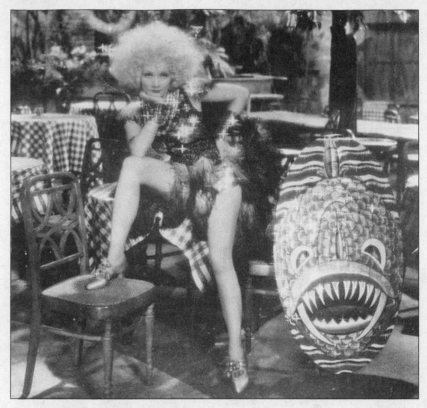

MARLENE DIETRICH IN *BLONDE VENUS*

DIETRICH, Marlene (1901–1992). German actress.

All claims for Greta Garbo to the contrary, Marlene Dietrich emerged as the archetypal sexual temptress of the twentieth century. Garbo was frosty and distant, a snow queen, but snow, once excavated, reveals only more snow, whereas one knew that Dietrich's persona, sometimes enigmatic, sometimes bantering and scornful, was a costume she could put off at will to expose a passionate being—a fact dramatized by Josef von Sternberg, her masochistic director and lover, in their 1931 film *Blonde Venus*. Led onstage in a gorilla suit by a chain of half-naked chorus girls in blackface, she lifts off the ape head and sleepily shakes out her tousled hair before donning a curly blonde wig to growl "Hot Voodoo," an anthem to animal passion.

Dietrich made no secret of the fact that she preferred oral to penetrative sex. (One male lover, she joked to friends, had been so ignorant that he thought "cunnilingus" was an Irish airline.) During *Blonde Venus,* she had Max Factor dust her wigs with gold dust, at sixty dollars an ounce, to give them greater shimmer. Tallulah Bankhead, working on an adjoining lot, displayed her pubic hair speckled with the same gold, and preeningly enquired, "Guess where this came from?" While there's no evidence that these two flagrant bisexuals ever consorted, Dietrich did share Mercedes de Acosta with Greta Garbo. Other lovers included singer Edith Piaf; actors John Gilbert, Maurice Chevalier,

Douglas Fairbanks, Jr., George Raft, Jean Gabin, Yul Brynner, John Wayne, Frank Sinatra, and Gary Cooper; novelist Erich Maria Remarque; broadcaster Edward R. Murrow; baseball star Joe DiMaggio; and, if rumor can be believed, JOHN F. KENNEDY, who seized the occasion of Dietrich's visit to the White House in 1962 for a quickie, though not before enquiring casually if there was any truth in the rumor that she'd also slept with his father. (She said not.)

Unlike Garbo, who fled from her legend, Dietrich, like Judy Garland, lived off hers, purveying the illusion in tireless cabaret tours that, like Garland's orgies of adulation, catered increasingly to her large and faithful gay audience. "In the culture, she had become a saint in the homosexual church," wrote David Thomson, "the wittiest example of gender crossover—whereas in life she had made love to women as well as men, quite naturally, because they were there, and what kind of impulse was sex if not applied universally, and with kindness?" See SEWING CIRCLE.

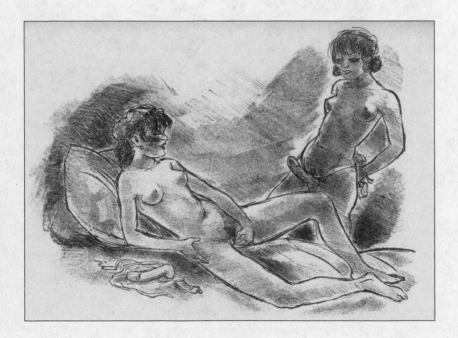

GIRLS USING STRAP-ON DILDOS, FRENCH, 1920S

DILDO (slang, international, 1800s–present) (Possibly from the Italian *diletto*, meaning "delight" or "darling"). Artificial penis, usually even though not always attached to a belt (STRAP-ON), and sometimes double-ended, for use by lesbian couples.

Originally of metal, kapok-filled leather, ceramic, or even wood, the dildo blossomed with twentieth-century technology, emerging in fleshlike plastics, sometimes transparent, and adapted to use in both vagina and rectum, with the added refinement of one or more built-in vibrators. It could also be cast in ice. *Dildo*, also a synonym for a fool, is notionally the source of the Australian epithet *dill*. See also STEELY DAN; BUTT PLUG; SYBIAN; VIBRATOR.

DIRTY DANCING (1960s–present). Omnibus term for mainly Latin dances such as the paso doble, tango, and merengue, which demand erotic body contact.

First brought to public attention in *West Side Story*, where the "Dance at the Gym" sequence used rival styles of dance to delineate the cultural differences between Hispanics and Anglo-Saxons.

ALSO
DIRTY DANCING (1987). U.S. film. Directed by Emile Ardolino.

Set in 1963 in a primarily Jewish resort in the Catskills, the film shows a middle-class doctor's daughter falling for the lead dancer in the resort's stage shows, and learning the "dirty" dances the staff perform for their own amusement. Subsequently a stage musical.

DIRTY SANCHEZ (gay slang, U.S., 1970s–present). Smearing excrement across the upper lip to create the effect of a moustache.

DISNEY, Walter ("Walt") Elias (1901–1966). U.S. animator, film producer, and entrepreneur.

Raised in the conservative Midwest, Disney was well qualified to produce films to which no censor or parent could object. Nevertheless, he was powerless to suppress his own adolescent tastes, which ran to near-breastless, barely pubescent girls and a gleeful anality, manifested in the frequent appearance, at least in his early cartoons, of outhouses, plump-buttocked cherubs, fat-uddered cows, and pink pigs with human-looking haunches. Pressed for an adjective to describe Walt's sexual tastes, Jack Cutting, one of his animators, diplomatically proposed "rural."

Disney's preoccupations made headlines in 1976 when Dr. Michael Brody chose the 128th Convention of the American Psychiatric Association, held in Anaheim, next door to Disneyland, to present a paper called "The Wonderful World of Disney: Its Psychological Appeal." Brody's modest suggestion of Freudian significance in the exaggerated buttocks of *Peter Pan*'s Tinkerbell, the spanking machine that punishes the Big Bad Wolf, and the way *Pinocchio*'s Jiminy Cricket is repeatedly kicked in the rump ignited a furor among fans. Columnist Jack Smith commented wryly, "I've always known that Disneyland was a Sodom of oral, anal, castration and obsessive themes, but at least you're out in the fresh air."

Disney shrugged off such sniping, but could be fanatical in protecting the innocence of his products. All animators make porn, mostly for their own amusement. A group at Disney in the 1930s created a porn version of Mickey Mouse, a joke they assumed the boss would enjoy. Walt laughed as loudly as anyone—then fired them all, an illustration of what became known as "Disney Law #1: Don't Fuck with the Mouse." But this didn't stop many other visual artists from building Disney characters into their fantasies.

DIVER (U.S. slang, 1920s). Person who enjoys administering oral sex.

According to F. Scott Fitzgerald scholar Matthew Bruccoli, the author's choice of the surname Diver for the main character in *Tender Is the Night* "reveals the ambivalence of Fitzgerald's feelings both about the hero and about himself. Dick Diver is of course the man who plunges from great promise to disgraced failure, but the name also has the slang meaning 'cocksucker.' " See MUFF DIVER.

DOG FUCK. Also *Dogfucker* and *Dogarama* (c. 1969). U.S. film. Directed by Bob Wolfe.

LINDA LOVELACE initially denied appearing in this film in which she has sex with a dog, and she accused AL GOLDSTEIN of faking the stills from the film published in *SCREW*. In her memoirs, however, she acknowledges her part in the film, but claims manager/husband CHUCK TRAYNOR literally held a gun on her while she performed.

Dog Fuck is, in its technique and setting, modestly up-market. The set imitates—or actually is?—a hippie-style apartment, with a calfskin rug, a Chinese trunk, wall hangings, and a low bed with a colorful cover. Lovelace, naked but for a long string of beads and much jewelry, has seldom looked more beautiful. Her long black hair is elaborately curled, her false nails lacquered an unchipped black.

There is even a plot, of sorts. At the opening, Lovelace, who appears cheerful and energetic throughout, is having sex with veteran porn stud Eric Edwards. When he leaves, Lovelace, unsatisfied, begins romping with a large and affectionate dog. Over the next ten minutes she masturbates and fellates the animal, then encourages it to mount her twice from behind. It's obviously difficult to keep it positioned and aroused, but the filmmaker devotes considerable effort to showing the acts in detail, shooting from a number of angles and moving in frequently for close-ups.

Filming must have taken at least a day. Since at no point does Lovelace appear under pressure, but instead smiles, moves sensuously, and visibly conveys pleasure in the act, showing no fear or distress, one must discount her tales of coercion. Being done by a dog while the world watched? For an ascetic such as Lovelace, it was probably no big thing.

For a 1970s porn film, DIFFERENT STROKES, *the filmmaker persuaded a dog to perform cunnilingus by stuffing the actress's vagina with peppermint candy.*

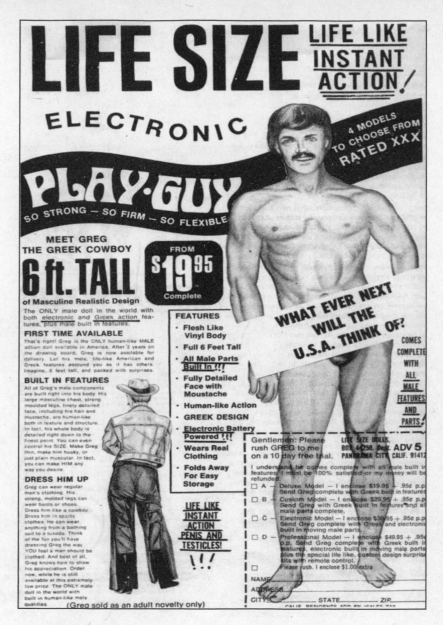

AD FOR MALE SEX DOLL

DOLL. Artificial human.

"Doll Tearsheet" appears as a character in Shakespeare's *Henry V,* but *doll* to describe an attractive woman entered general use in Britain only in the mid-nineteenth century.

The female doll that comes to life is as old as the legend of the sculptor Pygmalion and his statue of Galatea, so beautiful that he falls in love with it. Sculptors frequently worked in wax, the translucency and fleshlike texture of which led to life-size waxworks, often realistically colored and sometimes animated by clockwork. Casanova describes seeing such an automaton, made for sex, but being aged sixty-eight at the time, he never tried it out. In *Fellini's Casanova*, however, scriptwriter Bernardino Zapponi had the title character encounter the machine in his randy middle years. Skillfully mimed by Adele Angela Lojodice, the doll, despite its expressionless face, jerky movements, and a soft clack of hidden mechanisms, beguiles Casanova, offering sexual satisfaction without the demands of a relationship.

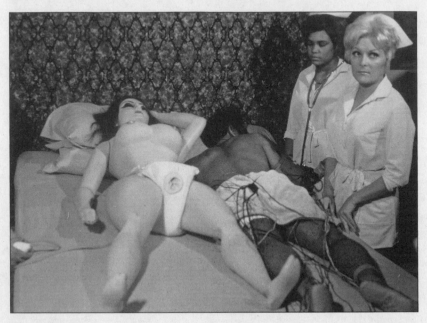

FEMALE SEX DOLL

In 1920, Austrian painter Oskar Kokoschka paid the Dresden dressmaker of his departed lover, Alma Mahler, to re-create her in effigy. He dressed the figure in real lingerie and clothing and took it for rides in his carriage and to the opera, where it prominently shared his box. Asked whether he also had sex with it, Kokoschka responded evasively. Finally, he held a party at which the doll was doused with wine, and partly dismembered.

Wax shop-window dummies first appeared in 1902, and gradually became more anatomically accurate and alluring. In the 1930s, Cora Scovill manufactured them with stuffed cloth bodies, and faces based on Hollywood stars such as Greta Garbo and JOAN CRAWFORD, while Lester Gaba modeled his figures on young New York socialites, creating an archetype called "Cynthia," which accompanied him to parades and parties.

Dolls inspired the SURREALISTS. Hans Bellmer made jointed dolls in the form of adolescent girls, and photographed them in erotic poses. In 1938, a surrealist exhibition presented mannequins as *apparitions d'êtres-objets* (phantom object-beings). André Masson's creation was typical. Her head is imprisoned in a birdcage, her face caught exactly within the cage door, and her mouth masked, with a pansy directly over the opening. Salvador Dalí designed shop window displays for Bonwit Teller, in New York, in 1936 and again in 1939, and André Breton and Marcel Duchamp, exiled in New York during World War II, collaborated on the design for the window of the Gotham Book Mart in 1944, which included a headless mannequin reading a book. The main character of Luis Buñuel's *The Criminal Life of Archibaldo de la Cruz* (1954) is obsessed with a mannequin.

Plastic technology increased the ubiquity of sex dolls, which began as simple inflatables, widely mocked for their wide-eyed, stylized faces and gaping mouths. So broadly were sex dolls accepted that the TV series *Ally McBeal* (1997) showed Boston lawyer Ally and her flatmate Renee competing to cuddle up to a life-size male inflatable. Dolls blossomed with lifelike genitalia, both male and female, often incorporating vibrators. Solid dolls or "gynoids," marketed as RealDolls or Andy Dolls and costing up to $50,000, featured warm skin and a variable heartbeat offered a wide range of hair and skin color and a choice of two hundred breast and vagina forms.

Lawrence Kasdan foreshadowed further sophistication in his 1999 film *Mumford*, in which a small-town computer genius creates a "Humanoid Life-Like Gender-Specific Anatomically Functioning Sexual Surrogate/Companion," i.e., an automaton that looks, feels, moves, talks, and fucks like a woman. He abandons his research when he discovers real sex, but his confidante psychologist is impressed; such a doll is sorely needed.

"All my ancestors went wrong here in the head. My father also. He was a great womaniser. When he was very old, he had a model of the perfect woman built in rubber—life-size. She could be filled with hot water in the winter. She was strikingly beautiful. He called her Sabina after his mother, and took her everywhere. He had a passion for travelling on ocean liners and actually lived on one for the last two years of his life, travelling backwards and forwards to New York. Sabina had a wonderful wardrobe. It was a sight to see them come into the dining room, dressed for dinner. He'd travelled with his keeper, a manservant called Kelly. Between them, held on each side like a beautiful drunkard, walked Sabina in her marvellous evening clothes. The night he died, he said to Kelly, 'Send Demetrius a telegram and tell him that Sabina died in my arms tonight without any pain.' She was buried with him off Naples."

—LAWRENCE DURRELL,
  JUSTINE (1957)

In Russia, the Bubble Baba Challenge tournament, held near St. Petersburg, invited contestants to cross the Vuoska River on an inflated sex doll. In 2006, a contestant was disqualified for "abusing" his vessel. "It is supposed to be a fun tournament," said an organizer, "not a sex game."

DOLLY (UK, 1960s–present). Sexually attractive. Also DOLLY BIRD (UK, 1960s), a girl more noted for attractiveness than intelligence. A word inseparable from images of miniskirts, white stockings, and goo-goo makeup.

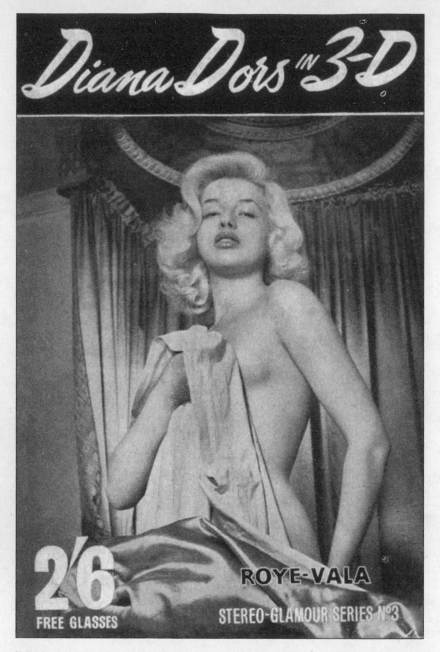

DORS, Diana (née Diana Mary Fluck) (1931–1984). British actress.

A part-time prostitute before entering movies, the bottle-blond and voluptuous Dors excelled in roles as a trashy moll, earning the label the "English Marilyn Monroe." Bisexual, she favored lovers such as porn star MARY MILLINGTON and men from the shady side of London's clubland. She married career criminal Alan Lake, and was a frequent guest of slumlord Peter Rachman at his country house, which was fitted out with one-way mirrors, hidden cameras, and tape recorders.

DOWN LOW, TO BE ON THE (U.S. slang, current). To indulge in clandestine behavior, usually homosexual. Sometimes abbreviated to DL, as in "On the DL."

Probably from hipster use of *down*, as in "Are you down?," i.e., "Can I trust you to keep this secret?" The term can cover heterosexual men who dabble in homosexuality, or any person who transgresses color, social, or sexual limits.

D.P. (Double penetration). Sex act in which a woman admits penises simultaneously to anus and vagina.

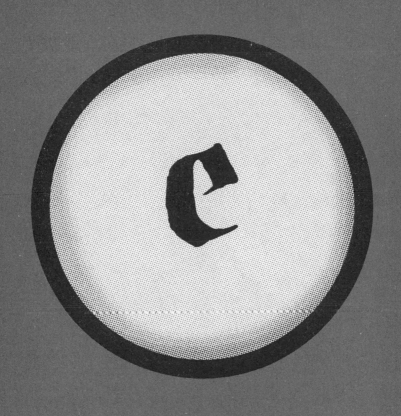

EAR. Underrated as an erogenous zone—except, not surprisingly, by Japanese men, who are apparently susceptible to the suggestion *"Hizakura so shite, mimi soo jisu shite ageru?"* ("Would you like to lie in my lap while I clean your ears with a pointed piece of bamboo?").

ECDYSIAST. Euphemism for stripteaser. From the Greek *ekdusis*, "to cast off or slough skin."

Coined by writer H. L. Mencken when intellectual stripper GYPSY ROSE LEE requested a more cultivated term to describe her profession.

EGGS. Popular sexual accessory because of their psychosexual relationship to birth.

During the 1930s, Paris's larger BROTHELS maintained restaurants, one function of which was to satisfy the popular fetish for an omelet to be slid, still hot, onto the naked flesh of clients. Some such demands were wildly surrealist. A man might ask to have a fried egg pinned to his lapel and watch a naked girl squirt ink at it from a fountain pen. In the Japanese film *Tampopo*, a couple transfers a raw egg yolk from mouth to mouth until it ruptures orgasmically in the woman's mouth, after which the white is placed in a bowl with a live crayfish, and the bowl upended on her bare stomach, where the crayfish scrabbles furiously, tickling her flesh and beating the egg white to a froth.

EKBERG, Anita (1931–). Swedish-born actress.

Heavy-breasted Ekberg, with long blond hair down to her waist, was an obvious candidate for the title of Miss Sweden, which she won in 1950. She moved to the United States, but failed at modeling and acting until Bob Hope, needing a voluptuous foil to enliven his tour of the war front in Korea, hired her. In 1956, she married failing British actor Anthony Steel, and moved with him to Rome, where she caught the eye of FEDERICO FELLINI. He cast her in *La Dolce Vita*, in which she parodied herself as visiting star Sylvia Rank, most notably in her first Italian press conference. When a journalist asks, "What was the happiest day of your life?" she has to consult her secretary for the scripted sexy answer —"It was a night, dear"—a line stolen from BRIGITTE BARDOT.

EMMANUELLE (1974). French film. Directed by Just Jaeckin.

Before he filmed this supposedly autobiographical novel by EMMANUELLE ARSAN, sex in movies, according to Just Jaeckin, was like "a hair in the soup," a disagreeable surprise that disturbed your appreciation. With *Emmanuelle*, the ex-fashion photographer aimed for a film in which characters, setting, costumes, locations, dialogue, and music immersed the viewer in sensuality—an archetype of the style that became known as SOPHISTIQUE SOFT. In such an environment, Jaeckin hoped, sex would arise naturally, shocking no one. The film's U.S. distributor agreed, merchandis-

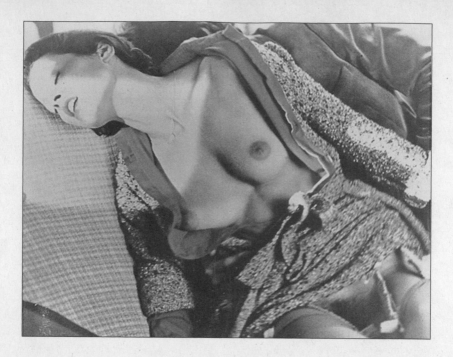

SYLVIA KRISTEL ENJOYING AIRBORNE SEX IN *EMMANUELLE*

ing *Emmanuelle* with the slogan "X Was Never Like This," and "The Film You Can See Without Being Guilty."

Though the real Arsan was of Thai extraction, Jaeckin shrewdly decided that Occidentals would relate more readily to the milky charm and open-mouthed wonder of twenty-year-old Dutch model SYLVIA KRISTEL, if not to her rabbity overbite and celery-stalk legs. He also reasoned it would prove more erotic for Occidentals to see such a woman melt in the Asian heat. Arsan herself refused to meet Kristel.

The film follows Emmanuelle, nineteen and inexperienced, as she flies to Bangkok to join her diplomat husband Jean (Daniel Sarky). After a vigorous reunion in their luxurious house, Emmanuelle is cast adrift in the society of bored embassy wives. "You may play tennis, golf, explore the canals," Jean tells her, "and you can make love." That she is ripe for sexual adventure is demonstrated in a flashback where she recalls fucking with her seatmate during lights-out on a 747. The sight so inflames another passenger that he hauls her into the lavatory for a second, cramped climax.

Hesitant about joining Bangkok's swinging set, Emmanuelle is seduced by precocious seventeen-year-old Marie-Ange (Christine Boisson), who concludes their morning meeting for coffee by masturbating to a magazine portrait of Paul Newman, and persuades her to do the same. Kristel shot the scene high on local Thai dope. Emboldened, Emmanuelle surrenders to lesbian Jeanne Coletin in the showers of the country club, and embarks on an affair with bossy archaeologist Bee (Marika Green). When she and Bee depart on an excursion to the interior, Jean, unexpectedly jealous, consoles himself by visiting a nightclub—an excuse to film a floorshow that includes nude girl-on-girl romps and a performer who puffs a cigarette with her vagina. Jaeckin was offered but declined an alternative act involving a ping pong ball.

When Emmanuelle returns, Jean, deciding she's now ripe for graduation, assigns her to Mario, the standard Older Man, embodied with suave reticence by veteran Alain Cuny. The star of *Les Visiteurs du Soir* plays a small but crucial role. As French porn producer Henri Zaphiratos pointed out, "Alain Cuny, perhaps the greatest of our actors, gives a facade of respectability. He reassures the conservative bourgeoise and right-thinking people, and it's those people who are going to see the film." That Cuny was also openly gay helped further to render *Emmanuelle* sexually neutral.

Mario takes Emmanuelle on his own unique Bangkok By Night tour. She is groped by a drunk chosen by him at random as they clop through the streets in an open carriage, experiments with hashish, is raped by two fellow smokers, and given as the prize in a Thai boxing match, after which she joins a trio with Mario and another man. The final shot of the film shows her primping before a mirror after her experience, now hard-eyed, heavily made up but, presumably, totally liberated. She's ready for *Emmanuelle II: L'Anti-Vierge* and its interminable sequels.

Emmanuelle sold a record 126,530 seats in its first week in Paris. It soon became the most popular erotic film of all time. The phenomenon baffled reviewers such as London's Alexander Walker, who called it "a fashion model's daydream of sex that simply transports the daydream to a travelogue setting." But to most Anglo-Saxons, the travelogue and the tourist brochure *were* the most familiar experience of "abroad." Barbet Schroeder's film of backpacker porn, *More*, had already put sex into the context of *Europe on $5 a Day*. *Emmanuelle* upgraded it to Club Méditerranée.

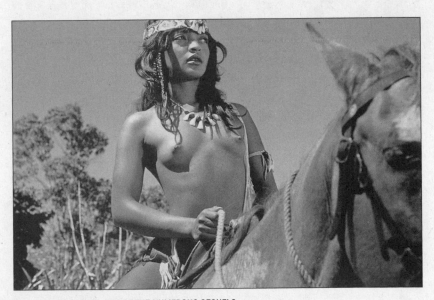

BLACK EMMANUELLE, ONE OF THE NUMEROUS SEQUELS

The film engendered a hundred imitations and rip-offs. In addition to the official and semi-official *Emmanuelles II* through *VI*, there was *Emmanuelle and Joanna; Emmanuelle the Queen of Sados; Emmanuelle on Taboo Island; The Joys of Emmanuelle; Emmanuelle Around the World*, a *Yellow* ... and *Black Emmanuelle* (*I* and *II*); *Emmanuelle in America*; ... *in Bangkok*; ... *in Soho; Goodbye, Emmanuelle*; and, inevitably, *Carry On, Emmanuelle*, which parodied the whole cycle.

> *"Emmanuelle is ... well, she's nothing, really."*
> —SYLVIA KRISTEL

EMPEROR'S CLUB V.I.P. (?-2008). New York–based online international prostitution service whose clients included New York State governor Eliot Spitzer, who was forced to resign when he was exposed as a regular customer of the agency's girls, whose prices ranged from $1,000 to $5,500 a "date."

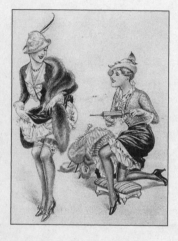

GIRL ABOUT TO ADMINISTER ENEMA
WITH CLYSTER

ENEMA. Voiding the lower bowel through colonic irrigation, usually with the use of warm soapy water, often administered with a hand pump called a clyster.

Enemas became popular in Victorian times as a "genteel" method of defecation, although long-term use weakened the sphincter. Among their adherents (and victims) were the writer Djuna Barnes and actress MAE WEST, who attributed her fine skin to a morning enema. Enemas were adopted by sensualists as a source of anal gratification, celebrated in pornographic films such as *WATERPOWER*.

ENEMA BANDIT, THE. Michael Kenyon, aka Gino Cordero, a serial rapist and burglar who forcibly administered enemas to his victims.

From April 1966, Kenyon, an accounting student, attacked a number of young women, beginning with two teenage sisters in Champaign, Illinois. He habitually entered the rooms of his victims at night, ski-masked and carrying a gun, a modus operandi which was to prove his downfall.

He continued his assaults around Champaign until 1969, when he graduated and joined first the army, then the Internal Revenue Service. Further attacks occurred in Los Angeles, Manhattan, Kansas, and in Norman, Oklahoma, as he was posted around the country. On one occasion he administered an enema to a girl in a train en route to Florida. In 1974 he attacked five sorority girls, inflicting enemas on four of them. He locked the fifth girl in a closet, after telling her she was too ugly. (She subsequently had to seek counseling for damage to her self-esteem.)

In April 1975, police arrested Kenyon near Champaign after noting that the style of breaking and entering in a spate of burglaries resembled that of the Enema Bandit. He served six years for armed robbery and battery, and was paroled in 1981.

Kenyon's exploits inspired Frank Zappa to write the song "The Illinois Enema Bandit," and pornographers to add him to their list of sexual grotesques. An audiotape of a mad doctor giving an enema to a helpless victim inspired the Gambino crime family to commission a similar film. The result was *WATERPOWER*, the star of which, JAMIE GILLIS, asked, as research, to interview Kenyon in prison, but was refused.

ESCORT AGENCIES. Agencies that provide paid companionship, usually but not always involving sex.

Escort work differs from prostitution mainly in its public element: escorts expect to be seen in public with the client, and may be chosen for their value as ARM CANDY as much as for sexual favors. In the TV series *The West Wing*, Lisa Edelstein plays a glamorous prostitute who, as a law student, is intelligent enough to accompany a visiting dignitary to a White House reception. The eponymous economist and part-time escort in Paul Theroux's novel *Doctor Slaughter* is in demand because she can hold her own in the conversation at the most elevated of dinner parties, but also later in the evening pedal an exercise bike naked while an Arab sheik records her on video.

"ESKIMO NELL, THE BALLAD OF." Bawdy poem of obscure origin and authorship, presumably U.S., 1940s.

One of the two best-known pornographic poems of the twentieth century, the other being "THE GOOD SHIP VENUS," "Eskimo Nell" tells the tale of Deadeye Dick and Mexican Pete, two horny gunslingers who, fed up with no sex partners except for

> a moose or two, and a caribou,
> And a bison cow or sow,

leave Dead Man's Creek to visit a WHOREHOUSE on the Rio Grande. They fornicate with a number of the women, but Pete is daunted by the appearance of Eskimo Nell.

> She blew the smoke of her cigarette
> All over his steaming knob.
> So utterly beat was Mexican Pete
> That he failed to do his job.

Dick does little better. Nell's sexual technique is so expert that

a squeeze of her thigh then sucked him dry
With the ease of a vacuum cleaner.

A furious Pete tries to avenge his friend's humiliation by firing his six-shooter into Nell's vagina.

> He rammed it hard to the trigger guard,
> Then fired two times three,
> But to his surprise, Nell closed her eyes
> And smiled in ecstasy.
> She rose to her feet with a smile so sweet,
> Then "Bully," she said, "for you.
> Though I might have guessed that that was the best
> That you two poor pimps could do."

Nell announces that she's returning to her home country, where the standards of sexual performance are more rigorous.

> "I'm going forth to the frozen North
> Where the peckers are hard and strong,
> Back to the land of the frozen stand
> Where the nights are six months long.
> Back to the land where they understand
> What it means to fornicate,
> Where even the dead sleep two in a bed
> And the babies masturbate."

GERSHON LEGMAN first recorded "Eskimo Nell" in songbooks compiled by South African students in the 1940s, but other references date it from the United States in the 1920s. Nell is evoked in various films, most oddly in the TV series *Ally McBeal*, where the character of Nell Porter (Portia de Rossi) is nicknamed "Iceberg Nell," presumably because the network censors wouldn't countenance "Eskimo Nell."

ALSO
ESKIMO NELL, THE BALLAD OF (1975). UK film. Directed by Martin Campbell.

A parody of SOFTCORE porn filmmaking. Three sexual innocents, beset by crooked producers, bickering backers, and their own incompetence, try to make a film based on the poem.

ESKIMO NELL, THE TRUE STORY OF (1975). Australian film. Directed by Richard Franklin.

Franklin transfers the story to the Australian outback, with an elaborate flashback, to Canada, to show how Deadeye Dick lost his eye. Dick and Pete seek the elusive lady in every corner of Australia, but without success, although Victoria Anoux makes a glamorous guest appearance as their fantasy Nell.

EVERYTHING YOU ALWAYS WANTED TO KNOW ABOUT SEX *BUT WERE AFRAID TO ASK* (1969). U.S. book by David Reuben.

Reuben, a San Diego psychiatrist holidaying in Acapulco, noted obvious signs of sexual ignorance among honeymooning couples. "They'd be laughing, dancing and sitting so close together that they'd only be using one chair," he recalled. "The next morning we'd see them at breakfast—angry, discouraged."

This behavior inspired Reuben to write the book he initially called *Beyond the Birds and the Bees*. Constructed as a series of answers to questions he'd been asked a thousand times, it began with one of the most common: "How big is the normal penis?" The book fulfilled perfectly the recipe for the later success of *People* magazine as articulated in Lawrence Kasdan's *The Big Chill*: nothing in it took longer to read than the average crap.

Initially the book was dismissed by the few papers that took any notice. Reviews frequently accused Reuben of over-simplification. Other writers, including Gore Vidal, charged homophobia and ignorance of homosexual practice. Fortunately for Reuben, Dick Cavett invited him on his TV talk show. As another guest lamented the increasing ubiquity of credit cards, Reuben volunteered that even CALL GIRLS now accepted plastic. This instantly caught audience interest.

The book spent thirty weeks on *The New York Times* bestseller list, was translated into twenty-two languages, and spawned a crowd of sequels. In 1971, *The Chronicle of Higher Education* listed it as number one among campus bestsellers, ahead of *Love Story*, *Future Shock*, *The Prophet*, and *The Godfather*. WOODY ALLEN, watching a later TV appearance by Reuben, was delighted when the psychiatrist, asked, "Is sex dirty?", responded, "It is, if you're doing it right"—a line from Allen's film *Take the Money and Run*. Allen acquired the rights to the book and set out to adapt it into a film.

ALSO
EVERYTHING YOU ALWAYS WANTED TO KNOW ABOUT SEX *BUT WERE AFRAID TO ASK* (1972). U.S. film. Directed by Woody Allen.

Written in collaboration with Marshall Brickman, Allen's film uses some of the questions posed by Reuben (and a few that are not) as pretexts for comic sequences that relate only tangentially to the book. Most successful is the futuristic "What happens during ejaculation?," in which Allen plays a sperm waiting to go "over the top."

EXOTIC DANCER (see STRIPTEASER).

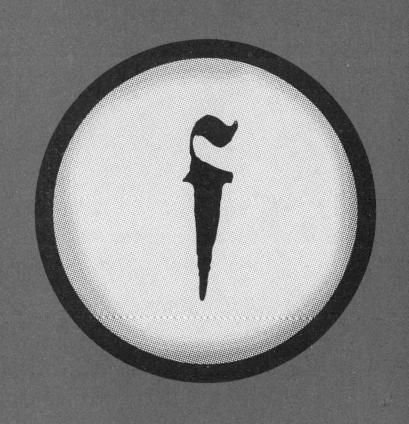

FACIAL (U.S. slang, 1990s-present). Photograph or film in which a man ejaculates in the face of his partner. See BUKKAKE.

FAGGOT or FAG (1920s-present). Derogatory term for male homosexual, in wide use until the advent of GAY in the early 1940s. Source obscure, but perhaps related to English public school custom of forcing new students to serve as "fags," or unpaid servants, for seniors, which often included sexual favors.

FAG HAG (U.S. slang, 1960s-present). Woman who prefers the society of male homosexuals.

FAIRY (UK slang, 1920s-present). Derogatory term for male homosexual. JEAN COCTEAU, unaware of the connotation, was initially flattered to be called "a fairy" by an English child, mistaking it for evidence of a charming national belief in the supernatural.

FALSIES (U.S. slang, 1950s-1960s). Pads for a padded brassiere.

In the 1960s, the pads were briefly replaced by sacs of compressed air.

FANG CHUNG. Chinese sexual technique. See SIMPSON, Wallis.

FARMER'S DAUGHTER. Stock character, habitually promiscuous, of dirty jokes, often involving a TRAVELING SALESMAN.

Both appeared frequently in 1920s films and plays, e.g., the lyrics of "Shuffle Off to Buffalo (1933). ("I'll bet that she's the farmer's daughter / And he's that well-known traveling man / He once stopped down at the farm house. / That's how the whole affair began."). The first version of the PRODUCTION CODE specifically banned references to either.

FARMING (UK slang, 1980s-present). Form of COPROPHAGY where enthusiasts haunt public lavatories for fresh feces.

FAROUK I (1920-1965). King of Egypt, deposed in 1952.

The cliché decadent monarch, Farouk accumulated a legendary library of erotica, seen only by a few intimates and by celebrities such as Errol Flynn. When Gamel Abdel Nasser deposed Farouk, invaders of his palace supposedly found that the collection consisted mainly of cheap paperbacks, though it's more likely the better items were misappropriated, or had already been sold off to support Farouk's lavish exile in Rome.

FEAR OF FLYING (1973). U.S. novel, by Erica Jong.

An ostensibly autobiographical novel in which the Jong character, Isadora Wing, a failed writer married to a psychiatrist, and terrified of flying, accompanies her husband to a conference in Vienna, where she is sexually liberated by a rival therapist who embodies for her the vision of the "zipless fuck"—defined as the spontaneous sexual encounter with a total stranger during which "zippers fell away like rose petals, [and] underwear blew off in one breath like dandelion fluff." The book, described somewhat vaguely by Jong as "a mock-memoir, *a la Moll Flanders* or *Robinson Crusoe*," sold twenty million copies worldwide, but aroused the anger of many, including Jong's sister, who repudiated the chapter in which Wing's brother-in-law climbs into her bed. Shrugging off the criticism, Jong justified any excesses as psychological self-medication. "If I didn't write that book, I would go mad and die."

FEGELE, sometimes FEGELAH. Effeminately homosexual. (From the Yiddish *foygl*, "a bird").

FELCHING (gay slang, 1980s-present). Practice, mainly of male homosexuals, of sucking semen from the anus after ejaculation.

Film director John Waters categorized felching as a "CONCEPTUAL" SEXUAL ACT, i.e., more talked about than actually practiced.

FELLINI, Federico (1920-1993). Italian film director.

The erotic tone of Fellini's largely autobiographical films, and the fact that he was married to actress Giulietta Masina, misled audiences into believing he enjoyed a rich heterosexual life. In fact, he was sexually ambivalent and, because of a chronic glandular deficiency, effectively impotent. The details of adolescent lust in *Amarcord* and of Rome's brothels in *Fellini Roma* were drawn from the experiences of schoolmates. For *Fellini Casanova*, he turned to Marcello Mastroianni and priapic novelist Georges Simenon and to screenwriter Bernardino Zapponi, a noted eroticist and author of a book on BETTIE PAGE. Zapponi also scripted Fellini's most overtly erotic film, *Fellini Satyricon*, the main characters of which—three bisexuals, one of them impotent—betray the director's true concerns.

While Fellini habitually chose intellectual young gays, among them Pier Paolo Pasolini, as confidants and companions, the relationships remained sexless. His own fantasies involved grotesquely overweight earth-mother figures such as "La Saraghina," in *Otto e Mezzo*.

In public, Fellini disapproved of porn, declaring, when it was suggested he try the form, "I have never found anyone who said, 'Ah, I have seen a beautiful porno film.' I have always understood that there were hideous women in them who make you feel you're in the morgue or the stockyards.' " This is ironic in light of revelations that, when he met with GROUCHO MARX in the hope that Marx would play the CROSS-

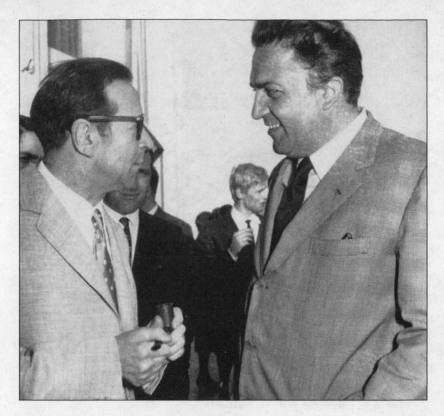

FEDERICO FELLINI (RIGHT), WITH GEORGES SIMENON

DRESSING Lichas in *Satyricon*, Marx introduced him to STAG FILMS, of which he became an enthusiastic collector.

The unique meeting, in Fellini's imagination, of infantile sexuality, fetishism, homophilia, and pornography created a distinctive vision of sex, typified by his masterpiece *La Dolce Vita*, inhabited by bored and decadent aristos who perform STRIPTEASE for their friends and borrow the beds of whores for assignations. The richest images of *Giulietta degli Spiriti* and *Fellini Satyricon* are sexual fantasies in which the nude Sandra Milo descends into her giant bath down a rococo slide and an impotent Martin Potter tours the BROTHELS of imperial Rome searching for his lost erection, with the help of whores who beat him with canes while a solemn elephant looks on. *Fellini Roma* recreated the whorehouses of World War II, showing his handsome alter ego besotted by a voluptuous prostitute whose fetishist costumes recall Cabiria, the heroine of his favorite movie melodrama of love and sacrifice in the Roman arena. The eunuchoid Fellini never experienced at firsthand any of these excesses, but his dreams seethed with them. As he put it, "my head hits the pillow, and the carnival begins."

FEMLIN. Miniature female, nude but for black stockings, created by artist LeRoy Neiman, who decorated the joke page of *PLAYBOY* magazine and featured in its advertising.

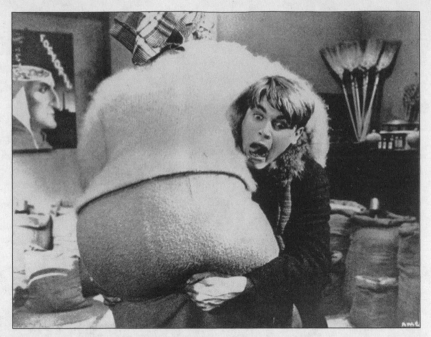

FELLINI'S FILM *AMARCORD*, GUESSING THE WEIGHT OF THE BAKER'S WIFE

FEMME PRODUCTIONS. U.S. porn production company, 1983–1999.

Launched in 1983 by porn star Candida Royalle with her husband, director/cameraman Per Sjostedt, and veteran performers Gloria Leonard, Veronica Hart, ANNIE SPRINKLE, and Veronica Vera, Femme Productions aimed to create video porn primarily for the female audience. In a calculated appeal to the same women who had taken NANCY FRIDAY's collection of sexual fantasies, *My Secret Garden*, through twenty-nine printings, Femme's films were mostly plotless successions of sexual episodes. In classic demonstrations of Erica Jong's ideal ZIPLESS FUCK, couples met and, without preliminary conversation, made love. Settings included art galleries, discos, and photo sessions, while the characters ranged from the archetypal fantasy stranger to the Avon lady, a popular figure of erotic fantasy.

Femme productions omitted the traditional MONEY and PINK SHOTS, the obligatory lesbian scenes, and the emphasis on male sexual supremacy. Often the studs remained limp throughout foreplay, putting their partners' pleasure before their own. Royalle also insisted that all performers who were not lovers off the set wear condoms, the only producer in the business to do so at that time.

While the industry applauded Femme's courage, the public, though briefly intrigued, quickly demonstrated a preference for stories whose characters occupied familiar fetishized roles. As X-rated distributor Steffani Martin remarked, "sensitivity is wonderful, but it's not grounds for arousal." The company was subsequently absorbed into the PLAYBOY empire.

FERRARI, Lolo (Eve Valois) (1963–2000). Porn actress.

French-born Ferrari possessed, according to *Guinness World Records,* the world's largest breasts, augmented by plastic surgery to a grotesque 56G. With a mane of bleached hair and lips swollen by further surgery, Ferrari appeared in five porn features and made numerous nightclub and TV appearances before being found dead of what was initially assumed to be an overdose of antidepressants, but was later identified as suffocation by one of her own mammaries. Her husband-manager was later jailed on charges connected with her death.

FETISH. Object or practice invested with mystic significance independent of its intended function. From Latin *facticius,* "artificial," and *facere,* "to make."

The term *fetish* was coined in the eighteenth century to describe ritual items in tribal cultures that the shaman invested with quasi-magical power. It migrated to psychology in 1887 when Alfred Binet applied it to the sexual admiration of an inanimate object. In 1912, Richard von Krafft-Ebing widened the definition to cover a preoccupation with parts of the body (for example, the tendency of some people to be aroused by feet).

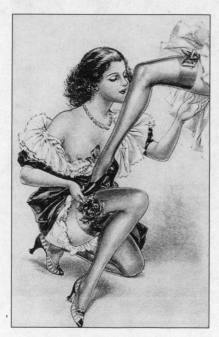

In 1927 SIGMUND FREUD suggested that all fetishism had its basis in childhood trauma, citing as an example the male child who, finding his mother lacked a penis, became preoccupied with that organ. Fetishism soon ceased to be considered a disorder, and was reassessed as an essential element of human sexuality. In France, the word *fetiche* was downgraded to mean any object, practice, or person consistently favored over others, e.g., Marcello Mastroianni was the *fetiche* actor of FEDERICO FELLINI.

Among the most commonly fetishized items in Western society are feet and shoes, hands and gloves, womens' legs and stockings, fur, rubber and LEATHER, urine and feces, and body hair. The fetishizing of SEMEN explains the importance of the MONEY SHOT in porn films. However, given special formative circumstances, almost anything can become fetishized. There are examples of men who've had sexual relations with paving stones and are excited by watching the changes in color of a handkerchief stuffed into an automobile exhaust pipe.

SHOE AND STOCKING FETISHISM

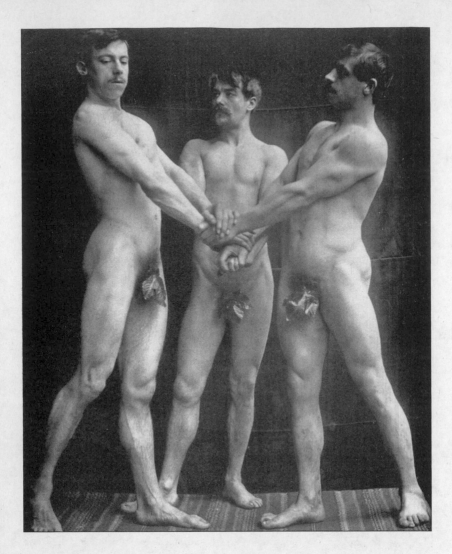

ARTISTS MODELS IN FIG LEAVES, 1902

FIG LEAF. Traditionally used by sculptors to cover the genitals of nude figures. In the book of Genesis, Adam and Eve cloak their nakedness with fig leaves when they're cast out of the GARDEN OF EDEN.

FINGER FUCKING (see FRIGGING).

FISTING (also FIST FUCKING). Inserting the hand and part of forearm into the rectum or vagina. The term is actually a misnomer, since the hand is not clenched into a fist until after insertion, and often not even then. Fisting requires much preparation, often involving multiple ENEMAS, the use of relaxants such as amyl nitrite, elbow-length gloves, lubricants, etc.

Though not intrinsically attractive on the aesthetic level, fisting was celebrated photographically by ROBERT MAPPLETHORPE. Two Australian lovers introduced a graphic element when one had a kookaburra tattooed adjacent to his anus while his partner had another inked on his forearm, the aim of a successful fisting being to bring the two birds together as if perched side by side.

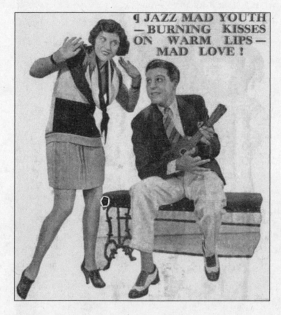

FLAMING YOUTH
(1923). U.S. novel by "Warner Fabian" (pseudonym of Samuel Hopkins Adams).

A negligible novel about an ennui-afflicted society of wealthy Americans drifting into divorce, drunkenness, and aimless hedonism, *Flaming Youth*, or at least its title, entered the popular imagination when it was filmed in 1923. Colleen Moore as the pleasure-seeking heroine was seen as emblematic of the Jazz Age. "I was the spark that lit up flaming youth," wrote Scott Fitzgerald. "Colleen Moore was the torch. What little things we are to have caused all that trouble."

FLASHING (British slang, 1920s-present). Publicly exposing nude body or genitals for shock effect.

The flasher is customarily depicted as a man, hands in pockets, flinging open a raincoat (normally described in Britain as "a dirty mac") to reveal his nudity. Systematic flashers modify clothing to facilitate their pleasure. Christopher Isherwood described one such outfit seen in Berlin: "Here were the lower halves of trouser-legs with elastic bands to hold them in position between knee and ankle. In these and nothing else but an overcoat and a pair of shoes, you could walk the streets and seem fully clothed, giving a camera-quick exposure whenever a suitable viewer appeared." Photographers such as HELMUT NEWTON adapted the practice for photo shoots with female models.

FLEISS, Heidi (née Heidi Lynne Fleiss) (1956–). U.S. madam.

During the late 1980s and early 1990s, Heidi Fleiss operated the most successful CALL GIRL service in Los Angeles, supplying beautiful women to the rich and famous for thousands of dollars a night. A sometime lover of financier Bernie Cornfeld, Fleiss developed a taste for the high life, which she could not sustain when the two broke up.

She became a prostitute for L.A. madam Elizabeth Adams, aka "Madam Alex," then took over Adams's business, managing it from various luxury homes she occupied with her friend Victoria Sellers, daughter of actor Peter Sellers and Britt Ekland.

Writing later, with the benefit of hindsight, Fleiss said, "If you're going to run an illegal business, you better be driving the best car, living in the biggest house, fucking the best-looking people, and spending every dollar you make, because sooner or later you're going to get caught." And caught she was, in 1993, when the "Japanese tourists" to whom she sent cocaine and girls turned out to be members of the Beverly Hills Police Department. Her trial was expected to expose numerous stars as her clients, but the only name to surface was that of Charlie Sheen, already known for his wild lifestyle and relationships with porn star GINGER LYNN and TRACI LORDS.

After spells in jail and "community service" in a soup kitchen, Fleiss, bankrupt and drug-dependent, tried to relaunch herself with memoirs, movies, and stints as a TV personality and proprietor of a line of underwear. In 2008, she resurfaced in Nevada, where she promised to open a male brothel exclusively for women.

FLESH GORDON (1976). U.S. film. Directed by Howard Ziehm and Michael Beneviste.

A SOFT-CORE spoof of the 1930s comic strip and its movie serial version, produced by LA LOOP king BILL OSCO. Ming the Merciless of Mongo became Wang the Perverted of planet Porno; Flash's girlfriend Dale Arden was transformed into Dale Ardor; his colleague Doctor Zarkoff into Flexi Jerkoff. Instead of directing onto earth a ray that induces earthquakes, Wang causes it to be overcome by an urge to copulate. Racing to Porno, Flesh, Dale, and Jerkoff save the world, but only at the expense of Flesh submitting to homosexual fellatio and Dale being raped by rampant lesbians.

Flesh Gordon began as a porn movie on a budget of $25,000, but expanded to a $500,000 production once a number of eager young special effects technicians became involved. These included nine-time Oscar winner Dennis Muren, later Steven Spielberg's right-hand man on *Star Wars*, *Indiana Jones*, and *Jurassic Park* films; and six-time Oscar-winning makeup man Rick Baker. "The porn scenes that we shot for the film were confiscated by the police," says Ziehm. "They confiscated the film's negative and I had to relinquish any hard-core in order to get the film back. By that time, I had decided not to make the film hard-core anyway." Osco, with typical *chutzpah*, won widespread publicity by claiming that the effects had been nominated for an Oscar, but that the Academy got cold feet at the last minute and substituted *The Poseidon Adventure*. He even hired pickets to protest at the Oscar ceremonies. In the resultant publicity, he cut the film's raunchier moments and won a limited general release in 1974.

FLUFF (U.S., 1960s–present). Girl employed on porn film sets to stimulate male performers during breaks in filming and help them retain their all-important erections, or WOOD.

FLYNT, Larry (né Larry Claxton Flynt) (1942–). U.S. publisher and free-speech activist.

During the 1970s, Flynt operated a number of strip clubs in Ohio, and published a newsletter promoting them. In 1974, he transformed this into the magazine *HUSTLER*, aimed at a blue-collar clientele, and containing graphic cartoons and raunchy photos. Flynt derided *PLAYBOY*'s policy of AIRBRUSHING nudes, in particular to disguise the labia. Instead, HUSTLER became the first mass-circulation porn magazine to feature PINK shots of women with spread legs and open vulvas. Circulation soared, particularly when Flynt transgressed other taboos, such as printing paparazzi shots of a nude Jackie Kennedy Onassis.

In 1978, Flynt and his lawyer were shot from ambush near the courthouse in Lawrenceville, Georgia. Flynt was paralyzed from the waist down. Undeterred, he built an empire that included more strip clubs, Hustler shops, a casino, and a second magazine, *Barely Legal*, featuring models who had just attained the AGE OF CONSENT. He was also often in court on obscenity, organized crime, and libel charges, and became notorious for labeling the U.S. Supreme Court "nothing but eight assholes and a token cunt." He was also jailed for wearing an American flag as a diaper. Milos Forman filmed Flynt's life story in 1996 as *The People vs. Larry Flynt*, which idealized him as a devoted husband and valiant protector of the right of free speech.

FOREVER AMBER (1944). U.S. novel, by Kathleen Winsor.

This BODICE RIPPER set in seventeenth-century England followed the adventurous Amber St. Clare, who schemes her way out of Newgate prison to become a mistress of Charles II. The book was banned in Boston after the Massachusetts attorney general discovered seventy references to sexual intercourse, thirty-nine illegitimate pregnancies, seven abortions, ten descriptions of women undressing in front of men, and forty-nine "miscellaneous objectionable passages."

ALSO
FOREVER AMBER (1948). U.S. film. Directed by Otto Preminger.

The scandal that got Winsor's novel banned in Boston helped promote this expensive but unremarkable film starring Linda Darnell as the eponymous heroine. Even a C rating, for "Condemned," by the LEAGUE OF DECENCY could not make the movie a hit.

FORTY THIEVES, THE. Collective term for the independent U.S. film distributors who, from the 1920s to the 1960s, circumvented Hollywood's self-imposed censorship by "road-showing" their films, i.e., sending them by car across the country and screening them at theaters hired for the night.

Typical were Dwain Esper, so-called "King of the Roadshows," whose releases exploited drug use (*Narcotic*), mental illness (*Maniac*), and sexually transmitted disease (*The Seventh Commandment*); and KROGER BABB, who made his fortune with the sex education film *MOM AND DAD*. The same methods were used by 1930s independent African American filmmaker Oscar Micheaux and 1970s porn producers such as BILL OSCO.

FOUFOUNE. French slang for "vagina." See also *BITE*.

FRANCIS, "Miss" Lee. Hollywood madam.

From the late 1920s through the early 1940s, Francis provided Hollywood's highest-class prostitutes, favoring those resembling movie stars. Her operation inspired James Ellroy's novel *L.A. Confidential* and Curtis Hanson's film version, starring Kim Basinger as a Veronica Lake lookalike. Many of her girls enjoyed minor movie careers. When Erich Von Stroheim, a stickler for realism, needed to show his character in the 1928 *The Wedding March* in an open car filled with the most beautiful whores, he simply hired the real thing from Lee Francis.

FRANKS AND BEANS (U.S. slang, 1980s–present). Police slang for male genitals. See also PICKLE; BEAVER.

FREDERICK'S OF HOLLYWOOD. Los Angeles lingerie store.

Frederick Mellinger, inventor of the push-up bra, opened his original store on Hollywood Boulevard in 1946. Unashamedly trashy, it catered to a clientele with whorehouse taste, specializing in wasp-waisted corsets, marabou-trimmed mules, and baby doll nighties. Many bondage models, including BETTIE PAGE, bought outfits from the boutique's catalogue. Frederick's dominated the market until supplanted in the 1980s by the more discreet Victoria's Secret.

FREE LOVE.

In Article 10 of the 1848 *Communist Manifesto*, Karl Marx and Friedrich Engels declared, "We have no need to introduce free love. It has existed almost from time immemorial. What we desire to introduce is an openly legalized system of free love." Quite what they meant was never spelled out in detail—understandably, since the concept of unregulated sexual arrangements between free individuals and among the members of groups threatened social institutions such as monogamous marriage and the laws of inheritance that were regarded as the foundations of society.

In theory, "free love" guaranteed the right of consenting adults to enter into polygamy, polyandry, serial marriage and divorce, and group marriage. Moreover, that right would be backed up by the force of law. In practice, the social effects threatened to be so disastrous that nobody dared apply it. When it was occasionally tried, as under the brief anarcho-socialist administration in Spain in 1936, the response of the largely peasant population was blank incomprehension.

The term speedily devolved into simple shorthand for promiscuity. As such, free love was practiced vigorously in the 1920s, particularly among the left-wing intellectuals of sophisticated societies such as those of Great Britain and the United States, and was revived with similar motives during the sexual revolution of the 1960s, when it dovetailed neatly with such slogans as MAKE LOVE, NOT WAR. Ironically, with the gradual acceptance of single parenthood, gay marriage, partnerships unsolemnized by religion, and the legal protection of children born outside wedlock, the "openly legalized system of free love" envisaged by Marx and Engels has almost come about. See COM-MUNISM.

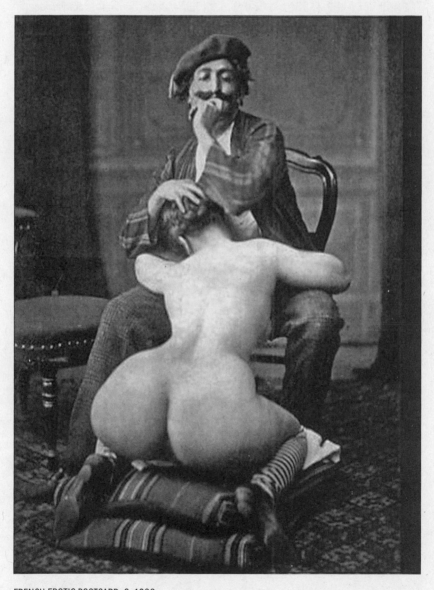

FRENCH EROTIC POSTCARD, C. 1900

FRENCHING (U.S. slang, 1890s–1950s). Fellatio or cunnilingus. Supplanted by BLOW JOB; GOING DOWN, etc.

FRENCH KISS (U.S. slang, 1880s–present). Ambiguous term that, like MAKING LOVE, changed its meaning during the century. Originally any kiss involving the tongue or open mouth, it developed into a synonym for oral sex.

FRENCH LETTER. See CONDOMS.

FRENCH TICKLER (1930s–1960s). CONDOM with a rough or irregular surface, designed to increase vaginal stimulation.

FREUD, Sigmund (Sigismund Schlomo Freud) (1856–1939). Czech psychologist.

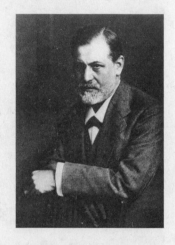

No school of thought exercised a more funda-mental influence over the twentieth century than that of Freud. His contention that sexual desire subconsciously motivated many of our actions, and that our needs, even if forbidden by conven-tional society, manifested themselves in dreams, suggested an entirely new way of viewing mankind and its actions. His work on sexual symbolism, his formulation of the OEDIPUS COMPLEX, his con-troversial theories of infantile sexuality, and above all his development of psychoanalysis as a method of revealing and dealing with hidden fears and desires swept away the prevailing belief, instilled by religion, in a fixed moral universe, substituting one centered in what Hannah Arendt defined in her 1958 book of the same name as "the human condition."

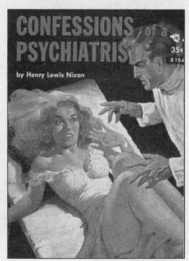

Freud gave us permission to be hu-man. That the permission was much abused doesn't invalidate his ideas, but simply em-phasizes the dangers of license and the val-ues of education and discrimination. Some of his theories do not bear scrutiny in the light of later research, but even though it was not he who joked, in relation to sexual symbol-ism, that "sometimes a cigar is just a cigar," the quip nevertheless represents his point of view. He was proposing a theory, not deliver-ing a decalogue. Nor, unlike such Hollywood films as Hitchcock's *Spellbound*, did he suggest that mental illness could be cured merely by unraveling the symbolism of a dream. "The purpose of psychoanalysis," he wrote bleakly, "is to go from hysterical misery to ordinary unhappiness." See FETISH; WOLF MAN.

FRIDAY, Nancy (1933–). U.S. author and editor. Best known for *My Secret Garden*, she produced bestselling collections of what are purported to be women's sexual fantasies.

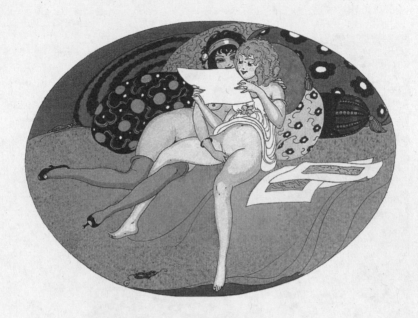

FRIGGING. GERDA WEGENER ILLUSTRATION, 1910S

FRIG (UK and U.S. slang, 1880s–1959s). To stimulate the vagina with the fingers. Also FINGER FUCKING.

FROG-TIED. Bondage position in which the subject's calves are tied to his thighs, imitating the rear legs of a frog. See also HOG-TIED.

FROTTAGE (from the French *frotter*, "to rub"). Deriving sexual pleasure from rubbing up against a person or object, often during dancing.

FRUIT (U.S. slang, 1920s–1970s). Derogatory term for male homosexual.

As far back as the sixth century, the *Kama Sutra* acknowledged that women in harems, deprived of regular sex, "use carrots, fruits and other objects to satisfy their desires." (Some may even have anticipated the advice of British birth-control pioneer Marie Stopes and employed the skin of half an orange as a contraceptive shield.) Later commentaries on Vatsyayana's manual mention the sexual use of "carrots, turnips, and fruit such as bananas, aubergines, roots like that of the sweet potato . . . marrows, cucumbers etc. Having cleaned the fruit, they grasp it and insert it in the organ, so as to cause a pleasurable feeling." In case their husbands should regard this as evidence of infidelity, the commentator reassured them, "this is merely a question of erotic amusements and does not involve feelings of love."

Fewer fruits are used sexually by men. In *PORTNOY'S COMPLAINT*, Philip Roth describes how his hero, on coring an apple, "ran off into the woods to fall upon the orifice of the fruit." Of all fruits, however, the melon boasts the richest sexual

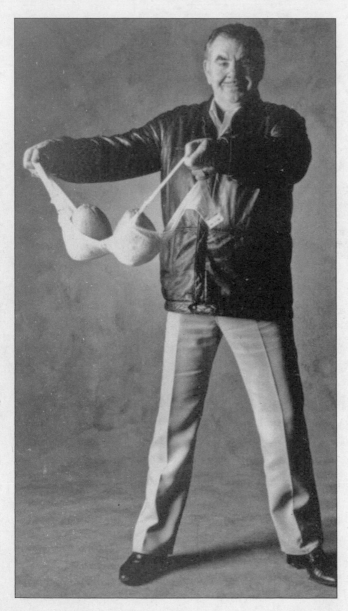

RUSS MEYER
DISPLAYS TWO
MELONS IN A
BRA TO INDICATE
HIS PREFERRED
DIMENSIONS IN A
WOMAN

mythology. A cantaloupe is the preferred metaphor for a heavy breast, while a hole cut in a ripe, sun-warmed watermelon has been since antiquity among the most satisfying vaginal surrogates, celebrated in the Turkish proverb "A woman for duty, a boy for pleasure, but a melon for ecstasy." See DENDROPHILIA.

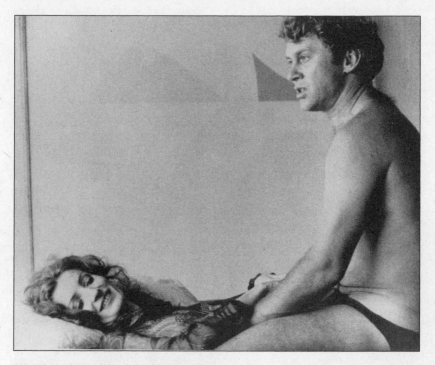

VIVA AND LOUIS WALDON IN *FUCK*, AKA *BLUE MOVIE*

FUCK (1969). Aka *BLUE MOVIE* and *LOUIS AND VIVA*. Directed by Andy Warhol.

Warhol has said, "I'd always wanted to do a movie that was pure fucking, nothing else, the way *Eat* had been just eating and *Sleep* had been just sleeping." The film was shot in October 1968 at David Bourdon's apartment in Greenwich Village. (It's unclear if Warhol was personally involved, since he was still recuperating from his near-fatal shooting by Valerie Solanas in June.) Viva and Louis Waldon do have intercourse for thirty-three minutes, but more screen time is spent discussing the Vietnam war, showering, and cooking a meal. Because the cameraman used the wrong film stock, *Fuck* has an overall blue tint, but censorship problems rather than this error dictated the change of title to *Blue Movie*.

The film had its first public screening on June 12, 1969, when Warhol ran all four spools, lasting about two hours, at the Elgin Cinema to benefit *Film Culture* magazine. In July 1969, a one-hundred-minute version opened at the New Andy Warhol Garrick Theater. It played to packed houses until the New York City Police seized it on July 31, 1969. Theater staff were arrested, and the manager fined $250.

FUCK BUDDY (U.S. slang, 1970s–present). A companion whom one meets occasionally for casual sex, without emotional commitment.

FUCKING MACHINES. See SEX MACHINES.

FUCK-ME SHOES. (sometimes FUCK-ME PUMPS [U.S. slang, 1960s–present]). Backless high-heeled shoes. So named because they can be easily kicked off in a sexual situation.

FUDGE PACKING, FUDGE PACKER (U.S. slang, 1940s–present). Derogatory term for male anal sex and those who practice it, suggesting that the penetrating penis "packs" or compresses "fudge," i.e., excrement.

FURVERT (sometimes FURRY or FURIENT; PLUSHY). Devotee of furversion, i.e., dressing as a furred animal.

Spun off from 1980s science fiction and fantasy convention masquerades, furversion was presaged in 1969 by "The Mouse Problem," a spoof exposé in *Monty Python's Flying Circus.* Furverts were shown meeting at establishments such as the Eek Eek Club and the Little White Rodent Room to dress as mice and eat cheese. In Stanley Kubrick's *The Shining* (1980), a couple in full fur suits is surprised in the midst of oral sex.

Furversion thrived as a sexual subculture, mainly U.S.-based but also popular in Japan, where it combined with *kemono*, the art of drawing and sculpting anthro-pomorphic creatures. Served by numer-

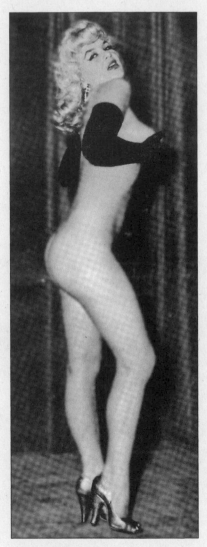

1950s FRENCH SHOWGIRL IN "FUCK-ME PUMPS"

ous websites and magazines, U.S. fur fandom holds its own conventions, initially called ConFURences but now known as Anthrocon, Califur, etc. Since 2001, the Ursa Major Awards have rewarded excellence in the area of Anthropomorphic Literature and Art.

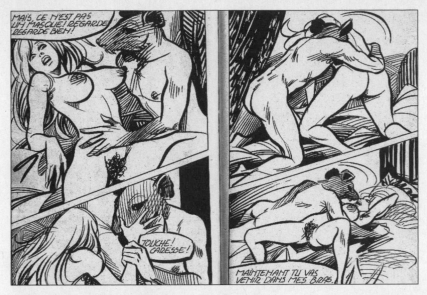

FRENCH FURVERT COMIC STRIP, 1960s

The furvert ideal, as reflected in its fiction and art, is slim, agile, and androgynous. Specialist costume makers create fur suits to measure. Foxes, cats, deer, bears, rabbits, wolves, squirrels, skunks, and horses predominate, though even dolphins are not unknown. Other costumes derive from fantasy fiction or animated films, e.g., the WALT DISNEY *Robin Hood*, where Robin and Marion are foxes. For strict authenticity, the suit should cover the entire body, including the face, and have "practical" elements, e.g., a twitching tail, mobile jaws with real teeth, or anatomically accurate genitalia.

Creating costumes and playing roles, often on virtual sites called MUCKs, provides the greatest satisfaction of Furversion, but sex in costume, while physically difficult, isn't unknown, and inspired a 2005 episode of *CSI Las Vegas*, set at a furvert convention. While the majority of furries are content with costumes and role-playing, the fetish also harbors a ZOOPHILIA contingent, who practice YIFF, i.e., sexual intercourse with real animals.

FUZOKU. Japanese. Omnibus term for the world of commercial sex, including PROSTITUTION, PORNOGRAPHY, voyeurism, etc.

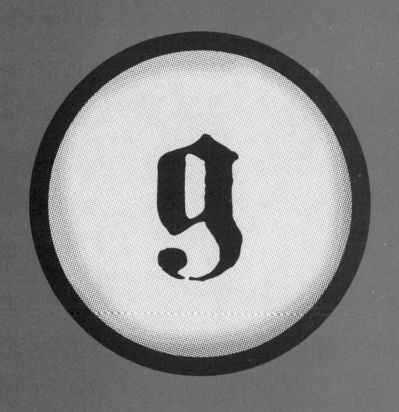

GARÇONNE (French, 1920s). Literally boy/girl but usually translated as "bachelor girl."

In this fashion fad, women, not necessarily lesbian, affected short haircuts and mannish suits, and adopted an aggressive male attitude to sex. The idea is celebrated in the 1922 novel *La Garçonne*, by Jean-Victor Margueritte, who is also credited with coining the term *PARTOUZE*. The novel's heroine, discovering that her fiancé is unfaithful, embarks on a life of excess, taking many lovers of both sexes and experimenting with OPIUM. The most vivid embodiment of the *garçonne* is the mysterious boyish actress Fano Messan in Luis Buñuel's *Un Chien Andalou*.

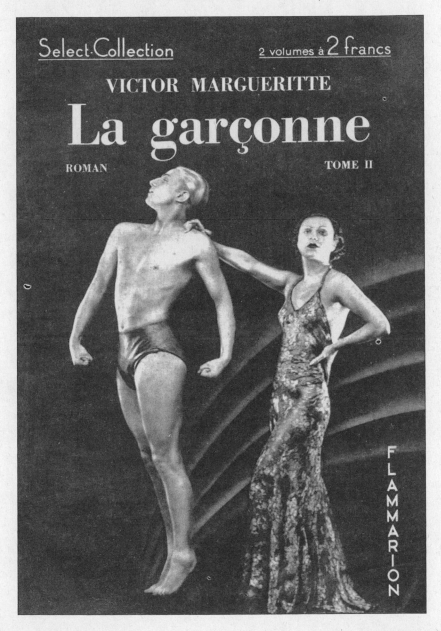

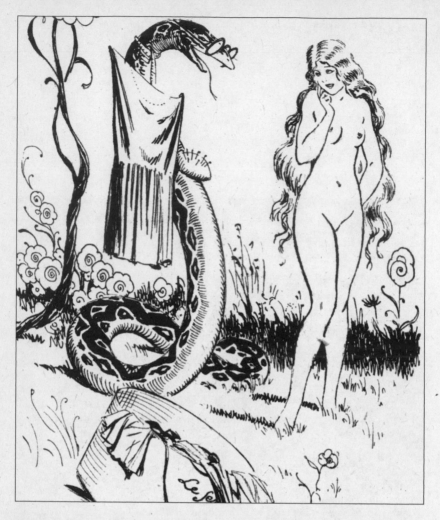

GARDEN OF EDEN. Popular setting for mid-twentieth-century films such as *The Bible: In the Beginning*, since it offered a religious pretext for the depiction of nudity.

In an unusual perspective on paradise, a PIMP interviewed by sociologists Richard and Christina Milner in 1972 asserted that "Adam was the first TRICK [and the] Snake was a PIMP."

ALSO

GARDEN OF EDEN (1955). U.S./Swedish film. Directed by Max Nosseck.

In 1955, the British Board of Film Censors, though busy with cutting or banning outright such threats to morality as *The Wild One, The Blackboard Jungle,* and *The Man with the Golden Arm*, took the time to axe *Garden of Eden*, by journeyman German director Max Nosseck. Featuring TV actress Jamie O'Hara as a young widow converted to NATURISM when she strays into a colony with her six-year-old daughter, the story was a framework on which to hang scenes of naked men and women, always discreetly photographed from behind or, if from the front, only from the waist up. In erotic charge, the film barely rivaled Nosseck's best-known previous work, the equine melodrama *Black Beauty.*

Distributor Nat Miller challenged the ban by inviting London's County Council to override it and permit screenings of the film in the capital alone. Not only did the LCC agree, but it also granted a U certificate, allowing even children to attend. Three hundred more local authorities licensed *Garden of Eden* over the next three years, but the BBFC remained adamant. Secretary Arthur T. Watkins wrote querulously to a protester, "Where are we to draw the line? . . . Long experience has convinced us that it is best to keep nudity off the screen . . . If we were led to depart from our general rule, we feel sure that we might soon be faced with a dangerous amount of exploitation which we should find it difficult to prevent."

Garden of Eden also became a cause célèbre in New York, where the State Education Department, then in charge of censorship, banned it. On July 3, 1957, the New York State Court of Appeals overturned the ban, since nudity itself wasn't illegal. A year later, the British Board reversed its stand, too, conferring a grudging A certificate on the film. But by then, the exploitation Watkins feared had taken place, and the nudist wave was upon them. See NUDIES.

GARFIELD, John (né Jacob Julius Garfinkle) (1913–1952). Tough-guy U.S. actor, famous in the sexual annals for having died of a heart attack while in the throes of sex. See also ROCKEFELLER, Nelson.

GATEWAYS, THE. London lesbian bar/club, 1930–1985.

The Gateways, on the Kings Road in Chelsea, opened in 1930 and quickly became a meeting place for London's lesbians. From 1967 to its closing in 1985, "The Gates," as it was called, maintained a women-only policy. Robert Aldrich used it to film a fifteen-minute sequence for his 1968 film, *The Killing of Sister George.* The fact that the club had a green door and that strangers were barred led to dubious suggestions that the establishment may have inspired the title of *BEHIND THE GREEN DOOR.*

GAY (slang, 1940s–present). Homosexual—at first male only, now applying also to lesbians. Originally, nineteenth-century slang for a female prostitute, cf., gey . . . or geyhouse, a synonym for a brothel.

Gay emerged as a synonym for male homosexuals during the early 1940s, gradually but not immediately supplanting *FAGGOT, FRUIT, FAIRY, QUEER, Nancy, SISSY,* etc. In the 1938 film *Bringing Up Baby,* Cary Grant (himself bisexual) explains his wearing a woman's nightgown with "Because I just went gay all of a sudden," but it's unlikely writers Dudley Nichols and Hagar Wilde knew the term. Writer Gavin Lambert confirms: "It was during the last winter of the war in Europe that I first heard the word 'gay,' from an American serviceman, but 'queer' was still the usual term when I left England twelve years later." *Gay* won public acceptance only with the STONEWALL RIOTS of June 1969.

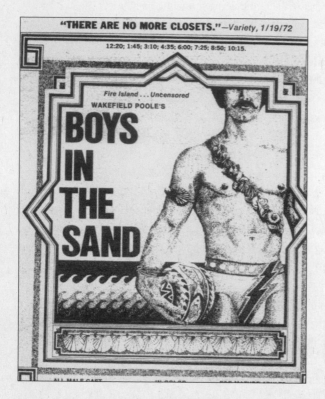

GAY FILMS OF THE 1970s:
BOYS IN THE SAND
AND *A BIGGER SPLASH*

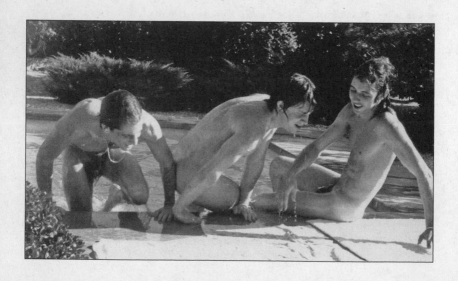

GAYDAR (1970s-present). Variant on *radar*. The ability to recognize a homosexual person, even if the inclination is disguised.

GAY LIBERATION FRONT. See STONEWALL RIOTS; MATTACHINE SOCIETY.

GENET, Jean (1910-1986). French writer.

The son of a prostitute who gave him up for adoption at the age of one, Genet rejected the values of his affectionate foster parents, who would have liked him to enter the Church, and became instead a not-very-accomplished thief. Committed to a juvenile prison run on the same strict discipline as a navy ship, he embraced its hierarchal culture, in which homosexuality and Catholicism blended in a homoerotic parody of religion. Jean-Paul Sartre was to christen the writer "St. Genet."

Thanks to JEAN COCTEAU, to whom Genet had shown the manuscript of his first book, *Our Lady of the Flowers*, Genet was saved from prison and launched on a career as memoirist, playwright, and, briefly, filmmaker, with the 1950 *Chant d'Amour*, which celebrated a cell as the setting for ecstatic masturbatory fantasies. He further explored the significance of ritual in plays such as *The Maids*, in which two servant sisters repeatedly act out, then commit, the murder of their mistress; and *The Balcony*, set in a brothel where clients can role-play figures of power such as generals and bishops. *Querelle de Brest*, filmed by Rainer Werner Fassbinder, celebrated the preoccupations of Genet's early reformatory years in a story about a gay SAILOR.

Genet was one of the first artists to reject the cliché image of the gay man as effeminate and fastidious, and to explore the contradictory aesthetic of grunge, sweat, and semen that underlies COTTAGING, the biker culture, and leads inevitably to BDSM. He significantly influenced the work of other gay writers such as William S. Burroughs and Edmund White, the latter of whom wrote a much-admired biography of Genet. See SAILORS; MAIDS.

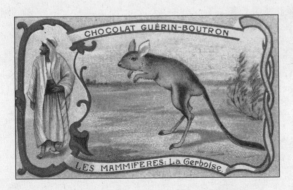

GERBIL. African rodent, typically between six and twelve inches long, and common as a pet.

Rumors of the sexual use of gerbils, mice, and hamsters first appeared about 1982, with stories of dead animals removed from the rectums of adventurous experimenters, in particular a Hollywood actor of ambivalent sexuality. In 1984, a Denver weekly claimed to have evidence of a gerbilectomy performed in a local emergency room. New York reports mentioned patients admitted with anal infections normally found only in rodents. In 1990, British crime writer Derek Raymond set part of his novel *I Was Dora Suarez* in London's imaginary Parallel Club, which featured rodent sex.

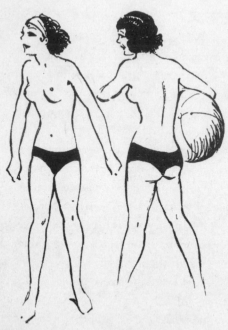

MONOKINI, IN A 1931 DRAWING BY RENE GIFFEY

GERNREICH, Rudi (1922–1985). Austrian-born couturier.

Gernreich, with varying degrees of truth, claimed credit for having invented those emblems of 1960s sexual chic, the topless swimsuit or "monokini"; the thong; the see-through shirt; the unboned lycra "no-bra"; the "pubikini"—the first swimsuit to expose pubic hair—and "cut-out" clothing, which omitted slices and circles of fabric (parodied by the 1981 film *So Fine*, in which garment maker Ryan O'Neal invents jeans with see-through discs over the buttocks). If Gernreich's creations remain memorable it's mostly due to the soup-bowl coiffeur and Betty Boop eyes of his longtime model Peggy Moffitt. On other women, his designs never looked as good. An active campaigner for homosexual rights, Gernreich helped found the MATTACHINE SOCIETY.

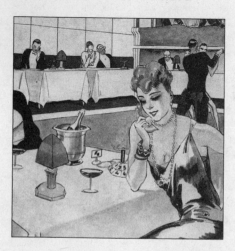

WOMAN RESERVING GIGOLO/DANCING PARTNER

GIGOLO (French, 1922–present). Male escort and paid lover. From French *gigole* or *gigolette*, a "dancing girl" or "prostitute."

By the late 1920s, gigolos were a commonplace of the European tourist scene, particularly in Paris. Most disguised the sexual transaction by posing as chauffeur, translator, or dance partner. In the film *Wonder Bar* (1934), Al Jolson's Paris club is staffed with dancer-gigolos skilled in conversational gambits such as "You are so kind. You remind me of my mother." In both Berlin and Paris, hotels catered to the market with "tea dances" at which handsome males sat at numbered tables, each with a telephone, and waited for lone females to call.

From the 1930s, the gigolo was conventionally represented as a melancholy figure, barred from romantic love, cf, songs such as "Just a Gigolo" (1930) and Al Dubin and Harry Warren's 1933 tune, *Boulevard of Broken Dreams*, subtitled *Gigolo and Gigolette*. The image persisted with Paul Schrader's film *American Gigolo* (1980), with Richard Gere playing a well-paid but exploited and finally tragic ESCORT in modern Los Angeles, a parable repeated with slight variations in Schrader's 2007 film *The Walker*. See also *MY HUSTLER; MIDNIGHT COWBOY*; RENT BOY.

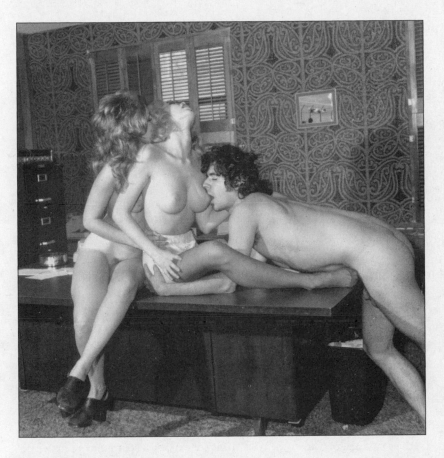

JAMIE GILLIS IN UNIDENTIFIED PORN FILM OF 1960s

GILLIS, Jamie (né James Ira Gurman). Aka Al Cianelli, James Gilles, Buster Hymen, James Kleeman, Ronny Morgan, James Rugman (1943–). U.S. actor.

One of the most distinctive presences in the classic porn cinema, Gillis came from the same Off-Broadway culture as HARRY REEMS, but in part because of his bisexuality and interest in BDSM, he staked out a territory on the dangerous edge of the porn business, which furnished a more enduring career. He appeared as the ENEMA BANDIT in *WATERPOWER*, and pioneered *On the Prowl*, the series evoked in *BOOGIE NIGHTS*, in which he cruised the city in a limousine with a female porn star, picking up amateur male partners at random and recording the resulting sex.

In the days of porn on film, Gillis appeared in a number of high-budget features, notably *The Private Afternoons of Pamela Mann* and *THE OPENING OF MISTY BEETHOVEN*, but is inevitably remembered for his live shows and own videos, some produced in France, which involved more extreme acts, including verbal abuse, FISTING, and COP-ROPHILIA. (In the 1990s he made four films in the series *Walking Toilet Bowl*.)

GINZBURG, Ralph (1929–2006). U.S. writer, publisher, and editor.

Brooklyn-born Ginzburg's 1958 book, *An Unhurried View of Erotica*, took an appreciative look at what he claimed were "the hard core of 2000 titles of classical erotica in the English language," held in secrecy by the world's libraries. In 1962, he launched *Eros*, an up-market hardcover quarterly of erotica, ranging from Bert Stern's suppressed nudes of MARILYN MONROE to a portfolio of Norman Lindsay to, most controversially, a photo feature by Ralph M. Hattersley, Jr., of biracial nude lovers.

Eros never made a profit, and published only four issues. Undeterred, Ginzburg launched *Avant Garde*, mixing contemporary erotica by Pablo Picasso and John Lennon with radical literature and political comment. A second magazine, *Fact*, promised "pants-down profiles and turn-'em-over-in-their-grave obituaries." In 1965, the U.S. courts judged *Eros* and two other Ginzburg publications obscene, a decision the publisher fought to the Supreme Court, which upheld it in 1972. He served eight months in prison, and although he retrieved his fortunes with other publications and remained active as writer and journalist, he never returned to the world of erotica—which, in any event, had by then been extensively liberated, due in part to pioneers like him.

GIRLS GONE WILD (1999–present). U.S. TV series.

Series, mainly sold on DVD by direct mail, for which camera crews trawl beaches and resorts, and encourage attractive young women to remove some or all of their clothing and otherwise behave in a sexually provocative manner, usually in return for nothing more than a "Girls Gone Wild" T-shirt or tank top. Extensively and sometimes unscrupulously plagiarized, the format has been hugely successful, though attacked as exploitative. Joseph Francis, GGW's producer, has been indicted on various charges, including failing to document the age of women appearing in his videos.

GIRODIAS, Maurice (1919–1990). Mainly Paris-based erotic publisher. See OLYMPIA PRESS; OBELISK PRESS.

GLORY HOLE (U.S., 1960s-present). Hole cut in a partition at hip-height, usually in PEEP SHOW booth or public toilet, through which a man pokes his penis, to be fellated or masturbated.

Anonymous sexual contact through a fence or other barrier is a staple of porn. In *The Goat*, a U.S. STAG FILM of the 1920s, a man, extorting sex as the price of returning the clothes of three girls he's surprised swimming nude, is tricked into penetrating a goat through a hole in a fence. A New York club in the early 1980s called the Glory Hole consisted of little more than two floors of partitions and holes. Around the same time, a SoHo gallery presented *Glory Holelujah*, a photographic exhibition of holes in public toilets.

Fiction has variously celebrated or deplored the practice; sometimes both at the same time. The heroes of T. Coraghessan Boyle's 1984 novel, *Budding Prospects*, scour San Francisco for sex, finding it in a backstreet garage, one end of which is walled off with plasterboard pierced by holes, on the other side of which mouths, sex undetermined, offer satisfaction. "This was crude, this was obscene, the ultimate in depravity, moral turpitude and plain bad taste," says the narrator, ". . . real anonymity, cold and soulless as an execution. I was repelled. But . . . I began to see the perverse allure of it too."

In Tony Fennelly's 1985 novel, *The Glory Hole Murders*, a New Orleans psychopath traps gays by skewering their penises with a hat pin on the other side of a glory hole. He then nips round to administer a fatally corrosive enema. But *Dancer from the Dance* (1978) by the (pseudonymously punning?) "Andrew Holleran," celebrates the practice. So does the French film *Liaisons Coupables* (Michel Ricaud, 1987). Chris Lerique and her equally beautiful companion, naked but for stockings and suspenders, take refuge from the denizens of a Paris sex club in the male urinal. Large holes have been drilled in the walls. As one penis, then another, pokes through, each wrapped in a large-denomination banknote, Lerique and her companion get to work.

GLYN, Elinor (née Elinor Sutherland) (1864-1943). English-born novelist and screenwriter.

Glyn's mediocre but sensational fantasies of bedroom athletics among European nobility paved the way for Jackie Collins, Danielle Steele, and Judith Krantz. Middle-aged and widowed, she resolved to crash the world of trash fiction, and in six weeks wrote *Three Weeks* (1907), the story of a twenty-one-day affair between an incognito princess and her English lover, who enjoy sex on animal skins and a bed upholstered in real roses. Overnight, Glyn became a sexual authority. Wrote one wit,

> Would you like to sin
> With Elinor Glyn
> On a tiger skin?

Or would you prefer
To err with her
On some other fur?

A flair for eye-catching sexual detail made Glyn a natural for movies. For the first time in Hollywood history, studio publicists were ordered, "Boom [i.e., promote] the author!" For the film of *His Hour* (1924), Glyn suggested that John Gilbert bestow a BUTTERFLY KISS on Aileen Pringle by brushing his eyelashes against her cheek, and would boast on *Beyond the Rocks* (1922), "[Rudolph] Valentino had never even thought of kissing the palm rather than the back of a woman's hand until I made him do it." Most influentially, Glyn coined the term "It" to describe that "strange magnetism that attracts both sexes." Her novel of the same name, about a shopgirl trying to win a wealthy lover, was filmed in 1927 with CLARA BOW, who instantly became known as the "It Girl."

GODIVA (c. 990–1067). Wife of Leofric, Duke of Mercia.

According to legend, the beautiful Lady Godiva protested the high taxes levied by her husband on the people of Coventry. He agreed to reduce them if she rode naked through the city. She did so, clothed only in her long hair, but demanded that all windows and shutters be kept closed. Only one person, a tailor named Tom, disobeyed, for which, traditionally, PEEPING TOM was struck blind. The tale, though probably apocryphal, proved durable, and has been the subject of numerous films and episodes in films. Maureen O'Hara played Godiva in *Lady Godiva of Coventry* (1955) and DIANA DORS appeared in *Lady Godiva Rides Again*, a contemporary comedy based on beauty contests. Godiva's story is also referenced in E. Y. Harburg's lyrics for the 1939 song "Lydia, the Tattooed Lady," whose tattoos include "Captain Spaulding exploring the Amazon River / Lady Godiva but with her pajamas on."

GO DOWN (U.S. slang, 1950s–present). To administer cunnilingus.

"It's Hanoi Hannah! Hannah, you slut. You've gone down on everything but the *Titanic*" (Robin Williams in *Good Morning, Vietnam*).

GO-GO DANCERS (1950s–1970s). Dancers, customarily placed on platforms or staircases above a dance floor, usually but not necessarily female, invariably lightly clothed, and occasionally TOPLESS or nude, who performed the SHIMMY, quivering or jerking frenziedly in place, fringed clothing added to the effect.

Go-go dancers featured in 1960s TV pop shows such as *Shindig* and *Hullabaloo*. In *Mantis in Lace*, the 1968 feature by WILLIAM ROTSLER, a topless go-go dancer crazed on LSD goes on a rampage with an ax and an ice pick. See also STONEWALL RIOTS.

GOING COMMANDO (U.S. slang, 1974–present). Dispensing with male underwear. Based on the U.S. Army Special Forces practice of wearing no underwear on combat missions to avoid "crotch rot."

GOING SLOPS (Australian slang, 1960s–1980s). In a group sex situation, entering a vagina already lubricated with the semen of previous partners. Also a metaphor for being third or fourth best in any situation.

GOLDEN SHOWER. See UROLAGNIA.

GOLDSTEIN, Al(vin) (1936–). U.S. writer, editor, producer.

Co-founder, with Jim Buckley, and longtime editor of the tabloid magazine *SCREW*, journal of record of the U.S. porn business, Goldstein also produced and presented the cable TV show *Midnight Blue* and made numerous appearances in movies, often as commentator on the careers of personalities such as ANNABEL CHONG, RON JEREMY, JOHN HOLMES, and LINDA LOVELACE.

Of his first encounter with Lovelace, Goldstein recalled, "We met in a small, cold $17-a-night hotel room, and it was the most difficult interview I ever conducted, because she's really inarticulate. . . . After the interview, I said, 'I'd like you to suck my cock,' . . . I ran the photos of her sucking my cock and my description of it. It was a paradigm of personal journalism."

Goldstein suffered worse than many in the backlash against pornography, filing for bankruptcy in 2004. "My life has turned to crap," he complained. "To go from being a millionaire and then living in a homeless shelter and being rejected by 98 percent of your friends is horrendous, but I'm a survivor." In 2007, he announced his candidacy for the U.S. presidency, running with the slogan "Support Al. He Likes It On Top." See LEVENSON, Larry.

"GOOD SHIP VENUS, THE." Bawdy ballad of obscure origin about licentious activities at sea, and customarily beginning:

> 'Twas on the good ship Venus,
> By Christ you should have seen us.
> The figurehead
> Was a whore in bed,
> And the mast a rampant penis

Because the words were seldom written down, the song exists in numerous versions. The last line of the first verse can appear as "sucking a dead man's penis," "sucking a red-hot penis," "and a mast of a phallic genus" or "and the mast the captain's penis," among many others. Some versions add a chorus:

There's frigging on the rigging,
Wanking on the planking,
Tossing on the crossing,
There was fuck all else to do.

GRINZING, TAKING THE STREETCAR TO . . . (Austrian slang, 1920s–present).
Mentioned by the philosopher, linguist, essayist, and novelist George Steiner in his sexual memoirs, and attributed to a Viennese lover. "She mapped her own opulent physique and that of her lover(s) with place names derived from the capital's varied districts and suburbs. Thus 'taking the streetcar to Grinzing' [a village on the outskirts of Vienna] signified a gentle, somewhat respectful anal access."

GROPE. To fondle, usually without permission.

GROUP GROPE. Collective NECKING or ORGY, usually consensual.

GROUPIE (U.S. slang, 1950s–present). A girl who attaches herself to the entourage of a performer, normally a male rock singer, and provides sexual favors to him and his colleagues.
I'm With the Band, by super-groupie Pamela des Barres, celebrated her exploits with everyone from Mick Jagger to Frank Zappa. Cameron Crowe depicts groupies sympathetically in *Almost Famous*, his film about his own days on the road as a teenage rock journalist. Groupies receive rougher treatment in *Alice's Restaurant*, where a girl sleeps with Arlo Guthrie "because you might be an album one day." While the overwhelming number of groupies are rock fans, a highly developed network of groupies followed jazz musicians touring Britain in the 1950s, while in WOODY ALLEN's *Stardust Memories*, a girl ambushes filmmaker Woody in his bed while her complaisant husband sleeps downstairs in their van.

GROUP SEX. There's much confusion about when group sex becomes an ORGY. The key may lie less in the numbers than in the types of persons involved. Traditionally, orgies had elements of religious observance, and indicated obesiance to a god or demon. No person was barred, no matter how ill-favored physically or of what sexual orientation. By this standard, any communal sexual activity that excludes the ugly, old, fat, or handicapped is no orgy. For examples of films calculatedly ecumenical orgies, see the MITCHELL BROTHERS' productions, e.g., *BEHIND THE GREEN DOOR*.

"Sex between two people is a beautiful thing; between five it's fantastic."
—WOODY ALLEN

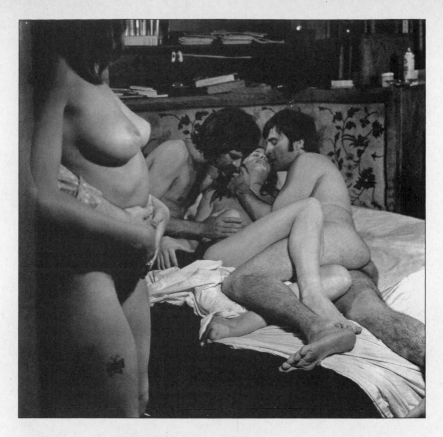

G-SPOT. Also GRAFENBERG SPOT. Area within the vagina that, when stimulated, supposedly yields powerful orgasms. It's claimed that women so aroused can "squirt" vaginal fluid in a form analogous to male ejaculation. Postulated by German gynecologist Ernst Gräfenberg in 1950, the existence of the G-spot has never been entirely accepted by the medical community.

G-STRING (U.S., 1890s–present). American term for the brief pubic covering originally known as a *cache sexe* (literally "hide sex"). More commonly called a thong.

G-STRING MURDERS, THE. See LEE, Gypsy Rose.

GUIDE ROSE (literally "pink guide") (French, 1890s–present). Booklet listing brothels, cafés, and bars where prostitutes can be found.

GUCCIONE, Bob (Robert Charles Joseph Edward Sabatini Guccione) (1930–). U.S. publisher and film producer. See *PENTHOUSE*.

GUN (U.S., 1940s–present). Synonym for penis.

As a punishment for referring to their rifles as "guns," U.S. Marine Corps recruits were required to parade naked with rifle in one hand and penis in the other, and recite the mantra "This is my rifle / This is my gun. / This is for fighting. / This is for fun."

GYNOID. See DOLL.

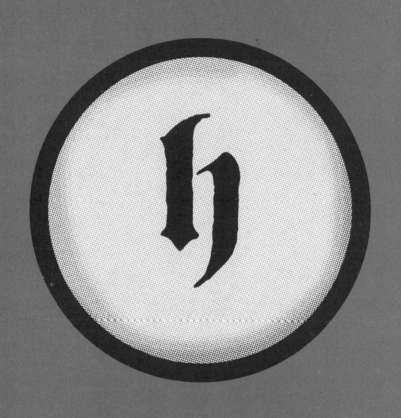

HAIR (1967). U.S. stage musical, by James Rado and Gerome Ragni (book and lyrics) and Galt McDermot (music).

A "tribe" of young people living communally confront the problems of interpersonal relationships and the looming threat of the Vietnam War and the draft. The first musical with a full rock score, the first to celebrate the hippie movement, and the first to feature group nudity, *Hair* premiered on October 17, 1967, at the Public Theatre in New York, then moved to Broadway, where it ran for 1,873 performances. A London production was equally successful.

For the first-act finale, the cast was invited, though not obliged, to appear naked. Cast members who went on to greater success were Melba Moore, Diane Keaton (who didn't strip), Ben Vereen, Johnnie Keyes (who appeared in *BEHIND THE GREEN DOOR*), Ted Neeley, Dolores Hall, Meat Loaf, Jennifer Warren, Paul Nicholas, Richard O'Brien, Elaine Paige, Tim Curry, and Donna Summer. Though audiences came to *Hair* for the nudity, its celebration of sex, including homosexuality and interracial relations, and its opposition to the Vietnam War charmed almost everyone, and many were moved to join the cast and dance. *Hair* is widely credited with ending theater censorship in the United States.

ALSO

HAIR (1979). U.S. film. Directed by Milos Forman.

An imaginative adaptation of the show, with a cast of young and little-known performers, including Treat Williams, John Savage, and Beverly D'Angelo. Forman had hoped *Hair* would be his first production after leaving Czechoslovakia in 1971, but the composer and writers consulted a guru, who after reading Tarot cards, advised against their assenting to his doing it at that time.

HAIR, PUBIC.

Some cultures find the female pubic "bush" sexually attractive. Shaving of pubic hair is a long-standing practice, particularly in Middle Eastern countries, and in prostitution, where the practice helped limit crab lice, but it became cosmetically popular in the West only during the mid-twentieth century, with the arrival of the BIKINI. After MARILYN CHAMBERS shaved her pubic hair, doing so became standard among female porn stars, though many preferred to retain a small patch, often decoratively shaped, below the navel. See also MERKIN.

HALL, Radclyffe (1880–1943). British novelist and lesbian activist. See *WELL OF LONELINESS, THE.*

HAMEDORI (Japanese, 1990s–present). Japanese porn films in which the cameraman films himself having sex, ideally with a first-time amateur performer.

HAMILTON, David (1933–). British-born photographer and filmmaker.

After establishing himself in Britain as a top advertising photographer, Hamilton relocated to the south of France, which became the setting for his images of nude adolescent girls in groupings or situations that hinted at lesbianism. Usually shot in locations with a rural element—haylofts, antique chateaux—his soft-focus, heavily filtered color photos flirted with child pornography, but in a style so drenched in greeting-card sweetness that most critics were disarmed.

In the 1970s, Hamilton ventured into movies with *Bilitis* (1977). Named for a group of supposedly antique lesbian poems forged by Pierre Louÿs, it followed "teenage schoolgirl" Patti D'Arbanville (actually twenty-six) as her presence on holiday in France drives her hostess Mona Kristensen (later Hamilton's wife) into her arms. Dismissed by critics, *Bilitis* was a commercial success. *Laura* (1979), *Tender Cousins* (1980), *First Desires* (1983), and *A Summer on St. Tropez* (1984) followed, each accompanied by a glossy photo book, which both Christian conservatives and the British police tried repeatedly but unsuccessfully to ban.

HAND. Common term in sexual language, often in regard to MASTURBATION, as in "give a hand" or HAND JOB, meaning to induce orgasm in a man with the use of the hand. "Wandering" or "busy" (hands) indicates GROPING. The appearance of hand in sex book titles—e.g., *The Intelligent Man's Guide to Handball, A Hand in the Bush, Trust: The Hand Book*—usually signals references to FISTING.

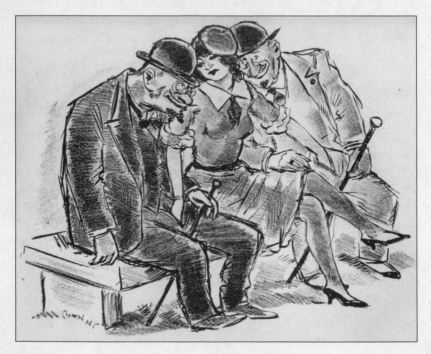

HAND JOB

HARD-CORE. Adjective denoting an intractably resistant or fundamental nature. Often applied to pornography, in contradistinction to SOFT-CORE. Generally, hard-core porn shows full frontal nudity and sexual penetration. Also:

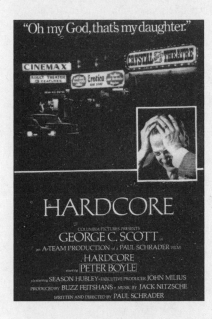

AD FOR PAUL SCHRADER'S *HARDCORE*

HARDCORE **(1979).** U.S. film. Directed by Paul Schrader.

Calvinist businessman George C. Scott infiltrates the world of Los Angeles porn searching for his runaway daughter. Schrader, who was raised in a similar fundamentalist community, extracts black humor from Scott dressing up in flower power gear to masquerade as a possible porn producer. There's excellent character playing from Season Hubley, as a cynical young prostitute, and Peter Boyle, as a sleazy private eye. When Scott asks about the source of the film in which his daughter appears, Boyle, in a concise encapsulation of porn's chronic anonymity, tells him, "Nobody makes it. Nobody shows it. Nobody sees it. It's like it doesn't even exist."

ALSO

HARDCORE (1977). UK film. Directed by James Kenelm Clarke.

Absurd "autobiography" of the British sex journalist Fiona Richmond, who, though then in her mid-thirties, insisted on playing herself, even as a seventeen-year-old in a school uniform. There are embarrassing appearances by has-been leading men Anthony Steel and former Batman Adam West.

HARLOW, Jean (née Harlean Harlow Carpenter) (1911–1937). U.S. movie actress.

Harlow was everyone's idea of the tart with a heart of gold—a role she played throughout her short career. With her white-blond "platinum" hair and untrained voice—diamond hard and irrepressibly vulgar—her flair for skin-tight satin evening dresses, her refusal to wear underwear, and her calculated seductiveness in bringing her nipples erect with ice cubes before each take, she could rouse the male audience to tumescence from her first appearance on-screen.

After some nude modeling and numerous BIMBO appearances in short comedies, including one with Laurel and Hardy, she found her level in Howard Hughes's World War I flying drama *Hell's Angels*, as the promiscuous Helen. While seducing Ben Lyon,

Harlow became the first actress to utter on film the classic cliché suggestion that she "slip into something more comfortable."

A TRAMP both off- and on-screen, Harlow was the lover of gangster Abner "Longy" Zwillman, who underwrote her movie career by loaning half a million dollars to Columbia Pictures. She also stood godmother to the daughter of "Bugsy" Siegel. However, in 1932, perhaps in a studio-instigated attempt to burnish her image, she married MGM producer Paul Bern. He was found dead two months later—supposedly a suicide. A note found near his body concluded, "You understand last night was only a comedy," sparking rumors that Bern had a small penis and on their wedding night had produced a grotesque DILDO, which Harlow derided. It seems more likely, however, that the note was faked by the studio publicity department, and that the killer was Bern's sometime lover who committed suicide the same day.

Harlow deserves to be remembered as the whore of *Red Dust*, competing with a wilting Mary Astor in the Malayan jungle for the affections of Clark Gable. She played the same character, cleaned up and poured into a satin evening gown, in *Dinner at Eight*, cooing baby talk to her thug of a husband, then sailing through the prejudices of the socialites with whom they dine. Summing up her career in a review of *Saratoga*, the film she was making when she died, GRAHAM GREENE commented, "there is no sign that her acting would ever have progressed beyond the scope of the restless shoulders and the protruberant breasts . . . she toted a breast like a man totes a gun."

HARRIS, Frank (né James Thomas Harris) (1856–1931). Irish author and journalist.

Opinionated, aggressive, and richly over-endowed with imagination, the bantam-sized Harris, with his well-oiled pompadour and bushy moustache, was an unignorable feature of British and French literary life for decades. A friend of Oscar Wilde and George Bernard Shaw, Harris wrote biographies of both—in Shaw's case, despite the subject's furious resistance. In 1922, after a series of attempts at playwriting, publishing, and editing, and a spell in prison, Harris retreated to the south of France, where he began writing and self-publishing *My Life and Loves*. Its four volumes included numerous seductions, which he described in documentary, if repetitive, detail. Since he inflated or falsified his autobiography—in particular his supposed life as a cowboy and his firsthand observation of the Great Chicago Fire—his bedroom exploits may also be invented, but since he was a skilled and colorful writer, the four volumes sold well, and remain the work for which he's best remembered.

Jack Kahane's OBELISK PRESS produced a four-volume edition of *My Life and Loves*, and in 1954 the OLYMPIA PRESS of Kahane's son MAURICE GIRODIAS published what Girodias claimed was the "fifth volume." In fact, Harris's wife Nellie, desperate for money, had sold the publisher her husband's notes, which Girodias paid Scots Beat poet Alexander Trocchi to expand, with liberal additions of sex. In 1967, with the imposture revealed, Girodias shamelessly reissued the forgery as *What Frank Harris Did Not*

Say, subtitled *The Tumultuous, Apocryphal Fifth Volume of My Life and Loves, as Embellished by Alexander Trocchi, with an Apologetic Preface by Maurice Girodias*. Harris's cowboy tales, described in *My Life on the Trail*, inspired the 1958 Western *Cowboy*, with Jack Lemmon as the young Harris buying his way into a cattle drive to pursue Mexican heiress Anna Kashfi.

HASKINS, Sam (1926–). South African photographer.

Haskins's playful erotic albums of chaste female nudes, uniformly slim, tall, and blond, notably *Five Girls* (1962) and *Cowboy Kate* (1964), influenced a generation of figure photographers and advertising directors.

HAT.

In the days of cinema porn, a hat in the lap was so common an accessory for frequenters of X-rated films that one producer, Bernard L. Sackett, producer of *Sweet Smell of Sex* and *Eroticon*, rated films as one-, two-, or three-hatters, signifying the number of times patrons could jerk off during them. In Mel Brooks's parody Western *Blazing Saddles*, Madeline Kahn, as saloon singer Lili Von Shtupp, notes the Stetson in a patron's lap and enquires, "Is that a ten-gallon hat, or are you just enjoying the show?"

HAVEN, Annette (1954–). U.S. actress.

The new middle-class taste for porn was reflected in the stars who made their debuts in the mid-1970s. Annette Haven, after working as a stripper at the MITCHELL BROTHERS' O'Farrell theater in San Francisco and as a MASSAGE PARLOR girl, appeared in her first X-film, ALEX DE RENZY'S *Lady Freaks*, in 1973, but was seen to better advantage the following year in *China Girl*. The most classically beautiful of all X stars, Haven, slim, with long straight hair, porcelain white skin and a look of well-bred disdain, won a huge following. Brian DePalma tried to cast her as porn actress Holly Body in *BODY DOUBLE*. He failed to convince the studio, but Haven acted as consultant on the film, which starred Melanie Griffith. Her character's list of requirements— "$500 a day, no WATER SPORTS, I don't work with animals, no S&M, and no coming in my face"—echoes that of Haven.

Born in Las Vegas, Haven came from the same repressive milieu that produces most porn stars. Her parents were both veterans of the Korean War, and the family had a background in Mormonism. Though she entered sex movies because of a natural aptitude, she soon adopted the proselytizing attitude that was to become better known in the 1980s through the advocacy of Nina Hartley and Candida Royalle of FEMME PRODUCTIONS, who saw adult movies as a route to sexual freedom for women.

In 1977, she received a Best Actress award for *A Coming of Angels* from the Adult Film Association of America, and was elevated to the X-Rated Critics Organization (XRCO) Hall of Fame for *Desires within Young Girls* and *Sex World*. She had a small mainstream acting role in Blake Edwards's "*10*," as a porn actress, but refused a part in Joe Dante's werewolf film *The Howling* because of the film's violence. Haven retired from erotic films in the late 1980s, although she reappeared in the mid-1990s to star in a couple of fetish videos with JAMIE GILLIS and dominatrix Kim Wylde.

HAYS OFFICE. See PRODUCTION CODE.

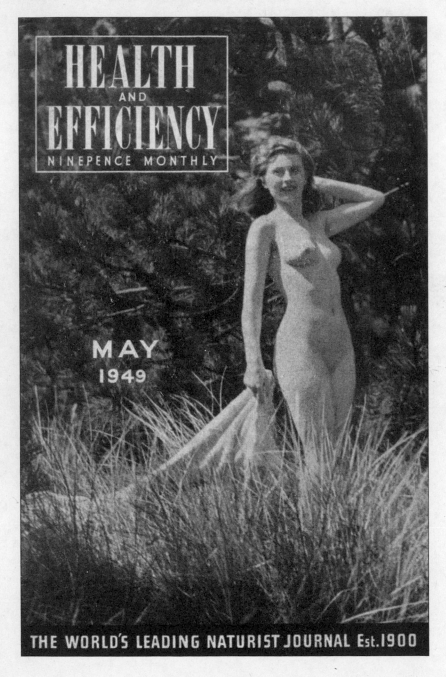

HEALTH AND EFFICIENCY (1890s-present). British NATURIST magazine, now called *HE Naturist*.

Charles Thompson, its first editor, labeled sex a debilitating force, insisting that the theory of "a physiological necessity for the exercise of the reproductive organs . . . is absolutely wrong." Masturbation, he believed, caused one to become "a moral imbecile." It's ironic, therefore, that, during the era of intensive censorship in the 1950s, when only *Health and Efficiency* and *National Geographic Magazine* were exempt from a blanket ban on showing female nudity, *H&E*'s scenes of happy naturists playing volleyball and tennis—albeit with the genitals AIRBRUSHED out—became a popular aid to "self-abuse." See NATURISM.

HEART-ONS (1985-1991). Awards given by the U.S. X-Rated Critics Organization (XRCO) honoring achievement in the adult film industry.

Beginning the year after it was formed, XRCO presented the Heart-Ons annually on Valentine's Day, at a ceremony in Los Angeles. The awards were intended to establish an objective standard by which to judge adult films, and supersede suspect competitions backed by publicists for the major producers. "We honor the meat, not the heat," said an XRCO spokesperson. The awards themselves, wooden hearts with the winners' names burned in, were designed by WILLIAM ROTSLER.

HEFNER, Hugh. See PLAYBOY.

HILBARD, John (né John Hilbert Larsen) (1923-2001). Screenwriter and director.

A prolific screenwriter and director of sex comedies in his native DENMARK, Hilbard, usually working with actor Ole Soltoft, directed the hugely successful *Bedroom Mazurka* (1970), *Danish Dentist on the Job* (1972), *Danish Bed and Board* (1972), and *Danish Pillow Talk* (1973). Most shared the same plot, of a naïve young woman who, convinced she's frigid, bumbles into sexual encounters with overweight captains of industry, horny schoolmasters, and randy politicians with dragon wives.

HIRSCHFELD, Magnus (1868-1935). German sexologist and gay rights activist.

During the first half of the twentieth century, Hirschfeld was in the forefront of the campaign to understand and decriminalize homosexuality. Following World War I, he won funding from the liberal Weimar government to open the Institut für Sexualwissenschaft (Institute for Sexual Research) in the palatial former home in BERLIN of the violinist Joseph Joachim. As well as pursuing research into sexuality, the institute housed Hirschfeld's huge library and a Museum of Sex, material from which appeared in the first film with a homosexual theme, *ANDERS ALS DIE ANDERN*.

Gay himself, Hirschfeld believed, misguidedly, that homosexual men, whom he called the "third sex," owed their condition to an imbalance of male and female hormones, and should be treated as handicapped. Many disagreed, but Hirschfeld was an energetic campaigner with a flair for raising money, and his views prevailed for many years. The fact that a number of deputies were homosexual led him to consider OUTING them, but he was dissuaded, although it's widely believed that much funding for his research came from public figures fearing they might be exposed.

Hirschfeld campaigned tirelessly for the removal of Paragraph 175 of the German Criminal Code, which criminalized homosexuality. He did get a bill introduced into the Reichstag, but it had the bad luck to coincide with the 1929 stock market crash, and was defeated. He continued to agitate for reform, even when harassed and assaulted by Nazi sympathizers, on one occasion being left for dead with a fractured skull. When the Nazis took power in May 1933, they destroyed the institute and burned the library. Archival films of Nazi book burnings usually show Hirschfeld's books feeding the flames. Absent on a speaking tour during this incident, Hirschfeld never returned to Germany. He died in Nice of a heart attack on his sixty-seventh birthday, in 1935, and is buried there.

HISTOIRE D'O (STORY OF O) (1955). French novel, attributed to Pauline Réage (aka Dominique Aury, aka ANNE DESCLOS).

A girl, identified only as "O," is persuaded by her lover René to submit to a group of wealthy sadists who convene in a château near the Paris satellite town of Roissy. During this and subsequent visits, O is whipped, sodomized, branded, and has her labia pierced for the insertion of a metal ring, but endures all out of love, even to being "given" by René to his friend Sir Stephen to use as he wishes. Subsequently, she seduces another girl, and persuades her to submit to the same regime.

With its combination of provocative content and high literary style—Graham Greene would call it "the only erotic book I know which is not in the least pornographic"— *Histoire d'O* was an immediate bestseller. In almost fifty years it has never been out of print. Insiders confidently identified "Pauline Réage" as *nouveau romancier* Alain Robbe-Grillet, scenarist of *L'Année Dernière à Marienbad* and, more to the point, writer-director of *Trans-Europ Express* (1967), which boasted erotic and bondage elements. If it was not by him, it was assumed the writer was his wife, Catherine, author, as "Jean de Berg," of a sadomasochistic novel, *L'Image*, for which Robbe-Grillet forged an introduction, signing it "P.R."

It took many years for Pauline Réage to be revealed as ANNE DESCLOS, long-time mistress of publisher Jean Paulhan, to fan whose ardor she wrote this hymn to submission. Although the fact that a woman had written it was initially an embarrassment to strict feminist critics, it's among women that the book has won its greatest acceptance. In many countries, sororities such as the Daughters of O meet to discuss and replicate the activities of O, while sadomasochist groups hold "O" weekends and even cruises. Their support appeared to be endorsed when it was posthumously revealed that Desclos was bisexual, and carried on a long affair with her friend Helen Thomas.

The book inspired a dozen films and TV series, numerous illustrated editions, also "sequels," pastiches, and imitations. Porn star MARILYN CHAMBERS was among the many women who had their labias pierced and rings inserted.

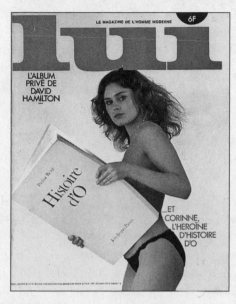

CORINNE CLERY, STAR OF THE FILM VERSION OF HISTOIRE D'O.

ALSO

HISTOIRE D'O (1975). French film. Directed by Just Jaeckin.

Parisian fashion photographer O is delivered by her lover René to a lonely chateau at Roissy, on the outskirts of Paris (these days the location of Aeroport Charles de Gaulle, and anything but secluded). There she's subjected to a regime intended to turn her into the perfect sexual partner. The girls of the chateau are forbidden to meet a man's eyes. They loiter, eyes downcast, dutifully on call, nude under their long dresses, which part front and back for the convenience of the male guests.

Periodically the women are beaten, though always with a thin dog whip, and never so violently as to leave permanent marks. In this fantasy world, scars and welts fade, and pain becomes pleasure. René reappears with an old friend, Sir Stephen, to whom he assigns O as his slave. She obeys, and is passed around among Sir Stephen's friends. Emerging from the experience confident and determined, she is able herself to seduce her friend and model Jacqueline, and introduce her into the Roissy regime. In a new climax written for the film, O accompanies Sir Stephen to a costume ball at which she chooses to appear nude except for a mask imitating a bird of prey. (The mask, copied from one designed and worn by beautiful Italian artist Leonor Fini, fueled rumors that she'd inspired O.)

Jaeckin shot *Histoire d'O* with all the blurring and soft focus of *EMMANUELLE* and a TV commercial's preoccupation with costume and décor. Réage's cruelty is understandably softened. No attempt is made to render the whippings with any accuracy. The branding is played down, and the labial piercing omitted entirely. There was no sexual penetration, so *Histoire d'O* didn't cross the line between SOPHISTIQUE SOFT and HARD CORE.

The script, by crime novelist Sebastian Japrisot, dispensed with the book's alternative narrative structures (a Robbe-Grilletian trick that fed the rumors of his

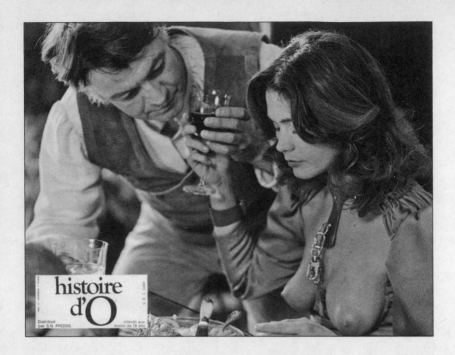

involvement). Nor was Japrisot any more interested than Réage in René and Sir Stephen. Udo Kier, the epicene Dracula and Dr. Frankenstein of ANDY WARHOL's camp versions, is hilariously miscast as René, while Sir Stephen (a role declined by Christopher Lee) is played by Anthony Steel, a British leading man of the 1950s working out his retirement in Eurotrash. All gray bouffant hair and tweeds, he's a milord out of a French whisky commercial. As O, ex-model Corinne Clery screams with vigor and pouts agreeably, but is no more effective than Sylvia Kristel at portraying a devoted sensualist.

HITE, Shere (1942–). American/German author and sexologist.

Hite's 1976 *The Hite Report: A Nationwide Study of Female Sexuality* challenged the conventional wisdom that women routinely achieved orgasm with penetrative sex. On the contrary, it seemed that, according to three thousand questionnaires completed by American women for her study, many were faking it. Hite urged a reassessment of sex roles and in particular a wider use of masturbation. The book sold fifty million copies.

HIZA-MAKURA. See EARS.

HO, sometimes HOE. See WHORE.

HOG-TIED. Bondage pose in which wrists, or sometimes forearms, of a subject are roped to the ankles behind his or her back. See also FROG-TIED.

HOLLYWOOD BABYLON. Compendium of reportage and rumor about vice in the world's film capital, written by underground filmmaker and former child actor KENNETH ANGER.

Beginning as a serial in the French film magazine *Cahiers du Cinema*, it was published in book form in France by Jean-Jacques Pauvert in 1959 and enjoyed a steady sale for many years in Europe until, most of the subjects having died, it was given hardcover publication, where it became a bestseller, followed by *Hollywood Babylon II*. Among other revelations, the book "outed" homosexual actors such as Greta Garbo, RUDOLPH VALENTINO, and Ramon Navarro, and tennis star Bill Tilden; claimed JOAN CRAWFORD had appeared in pornographic films; probed the clandestine relationship of Marion Davies and media mogul William Randolph Hearst; and accused Hearst of having shot film director Thomas Ince, mistaking him for Charlie Chaplin, whom he believed to be Davies's lover.

ALSO

HOLLYWOOD BABYLON (1972). U.S. film. Directed by Van Guylder.

Fumbling attempt to re-create some incidents from Hollywood's erotic history, e.g., the supposed on-set orgies of Erich von Stroheim. Includes Uschi Digard playing a lesbian MARLENE DIETRICH.

HOLMES, John C. (né John Curtis Estes) (aka Johnny Wadd, John Duval, Big John Fallus, John Helms, Big John Holmes, John Curtis Holmes, Bigg John, John Rey) (1944–1988). American adult film actor.

Holmes was the preeminent male porn performer of the 1970s. In *Around the World with Johnny Wadd* (1975), he brags, "I'm one of the wonders of the world. I have the biggest cock in the world, and I've been using it since I was seven years old. It's been inside 10,000 women at least, and none of them has been unsatisfied." He went on: "My cock is my responsibility. I must use it. Fortunately I can fuck four or five hours a day, but I'm still looking for that special woman who can make my cock disappear in her mouth, cunt and ass."

Estimates of his dimensions varied. His first wife described coming home to find him measuring his penis. "It goes from five inches to ten," he told her. "Ten inches long! Four inches around!" Later the figure was inflated to twelve inches, then thirteen and a half.

Holmes was the son of an alcoholic Ohio carpenter and a devout Baptist mother. An older friend of his mother seduced him when he was twelve. Moving to Los Angeles, he became an ambulance driver. In 1968, he was "discovered" in the men's room of a poker club in Gardena, a Los Angeles suburb, by a professional photographer who recruited him for porn stills, stripping, and finally movie LOOPS.

With his first money, Holmes bought the diamond ring he wore in all his films, and designed a belt buckle showing a mother whale and her baby; much as the MITCHELL

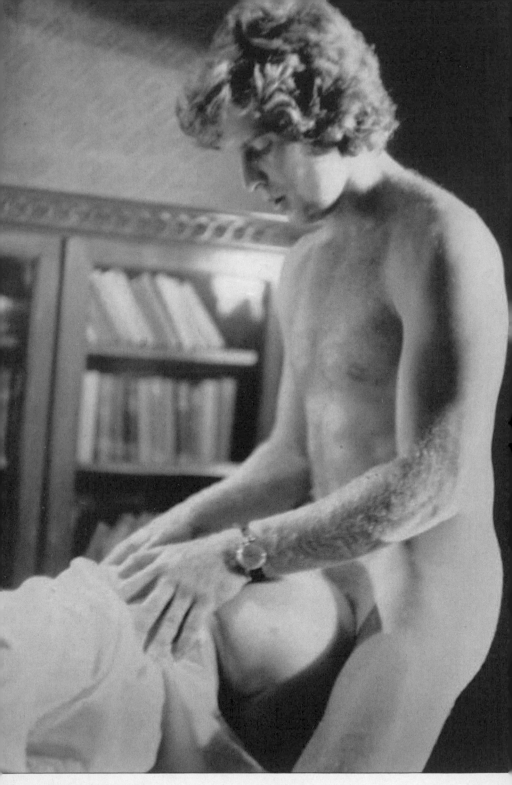

JOHN HOLMES IN HIS PRIME

BROTHERS, he saw himself as environmentally friendly, devoted to celebrating the joy of living.

Holmes is said to have made a thousand loops before he met producer-directors Bob Chinn and Richard Aldrich, who transformed his image. They invented "Johnny Wadd," a private detective and adventurer. In *Tell Them Johnny Wadd Is Here*, *Liquid Lips* (both 1976), *Jade Pussycat* (1977), *China Cat* (1978), and *Blonde Fire* (1979), Holmes's search for some jewel or curio is a pretext for sex with a variety of women.

Rare in porn films, Holmes—tall, slim, and classically handsome, with wavy hair—could carry off costume roles. In *The Spirit of '76*, he plays John Smith, telling Pocahontas, "Boy! You've got great tits!" *The New Erotic Adventures of Casanova* (1979) featured him as the eighteenth-century lover—at least for two reels, apparently all the time its producers could afford to rent the costumes. After that, the action reverts to contemporary California.

Women found Holmes's easy insolence both infuriating and attractive. One critic called him "everyman's gigolo, a polyester smoothy with a sparse moustache, a flying collar, and lots of buttons undone." Never moving faster than a stroll, he ambled into scenes, settled back, put his arms along the back of the couch, and let himself be pleasured. Like most porn stars, he improvised many of his moves, some of them hilariously arrogant. He was quite capable, after sliding his penis into a girl busy fellating another stud on her hands and knees, of reaching over her back and shaking hands with his companion.

In 1980, Holmes featured in MARILYN CHAMBERS's *Insatiable*, playing her publicist and, inevitably, lover. He was at the top of the porn heap. But when she made *Insatiable II* in 1984, which contained some footage from the earlier film, his name, now a liability, was crudely scratched off the negative.

Holmes, like most of Hollywood, was free-basing cocaine, but lacked the money to feed his habit. Instead, he hung out with dealers, notably a group called the Wonderland Gang. On July 1, 1981, addled by drugs, Holmes was peripherally involved in the murders of four people who'd incurred the wrath of gangster Eddie Nash. Terrified to testify against Nash, Holmes went on the run for six months. Finally tried for all four murders, he was acquitted, although he remained in jail on burglary and contempt-of-court charges until November 1982.

After prison, Holmes took any work he could find, including gay porn. In 1985 he tested positive for HIV. He died in 1988, of AIDS-related colon cancer. He was cremated, but not until friends, at his final request, had inspected his body to see that it was intact. "He didn't want any part of him ending up in a jar," said one. His ashes were scattered over the Pacific.

Holmes's life and death inspired the films *BOOGIE NIGHTS* and *Wonderland*, but his most succinct epitaph was penned by AL GOLDSTEIN, editor and publisher of *SCREW*, who called him "a sociopath and a liar. In effect, every manifestation of this man's life was a lie, a distortion, duplicity, a quagmire of deceit. The only truth was, he had a big dick."

HONEY SWEAT. (1957). The sweat after sex on hot tropic afternoons.

Coined by Lawrence Durrell in *JUSTINE*: "...those sun-tormented afternoons, 'honey-sweating', as Pombal called them—when we lay together, bemused by the silence."

HONEY TRAP. Espionage term for the recruitment or blackmail of an "asset" through the offering of sexual favors.

HOOCHIE-COOCHIE. See SHIMMY.

HOOKER (mid-1800s–present). Female prostitute.

Falsely believed to be inspired by the whores and camp followers who gravitated toward the headquarters of U.S. Civil War general Joseph "Fighting Joe" Hooker, the term appears in print as early as 1845, and probably derives from the practice of street prostitutes grabbing prospective clients by hooking arms with them.

HOT DATE (U.S./UK 1960s–present). Assignation expected to conclude with sex.

HOTEL DE PASSE. French. Hotel that rents rooms by the hour, usually to prostitutes. See RICHARD, Marthe.

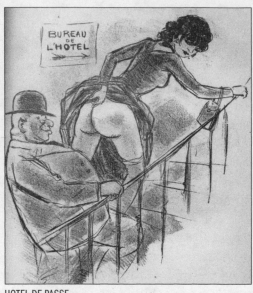

HOTEL DE PASSE

HOT LUNCH (Prostitute's slang, 1980s–present). A midday sexual encounter. Also COFFEE BREAK: a similar assignation at midmorning or mid-afternoon.

HOT PANTS (U.S. slang, 1920s–1980s). For a woman to "have hot pants" indicated heightened sexual desire.

ALSO

HOT PANTS (1970S–1990S). Tight, abbreviated female shorts that appeared in the early 1970s as successor to the MINISKIRT, and have never entirely been out of fashion since, particularly with street prostitutes.

HUMMER (U.S., 1970s–present). Oral sex given additional effect by vibrating the lips and mouth.

HUNG (U.S. 1960s–present). Calibration of penis size, the degree of "hungness" ranging from "well" or "enormously hung" or "hung like a horse" to disparaging similes such as "hung like a hamster." W. H. AUDEN is credited with the most often quoted literary use of the term:

> As the poets have mournfully sung,
> Death takes the innocent young,
> The rolling in money,
> The screamingly-funny,
> And those who are very well hung.

During the 1970s, in New York, a group called the Hung Jury convened informally to assess the dimensions of new arrivals on the gay scene. By extension, *hung* can be a synonym for the kind of sexual power conferred by the possession of a giant penis. In Jules Feiffer's *Carnal Knowledge* (1971), his womanizing character Jonathan complains, "Women today are better-hung than the men."

HUSTLER (U.S., 1930s–present). Sexually, a PROSTITUTE, though, more generally, anyone who strives aggressively to achieve, e.g., the pool player "Fast Eddie" Felson in William Tevis's novels *The Hustler* and *The Color of Money*.

ALSO
HUSTLER (MAGAZINE). See FLYNT, Larry.

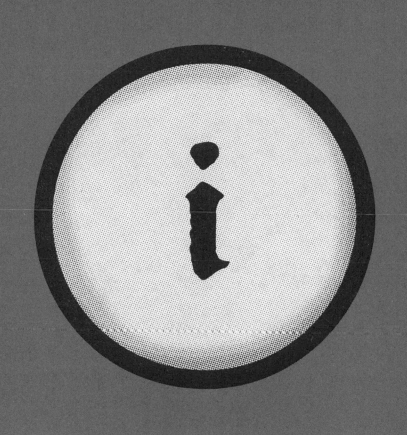

ICE.

An ice cube held in the mouth during oral sex can increase the sensation. Ice was also used by models and actresses such as JEAN HARLOW to make their nipples erect for photo shoots. In his 1961 guide *The Marriage Art*, John E. Eichenlaub, M.D., suggests filling a plastic bag with crushed ice and applying it to the testicles at the moment of orgasm. (Prior warning that you're going to use this technique is probably advisable.)

IMMORAL MISTER TEAS, THE (1959). U.S. film. Directed by Russ Meyer.

This sex comedy, shot in four days, launched not only the career of its director, RUSS MEYER, but the whole field of SOFT-CORE porn.

As he bikes around Los Angeles, paunchy dental equipment salesman Bill Teas (a friend of Meyer, playing himself) imagines he can to see through women's clothing. Various busty girls appear to him—and to the audience—discreetly naked.

Meyer claims that a print of *Teas* was accidentally sent to a San Diego cinema as support for the dour Gary Cooper Western *The Hanging Tree*. Within twenty minutes, police were milling around the box office, and the film's success was assured. Six months later, Seattle, Washington, gave it a censorship certificate. It ran there for two years. In January 1960, when it opened in Los Angeles, even the *Los Angeles Times* took notice. "Last Friday evening," wrote Charles Stinson, "the PEEP SHOW finally moved across the tracks from Main Street, and to judge by the concourse of solid-looking citizens, presumably all aged eighteen or over, the film is going to be a *great* success."

Many states cut or banned *Teas*. Meyer fought such decisions, and in most cases, won. For more nervous locations, such as Australia and the state of Maryland, he produced a doctored version. Fake steam, snow, and rain crudely inked onto the negative obscured all but the broadest detail of the well-endowed cast. This device did, however, allow cinemas to advertise the film as "Complete and Uncut," and the profits continued to flow.

INTERNET SEX.

Every new technical development, from clockwork to the telephone, quickly acquires an erotic dimension, but few did so more speedily and with greater success than the Internet. The problems of delivery that have always plagued erotica, and placed control in the hands of the postal authorities, film censors, and the police, were miraculously erased by the Internet, which could furnish as many people as wanted it with the latest forbidden material: anonymous, private, and—so at least it seemed at the start—untraceable.

Sex, it has been argued, shaped the Internet. The demand for large color pictures and streamed video—aided just as much, it must be said, by the parallel requirements of gaming—fanned the market for new and better delivery systems capable of handling broadband video and downloading quickly and cheaply. The same software that put porn into the home also delivered online news. Chat rooms and e-mail drew new subscribers to services such as America Online, Google, and Yahoo, while methods of paying for downloads from porn movie sites fed the rise of the auction site eBay and its online bank, PayPal.

Arriving as it did at the dawn of the era of AIDS, when real sex ceased to be blithe fun and became life-threatening, the Internet and its unlimited supply of erotica provided an alternative source of sexual excitement, which most people grasped with guilty enthusiasm. The Net didn't entirely instigate the retreat from physical sex; erotica was already a mainstay of the DVD market, and PHONE SEX services provided the aural equivalent of a chat room. But the prospect of a service offering not only anonymous sexual conversation but pictures, video, and text, all for a few cents a minute, was irresistible.

A moral backlash was inevitable, as was the realization that one's privacy was not so inviolate as had been expected. CHICKEN HAWKS trawling for fresh meat gave chat rooms a rancid reputation, and the greed for newer and ever more different porn fare created a forest fire of the bizarre, with every oddity and obsession on show.

IRMA LA DOUCE (1956). French musical, by Alexandre Breffort (book and lyrics) and Marguerite Monnot (music).

Musical about a Parisian prostitute, Irma, and her PIMP, Nestor. An innocent ex-law student, Nestor becomes jealous of Irma's clients and, in order to reserve her for himself, disguises himself as a rich man who's prepared to pay her to become his exclusive mistress. After exhausting himself to maintain this fiction, Nestor kills off the imaginary sugar daddy, only to be convicted of the murder and sent to Devil's Island.

ALSO
IRMA LA DOUCE (1963). U.S. film. Directed by Billy Wilder.

What interested Billy Wilder about the French musical *Irma La Douce* wasn't the songs—which he discarded—but the figure of Nestor, a reincarnation of his favorite character, the sexual loser who sacrifices everything in the name of love. As in *The Apartment* and *The Fortune Cookie*, the man is played by Jack Lemmon. Wilder turns Nestor into a naïve young cop on the beat who's fired for interfering with the comfortable arrangement that exists between the police and the prostitutes around the now-demolished food markets of central Paris, Les Halles. The situation suited Wilder's salty humor.

Billy Wilder was asked if there was any project he hadn't been able to film. "Yes," he replied. "I want to make a story set at the time of the Crusades. The crusaders lock all their wives in chastity belts, then head for the Holy Land. The rest of the film revolves around the town locksmith, played by Cary Grant."

Asked by his secretary to buy her a real French bidet, he cabled her: "Bidet not available. Suggest handstand in shower."

IT. Euphemism for sexual attraction coined by ELINOR GLYN for her novel of the same name. *CLARA BOW* was christened the "It Girl."

ITALIAN GAY SLANG.

"Homosexuality had never been a problem in Mediterranean countries," explained film director Franco Zeffirelli, "because no one talked about it!" Yet the language has a vivid assortment of words describing homosexuality, and its acts and actors. Among the best known is *finocchio*, literally "fennel," for a homosexual man. Neapolitan equivalents include *frocio* and the milder *froscio*. In the 1980 play *Le cinque rose di Jennifer*, by the Neapolitan dramaturge and actor Annibale Ruccello, the transvestite protagonist, Jennifer, embodies the fusion between the *femmeniello*, a man with female characteristics considered a central, symbolic figure in Naples, and the *travestito*, a drag queen regarded as more of a sex object for sale. *Ricchione*, literally "big ear," means a gay man. In Naples, touching the back of one's ear and pushing it slightly forward with one's fingers signals that the person to whom the ear-turner refers is gay. *Frollo*, meaning "ripe and tender" when referring to meat, or "lethargic or weak" when referring to human beings, is also a synonym for *gay* (and gives a new subtext to the celibate but sexually obsessed character of Claude Frollo in *Notre Dame de Paris*). *Bucchinaro*, a man who performs BLOW JOBS, originates from *bocchino*, with its myriad meanings, e.g., cigarette holder, but also mouthpiece of a musical instrument. *Pompino*, or blow job, comes from the verb *pompare*, "to pump."

IUD. Intrauterine device.

Contraceptive method in which a metal object, sometimes called a "shield," "loop," or "spring," is inserted into the neck of the uterus. Largely discontinued in the 1990s because of health problems. There was a brief fad in the 1980s to wear gold-plated IUDs as earrings.

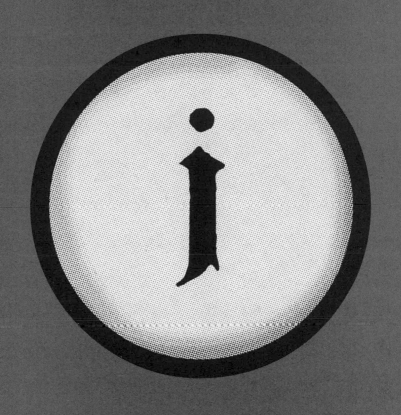

JAMESON, Jenna (née Jenna Massoli) (1974-). U.S. porn star.

Short, blond, and bisexual, Jenna Jameson is a sometime cocaine addict and victim of child molestation and adolescent rape, then underage stripper. She has a broken heart tattooed on one buttock, and her ballooning breasts are underpinned with two sets of implants. Jackie Collins could not have written a better version of the cliché porn performer—a fact Jameson exploited by publishing a lurid bestselling 2004 autobiography, *How to Make Love Like a Porn Star: A Cautionary Tale*.

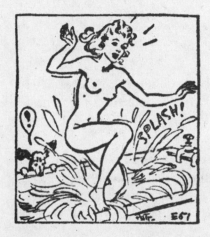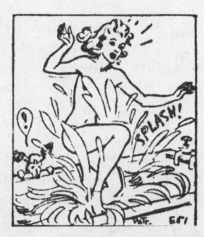

JANE NAKED AS NATURE INTENDED, THEN CENSORED FOR GENERAL CONSUMPTION

JANE (1930s-1960s). British comic strip. Also stage show.

Norman Pett's *Jane*, originally entitled *Jane's Journal—Or the Diary of a Bright Young Thing*, debuted in the British daily newspaper the *Mirror* in 1932. A slim, pretty blonde always being surprised without her clothes, Jane won a huge following, particularly during World War II. Pett's real-life model, Christabel Leighton-Porter, played Jane in a wartime stage comedy, reprised in a film version.

ALSO
JANE (U.S. slang). Term for girl, popularized by Damon Runyon in his stories of semi-criminal New York.

Mostly 1950s, though in *Pattern Recognition* (2003), by William Gibson, the lover of its very up-to-date heroine asks her to "make . . . like, those Jane faces" during sex.

JAZZ (sometimes JASS or "THE JASS" (U.S. slang, 1890s–present).
Originally a term used in the South for sex, "jazz" became attached to the syncopated music of New Orleans through association with pimps and brothel piano players like Ferdinand Joseph Lamothe, aka "JELLY ROLL Morton."

> *"The word jazz,in its progress toward respectability has meant first sex, then dancing, then music. It is associated with a state of nervous stimulation, not unlike that of big cities behind the lines of a war."*
>
> —F. SCOTT FITZGERALD, *ECHOES OF THE JAZZ AGE*

JELLY ROLL (U.S. slang, 1900s-1940s). Euphemism for *vagina*, used in the lyrics of many early blues songs.

> I ain't gonna give nobody none of my jelly roll
> I wouldn't give you a piece of my cake to save your soul.

Later abbreviated to *Jelly*, as in "It Must Be Jelly ('Cause Jam Don't Shake Like That)." Adopted as a nickname by musician Ferdinand "Jelly Roll" Morton, who claimed to be the "inventor" of JAZZ. See PIG FOOT.

JEREMY, Ron (né Ronald Jeremy Hyatt), aka B. Blackman, Bill Blackman, Lolita Brooklyn, David Elliot, Ron Gerimiah, Ron Hedge, Ron Hiatt, Ronald Hyatt, Ron Hywatt, Ron Jeremi, Lulu Latouche, Nicholas L. Pera, Norm L. Pera, Ron Prestissimo (1953-). U.S. porn performer and director.

Enduring, prolific, and opinionated performer, producer, director, and spokesperson for porn, the squat, overweight, balding, olive-skinned Jeremy, hairy as a hearth rug, deserves his nickname "the Hedgehog." Entering porn in 1978 after abandoning a career as schoolteacher, he has never been off-screen since, and holds the record for the largest number of porn appearances; well over a thousand. He has also directed or written hundreds of films, none of them impressive. "He does as many as two [videos] in two days," charged WILLIAM ROTSLER. "He's done *three* in two days. It's nothing but people on a couch. There's no plot, and usually they're not even well written. The only question you ask with these films is, 'How many times can a man have an orgasm in a day?'" Jeremy also directed such milestones of bad taste as *John Wayne Bobbitt Uncut* (1994). See BOBBITT, John Wayne

JOENSON, Bodil (1944-1985?). Danish performer in animal pornography.

With her horse Dreamlight, her pig, and her German Shepherd bitch Smut, Joenson featured in most of Copenhagen's and Stockholm's live sex shows, and in numerous magazines. All the animals used in her films were raised by Joenson on her farm in the north of Zeeland. Her stock included cattle, twelve pigs, four cats, two horses, two dogs, some geese, and a hamster. Not all, she reassured visitors, were sex partners, although she insisted she preferred animals to people. "When we made the last porno magazine," she said, "they gave me a new partner, a man I didn't know, and it was *awful!*" See DENMARK; ZOOPHILIA.

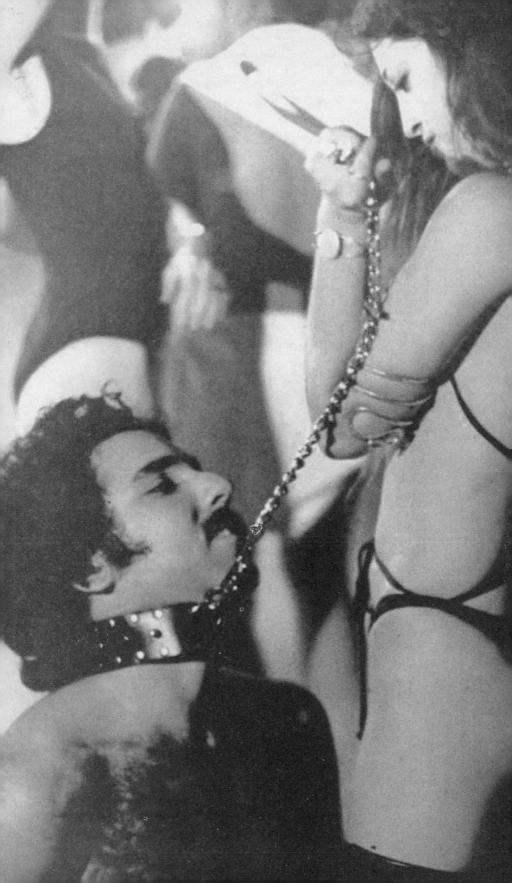

JOY.

In the wake of *EMMANUELLE*, Joy Laurey's frankly imitative novel *Joy* also triggered a series of films (e.g., *Joy and Joan, Joy in Africa*), in which the eponymous fashion-model heroine, fleeing from an unhappy love affair, rebounds around the beds of a dozen exotic locales. Some of these featured BRIGITTE LAHAIE, the most sophisticated of France's X-rated stars, whose serious, absorbed face and husky voice gave class to the trashy stories, but they couldn't hope to compete with *EMMANUELLE*'s extraordinary success.

JOY OF SEX, THE (Also MORE JOY OF SEX, NEW JOY OF SEX, POCKET JOY OF SEX, etc). Popular series of sex manuals by ALEX COMFORT.

The Joy of Sex, subtitled *A Gourmet Guide to Lovemaking*, was first published in Britain in 1972 by James Mitchell, who had suggested to his friend Comfort, a gerontologist, political activist, minor poet, and novelist, that he compile a book on fornication as a leisure activity. Though Comfort's original title, *Cordon Bleu Sex*, had to be discarded when the cookery school objected, culinary echoes survive in the chapter titles: "Starters," "Main Courses," "Sauces and Pickles," etc. Comfort completed the book in two weeks, drawing on personal experience, augmented by such Eastern manuals as the *Koka Shastra*. As a result, the text reflected his own sexual tastes, among them an enthusiasm for the sexual use of TOES (at fourteen, he'd lost the fingers of his left hand). He also recommended some mild BONDAGE, though this was removed from later editions. The books made Comfort rich and famous. He accepted various teaching positions in California, and became semi-resident at the SWINGERS' retreat SANDSTONE RANCH.

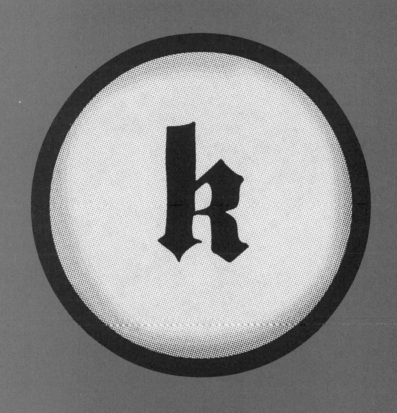

KAMA SUTRA CHAIR (sometimes TANTRA CHAIR, 1990s–present). Narrow padded platform of undulating profile, designed exclusively for sexual use. This ingenious adaptation by various designers of the traditional couch and footstool showed American know-how applied to meeting the physical demands posed by the increasingly taxing movements and acrobatic positions of contemporary sexual intercourse.

KEFAUVER COMMITTEE.
Convened by the U.S. Senate in the early 1950s, the Subcommittee on Juvenile Delinquency was initially chaired by Senator Robert Hendrickson, but became better known under the name of his replacement, Minnesota senator Carey Estes Kefauver, who had become nationally famous when, as chairman of another committee, investigating organized crime, he publicly exposed the existence of the Mafia.

The Juvenile Delinquency investigation was inspired in part by writings such as Frederick Wertham's *Seduction of the Innocent,* which claimed that comic books and pulp magazines were root causes of crime. Lawmen from FBI director J. Edgar Hoover on down solemnly testified that "lewd photographs and magazines stimulate latent sexual desires among adolescents, and tend to trigger serious sex crimes. One police officer could not recall a single arrest in a juvenile sex case in which quantities of pornography were not found in the offender's possession."

The committee probed the suggestive small ads that clogged the back pages of pulp magazines. A New York "Movie Club" would sell you "four tantalizing movies on one big reel for $9.99," but what one got, complained a disgruntled buyer, was "three minutes and fifty seconds of children's magic shows, animal pictures and travelogues, with a concluding ten-second shot of an alluring dame."

To avoid conflict with the free-speech provisions of the Constitution, the committee, like the nineteenth century censorship campaigns of Anthony Comstock, recommended removing the right of guilty publishers to send their products through the mail. In response, the comic book industry introduced the self-regulatory Comics Code Authority, similar to the system adopted by Hollywood. However, producers and distributors of visual porn, such as IRVING KLAW, were put out of business.

KENNEDY, John Fitzgerald (1917–1963). Politician.
The White House was no stranger to sex, Warren Harding, Franklin Roosevelt, and Dwight Eisenhower all having enjoyed extramarital relations while in or headed for presidential office, but before BILL CLINTON, Kennedy was the most sexually active of all American presidents, entertaining such regular sex partners as MARILYN MONROE, Angie Dickinson, Judith Campbell Exner, Jayne Mansfield, and, according to KENNETH TYNAN, MARLENE DIETRICH, although her family denies this. Kennedy is also reliably believed to have had an illegitimate son before his election.

KEPT WOMAN (1800s–present). A woman who reserves sexual favors for one person in return for financial or other advantages, traditionally an apartment or house, a car, etc. See *BETTAKU*.

KIKI OF MONTPARNASSE (née Alice Ernestine Prin) (1901–1953). Model, writer, and painter.

Kiki came to Paris at twelve, and immediately found her level in the easy morality of Montparnasse. Despite a bottom-heavy body and small breasts, she flourished as a model, trading on her dirty mouth and frank sexuality: she never wore underwear, and was rumored, erroneously, to shave her pubic hair. Among those whom she served as model and/or lover were Chaim Soutine, Tsuguharu Foujita, Francis Picabia, JEAN COCTEAU, Alexander Calder, Per Krohg, Hermine David, and Pablo Gargallo.

Introducing herself to MAN RAY shortly after he arrived in Paris in 1921, she became his mistress and model. Ray's photographs made her famous. He encouraged her to shave her eyebrows, drawing them back in an exaggerated double curve, like the Spanish diacritical mark the tilde. According to Kay Boyle, he applied her makeup himself, "putting other eyebrows back, in any color he might have selected for her mask that day . . . Her heavy eyelids might be done in copper one day and in royal blue another, or else in silver or jade."

So impressive was Kiki that the guests at a 1929 gala to raise money for starving artists declared her "Queen of Montparnasse." Louis Broca, publisher of a magazine to which Man Ray contributed erotic photographs, persuaded her to write her memoirs. Little more than a succession of vague reminiscences, which she illustrated with draw-

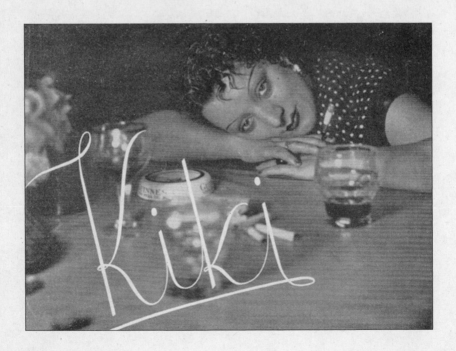

ings and photographs made of her by various artists, as well as her own naïve paintings, the book sold well. Ernest Hemingway, asserting that Kiki "dominated the era of Montparnasse more than Queen Victoria ever dominated the Victorian era," wrote the introduction to an English-language edition, which the United States duly banned.

A resentful Ray took up with Lee Miller, an ambitious young American, while Kiki reveled in her notoriety, singing in cabaret, exhibiting her paintings, and making an abortive attempt at an American movie career. But drugs and alcohol ruined her health. When she returned to Paris in 1945, having fled the German occupation, she haunted the cafés, amusing tourists, and borrowing money to buy cocaine. She died broke, with the café owners of Montparnasse paying for her funeral.

KINBAKU (Japanese, 1990s-present). Japanese bondage porn, featuring models bound in quantities of heavy rope, often suspended in awkward and painful positions, and sometimes with scatalogical elements, e.g., signs that the prisoner has urinated or defecated.

KINSEY, Alfred Charles (1894-1956). Biologist, sex researcher, and author.
At the behest of his highly religious and authoritarian father, Kinsey first studied engineering, and took up his first love, biology, at the cost of a rift between them that was never repaired. He did his first research on gall wasps, becoming a world expert, but then turned his interest to human sexuality, a subject that, as a bisexual with an enthusiasm for bondage and group sex, he was uniquely qualified to investigate. In private, Kinsey indulged in masochistic masturbatory practices, jumping from a chair with a cord tied around his genitals and forcing foreign objects into his urethra, including a toothbrush, bristle end first. He also recruited his wife and fellow researchers into group sex, wife swapping, and forms of exhibitionism, some of which were filmed in the interests of research.

Beginning around 1933, and in association with colleague Robert Kroc, he began collecting data on the sex habits of Americans. In 1935, he revealed some of his findings at a seminar at Indiana University, where he attacked the widespread ignorance of sexual practice and physiology among the general public. In 1938, the university agreed to let him teach a course on marriage, as a part of which he offered advice on sexual matters to his students but also asked them to complete questionnaires about their sexual experience.

In 1940, the university proposed he concentrate on his sexuality research full time. Funded by the Rockefeller Foundation, the Kinsey team systematically interviewed eighteen thousand people, encouraging them to discuss their sex lives, and rating the sexuality of each on a scale of zero to six, with zero representing heterosexuality and six homosexuality. Kinsey also accumulated, with the help of scholars such as GERSHON LEGMAN, a library of pornography and erotica still regarded as one of the most comprehensive in the world.

Published in 1948, *Sexual Behavior in the Human Male*, usually referred to as *The Kinsey Report*, immediately became a bestseller. *Sexual Behavior in the Human Female* followed in 1953. Americans were startled to learn that 37 percent of them had had some homosexual experience, that 50 percent of men and 26 percent of women had experienced sex outside marriage, and that 12 percent of women and 22 percent of men found sadomasochistic material stimulating.

Not everyone welcomed Kinsey's methods. In the interests of expediency, his staff interviewed groups of people who were not representative of the population as a whole; for instance, 25 percent were convicted criminals, including pedophiles, whose diaries provided part of the research material. His interviewers also asked what some saw as intrusively direct questions—not "Have you ever had extramarital sex?" but "When did you first have extramarital sex?" However, when later researchers "cleansed" the Kinsey data of what were seen as distorting factors, the findings were unchanged.

His report turned Kinsey into an international celebrity, but his punishing lifestyle and heavy use of barbiturates impaired his health, as did attacks on his work as "communistic." He died of a heart attack at sixty-two. The Kinsey Institute for Research in Sex, Gender and Reproduction at Indiana University continues his work.

Kinsey's life was the subject of *KINSEY*, a film directed and written in 2004 by Bill Condon, and starring Liam Neeson.

KLAW, Irving (1910–1966). U.S. publisher and film producer. The United States' first professional fetish pornographer.

In 1947, Klaw and his sister Paula operated Movie Star News from a warehouse in Manhattan, selling black-and-white movie stills for twenty-five cents each. When a client who bought only stills showing girls in ropes, chains, or corsets offered to finance the creation of some original pictures of the same type, Klaw rented a studio and, in 1947, shot what he claimed was the world's first commercial bondage photograph: a black-and-white image of model Lilli Dawn in black corset, suspenders, stockings, and heels, gagged, with her hands tied above her head.

Within two years, Klaw had become a one-man industry. As Movie Star News, he sold fetish pinups of Lilli Dawn, BETTIE PAGE, and other models. As Beautiful Productions, Inc., he produced two feature films, *Variatease* and *Teasarama*, featuring strippers such as Tempest Storm and LILI ST. CYR, with Page taking second billing. NUTRIX merchandised 16mm and 8mm STRIPTEASE and FETISH films, and published novels and magazines for the bondage market, often illustrated by artists such as ERIC STANTON. At a time when it was rare for a sex film maker to make even a handful of productions—the 1970 Presidential Commission found only fifty-one individuals or groups who'd done more than five—Klaw turned out scores of them.

Short, plump, and balding, Klaw needed only a cigar and three days' stubble to fit everyone's image of the pornographer. Nothing, however, suggests he was anything

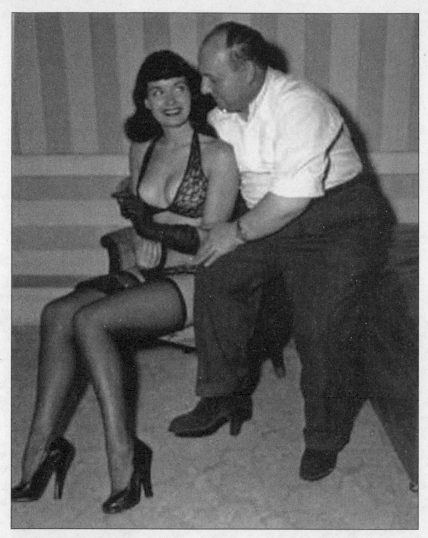

IRVING KLAW, WITH BETTIE PAGE

but a conscientious employer. Photographs show him as an amiable presence on the set, sharing coffee and doughnuts with his smiling employees. His sister Paula acted as chaperone and studio manager, and designed the gadgets in which Page and her fellow models were trussed up.

About Paula Klaw's bondage furniture of racks, pulleys, and ropes, admirers were positively avuncular. In his book on Page, Bernardino Zapponi, screenwriter for FEDERICO FELLINI, fantasized about Paula conceiving "torture devices that even a child could duplicate, tying her little sister [Page] upside down from the swing, her little butt well exposed." Zapponi detected therapeutic value in the books and pictures. "Looking at Bettie and her colleagues, even a Minnesota farmer come to town to buy some tools discovered he could buy a rope for his wife."

The KEFAUVER COMMITTEE put Klaw out of business. BETTIE PAGE was called by the committee to testify, and defended Klaw, but the sententious Kefauver, apparently incensed that America's most popular pinup should be from his home state, responded with a lecture about the evils of the life she had chosen. Klaw's stock was seized, and an attempt to move his operation to New Jersey failed. Indicted for mail fraud and publishing obscene literature, he burned almost all his negatives, though Paula Klaw retained enough to ensure that her brother's legacy was preserved.

KLEIN, Yves (1928–1962). French painter.

Notable mainly for his "anthropometry" paintings, for which nude models either painted their bodies with his trademark deep blue paint or rolled in baths of it, before pressing themselves to white canvas, while a live orchestra played a symphony consisting of a single note. See BODYPAINTING.

KNEE-TREMBLER (British, 1920s–present). Sex while standing, usually with the female partner leaning against a wall with legs locked around the male, the extra weight placing a strain on the knees.

ALSO

Dessert featured by the London restaurant School Dinners. Made from jelly and whipped cream, and decorated with color sprinkles, it was spoon-fed to the customer by a waitress dressed as a schoolgirl.

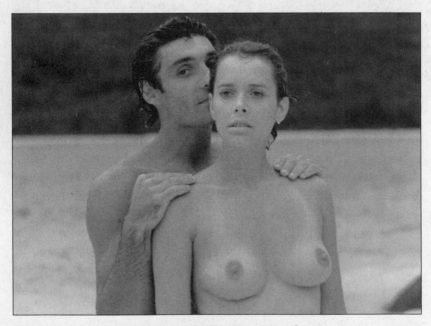

SYLVIA KRISTEL AND NICHOLAS CLAY IN *LADY CHATTERLEY'S LOVER* (1981)

KRISTEL, Sylvia (1952-). Dutch-born model and actress.

A "Miss TV Europe" title won Kristel a modeling and film career, notably in *EMMANUELLE* (1974) and its sequels. Tall, pale, small-breasted, with long, sometimes awkward limbs, Kristel was an unlikely candidate for sexual stardom, never transcending her Calvinist upbringing. For the sex scenes on *Mata Hari* (1985), a film for which she was woefully out of physical shape, she insisted on covering her pubic area and required that black velvet curtains be installed and the set cleared of all but the essential unit. She also played the scenes in dead silence, telling director Curtis Harrington, "I presume you will have someone put in the breathing."

In 1979, American producer Jennings Lang, whose sense of humor, not to mention his sexuality, had survived his being shot in the testicles by fellow producer Walter Wanger in a fracas over Wanger's wife, Joan Bennett, cast Kristel as a STEWARDESS in *The Concorde: Airport '79*, but hopes of an *EMMANUELLE* replay at supersonic speed with Hollywood production values were unfulfilled. She did enjoy some success with *Private Lessons* (1981), playing a housemaid who sexually initiates her fifteen-year-old charge, but otherwise it is as the gawky, shy but salacious Emmanuelle for which she'll be remembered.

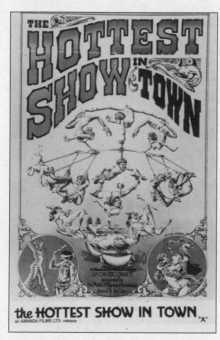

POSTER FOR AMERICAN VERSION OF *LA FOIRE AUX SEXES*

KRONHAUSEN, Phyllis (1929-) and Eberhardt (1915-). Psychologists.

The German-born Kronhausens held only minor degrees in psychology and marriage and family life education from the Teachers College of Columbia University, but took maximum advantage of them to exploit the new interest in sexual behavior that dominated the 1960s. Their dramatized documentary *Freedom to Love* (1969) followed four case histories, suggesting, among other things, that SWINGING can relieve domestic tensions. For thirty years, they churned out films, books, and essays, and added their dour presence and pedantic commentary to marriage manuals, collections of erotic art, filmed documentaries, and even some dramatic features.

In an Anglophone market hungry for erotica, the Kronhausens' films and others like them received wide circulation. Most audiences, however, left disappointed. Sexual positions were demonstrated with numbing attention to detail, and more information was offered about sexually transmitted disease and impotence than the audience really wanted to hear. Sex for the handicapped was discussed. Men were cautioned to wash under their foreskins after intercourse. When, in the course of one such film, an audience in London was offered, for the worthiest of purposes, a split-screen display of fifty vaginas, even the stony British moviegoer was appalled. From the darkness came the weary comment "Not a pretty sight."

In 1968 and 1969, the Kronhausens curated exhibitions of erotic art in Denmark and Sweden, the contents of which made up the International Museum of Erotic Art in San Francisco, opened in 1973. The same year, they returned to movies with a New Wave–influenced satire, *La Foire Aux Sexes* (*The Sex Fair*). The owner of a small bankrupt circus notes the interest with which his performers watch two dogs fornicating, and decides to offer sexual performances instead of juggling and lion taming. These include a nude knife-throwing act, two clowns copulating with an acrobat, a sex display by dwarves, and a mime who stands naked in front of a revolving wheel, to which numerous cows' tongues have been nailed, each one of which licks her vagina as it passes. Even with such an array of delights, and despite being renamed *The Hottest Show in Town* for U.S. distribution, the film failed at the box office.

In 1973, the Kronhausens stated confidently that "the era of pornography is coming to an end, for pornography is possible only where censorship exists." Once their optimism proved ill-founded, they turned their attention to nutrition, antioxidants, and longevity, compiling the bestselling guide *Formula for Life*. Retiring to Costa Rica, they opened a bed and breakfast.

LABIAL RING. A metal ring pierced through the labia minora and/or labia majora of the female genitalia.

This fad began with Pauline Réage's novel *HISTOIRE D'O.* To prove her subservience to a group of wealthy sadists, the heroine, O, agrees to be branded, then to have her labia pierced, and a ring inserted. Later, a metal tag is attached, and also a chain, by which she can be led on ceremonial occasions. Taken up in the 1960s by the PIERCING community, the practice became popular when adopted by MARILYN CHAMBERS.

LADY CHATTERLEY'S LOVER (1928). UK novel, by D. H. LAWRENCE.

The liaison between Lawrence's friend society, hostess Lady Ottoline Morrell, and a stonemason named "Tiger" working on her estate inspired *Lady Chatterley's Lover.* Constance, Lady Chatterley, is driven by the paralysis of her husband, wounded during World War I, to have an affair with Michaelis, an Irish playwright. Repelled by his cynicism, she takes up with their gamekeeper Oliver Mellors, who speaks in a broad Derbyshire accent, has a quaint turn of phrase—he calls his penis "John Thomas" and Connie's vagina "Lady Jane"—and embraces a primitive sexuality that celebrates nature and the earth. Even then, Connie is not entirely satisfied. While she enjoys the sex, she's more interested in having a child, which Mellors, knowing his place like any good family retainer, duly provides.

Lawrence wrote *Lady Chatterley's Lover* as an attack on the decline of British rural life, the encroachment of urban cynicism, and the arrogance of the aristocracy. The Olde England sexuality of Mellors and Connie, contrasted with the tight-lipped impotence of Clifford Chatterley, symbolizes what Britain lost in the Great War.

Chatterley first appeared in Florence in 1928 in a private printing, but by the time Lawrence died in 1930, it had become the most famous of all "dirty books," published in Paris by OBELISK PRESS and pirated everywhere else. No British or U.S. publisher would risk an unexpurgated edition until 1959, when Britain passed the Obscene Publications Act, which acknowledged that a work that outraged COMMUNITY STANDARDS might nevertheless have "redeeming artistic merit."

In 1960, John Lane of Penguin Books printed and stored two hundred thousand copies, and sent twelve to the director of public prosecutions, challenging him to prosecute. At the six-day trial in October, Penguin's parade of expert witnesses, including novelists, religious figures, and language experts, flummoxed the prosecution. Sounding like the reincarnation of Lord Clifford, prosecutor Mervyn Griffith-Jones, an old Etonian and former member of the Coldstream Guards, asked the jury, "Is it a book you would wish your wife or servants to read?" ("I don't know about my wife," joked one aristocrat, "but I wouldn't show it to my *gamekeeper*.") Penguin could not have wished for better publicity. Once the case was decided in its favor, queues formed at every bookstore. By the end of the first day of publication, one hundred thousand copies were sold.

LAHAIE, Brigitte (née Brigade Van Meerhaegue) (1955–). French actress.

Pale, blond, and slim, Lahaie was the classiest of French porn stars, with a solemn, long-faced, streamlined beauty reminiscent of 1920s art deco statuary. She has a brief but memorable cameo in Phil Kaufman's film about the affair of HENRY MILLER and Anaïs Nin, *Henry and June*, as the prostitute who, about to have sex with some friends of Miller's, suggests coolly "you may join in, if you wish." See JOY.

LAP DANCING (also TABLE DANCING). Erotic dance in which the woman performs close enough for the client to touch her (though, customarily, he's forbidden to do so).

With the end of BURLESQUE, sex shows moved out of theaters and into bars and clubs. Working on a bar or catwalk brought dancers close enough for clients to stuff money into their G-STRINGS. In wilder bars, women worked naked, and squatted to pick up coins with their vaginas—in WOODY ALLEN's *Bullets Over Broadway* this is the former speciality of the gang boss's mistress, played by Jennifer Tilly. To increase the take, some owners introduced "Mardi Gras," in which dancers perched on the edge of the bar and offered licks of their vagina for one dollar, wiping off with a medicated tissue between clients.

Higher-class establishments compromised, first with table dancing, in which the performer danced for one table or booth, then lap dancing, where she focused on a single client, who was permitted limited touching. The first such club in Britain, For Your Eyes Only, opened in 1994, offering nude table-side dancing. It was soon followed by THE WINDMILL, Stringfellow's, and Cabaret of Angels. Lap dancing also featured in Paul Verhoeven's film *Showgirls* and Atom Egoyan's *Exotica*.

***LAST TANGO IN PARIS* (1972).** Italian/French film. Directed by Bernardo Bertolucci.

A U.S. expatriate in Paris whose wife has committed suicide encounters a girl in an empty apartment that both are trying to rent. They begin an anonymous, carnal affair, meeting only in the apartment, and never revealing their names to each other.

Rumors circulated that Bertolucci originally intended the encounter to be homosexual, but he never confirmed this. Jean-Louis Trintignant, the reticent, tentative star of *A Man and a Woman*, one of France's few world-class box office hits, had been cast as the bereaved hero, but withdrew at the last minute, panicked by its nudity and simulated sex. Bertolucci's first choice for the girl, patrician Dominique Sanda, also bailed, and was replaced by the druggy but carnal Maria Schneider.

Marlon Brando, six years older than Trintignant, much heavier, and with a more flamboyant acting style, shifted the film toward the baroque. What had begun as another step by the self-absorbed Bertolucci in his screen self-psychoanalysis moved closer to Hemingway than to Freud, with Brando, the wounded lion, licking his wounds and burying his pain in an obliging younger member of the pride.

Bertolucci allowed Brando to improvise much of his dialogue from his own experience. New scenes were inserted, including the most sensational, in which Brando sodomizes Schneider with the help of a handful of butter. Schneider claims she knew nothing of his intention until they started shooting, and insists that, though the sodomy is simulated, her distress is not. Subsequently, she referred to Bertolucci as "a gangster," and refused to speak to him.

The butter scene was cut almost everywhere. In Italy, Bertolucci and the principals even faced criminal charges, later dismissed. Meanwhile, the film's reputation grew, to the extent that it is now regarded as central to the period, and to Brando's career.

LAVENDER MARRIAGE (U.S. 1930s–present). Anglo-Saxon version of the French *mariage blanc*—white marriage. Marriage of convenience, intended to obscure the homosexuality of one or both partners. Common in Hollywood, cf., Rock Hudson and Phyllis Gates; Robert Taylor and Barbara Stanwyck; Charles Laughton and Elsa Lanchester; and in show business generally, e.g., Cole Porter and Linda Lee Thomas.

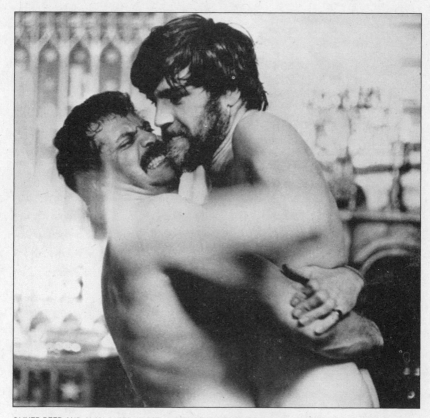

OLIVER REED AND ALAN BATES WRESTLING NUDE IN KEN RUSSELL'S FILM OF *WOMEN IN LOVE*

LAWRENCE, D(avid) H(erbert) (1885–1930). English writer.

Like the composer Frederick Delius, who railed against his native Britain while writing some of its most swooningly sensual music, D. H. Lawrence detested the provincialism of England while drawing his greatest inspiration from it. The son of a miner and a schoolmistress, he grew up in conservative Nottingham, where, though essentially heterosexual, he briefly rebelled against conventional sexuality by enjoying a brief homosexual relationship at sixteen with a young miner that he later described as "the nearest I've come to perfect love." Homoeroticism appears frequently in his novels, notably *Women in Love*, where the aristocratic Gerald Crich and his schoolteacher friend Rupert Birkin wrestle naked—an incident memorably re-created by Oliver Reed and Alan Bates in Ken Russell's 1969 film.

Despite chronic illness and a life spent almost entirely in exile in Italy, the United States, and Australia, Lawrence fought tirelessly for greater realism in literature and art. At a time when most artists occupied themselves with society and politics, he celebrated natural beauty, robust physicality, and powerful emotions, particularly sexual desire. His erotic paintings were banned, and his writing, most notably *LADY CHATTERLEY'S LOVER*, attracted censorship and prosecution. He died as he lived: a bitter, underappreciated exile. Obituaries labeled him a pornographer—ironic, since the cheap erotica of popular fiction and of pornographic POSTCARDS were among his greatest detestations. "The human soul," he wrote, "needs actual beauty more than bread."

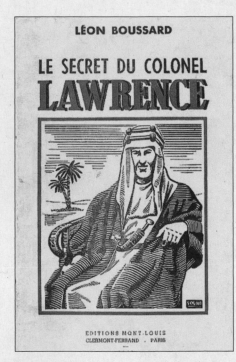

LÉON BOUSSARD

LE SECRET DU COLONEL LAWRENCE

EDITIONS MONT-LOUIS
CLERMONT-FERRAND . PARIS

LAWRENCE, T(homas) E(dward) (aka Lawrence of Arabia) (1888–1935). Soldier, statesman, and writer.

Little about Lawrence's life and death is entirely certain, least of all his sexuality, now generally agreed to be masochist. During World War I, he developed a romantic fascination with the Arabs, and in particular with Arab boys, though it's unlikely he had sex with them, or anyone else.

In his memoir *The Seven Pillars of Wisdom*, he claimed to have been captured in 1917 in the town of Deraa while disguised as an Arab, and subsequently flogged and sodomized by the Turkish *bey* and his men. No evidence was ever produced of this incident. Lawrence tore the page from his diary, and most scholars now believe it was a pornographic fantasy. However, the incident featured in David Lean's 1962 film and in the play *Ross*, where Terence Rattigan, himself homosexual, suggests a different scenario: that the beating and sodomy were inflicted by a Turkish general thoroughly aware of his prisoner's identity and intent on breaking him as leader of the Arab revolt.

After the war, Lawrence sought anonymity, enlisting in the British Army and Air Force under pseudonyms, and living frugally in a woodland cottage in Dorset. Clandestinely, he hired young servicemen to whip him, inventing a story about an uncle who insisted he prove his stamina. The men were required to write detailed descriptions of these beatings and Lawrence's reaction to them, and mail them to an address that proved to be that of Lawrence.

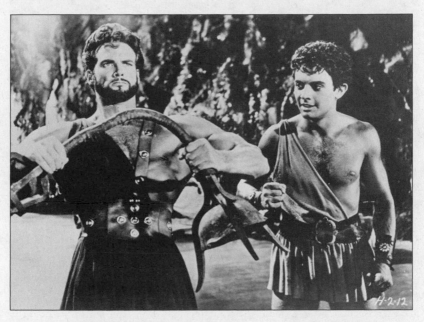

STEVE REEVES DEMONSTRATES THE VALUE OF A STRONG LEATHER ABDOMINAL SUPPORT

LEATHER.

Given its constricting and unyielding qualities, its use in belts, whips, and harness, its association with manual labor, the military and the police, and with such he-man pursuits as motorcycle riding and horsemanship, leather inevitably became a potent homosexual fetish. Even when advances in tanning and treatment made soft, thin, and pliable leather available for the fabrication of female clothes and shoes, it remained an essentially male gay interest. "Leather bars," patronized by ersatz bikers and construction workers, became a cliché of the gay landscape, parodied by the Village People pop group, the members of which dressed as a military man, a motorcycle cop, a cowboy, and a construction worker, with a fifth clad head to foot in black leather (and a sixth, puzzlingly, as an Indian chief).

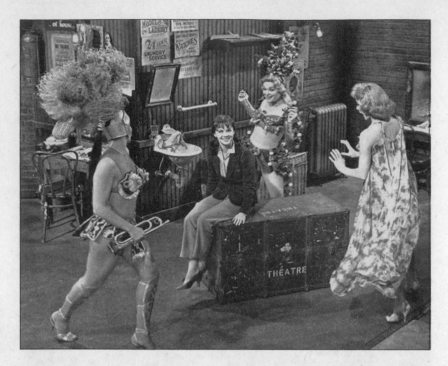

NATALIE WOOD AS THE YOUNG GYPSY ROSE LEE IS INITIATED INTO THE MYSTERIES OF STRIPTEASE BY MAZEPPA, ELECTRA, AND TESSIE TURA IN "YA GOTTA HAVE A GIMMICK," FROM THE 1962 FILM VERSION OF *GYPSY*

LEE, Gypsy Rose (née Rose Louise Hovick) (1911–1970). Actress, writer, and stripteaser.

Victims of a tyrannical stage mother, subsequently accused of child abuse and murder, Rose Louise Hovick and her sister June (later actress June Havoc) grew up on the road in a vaudeville child act. At fifteen, her mother bullied the less obviously talented Louise into striptease. As Gypsy Rose Lee, she proved a considerable success, not so much for what she stripped than for the tease that accompanied it.

Although a frequent headliner at Minsky's BURLESQUE, Lee was far from the average stripper. Flesh, she believed, "should be hinted at rather than hollered about." Intelligent and well-read, she collected modern art, put her name to a crime novel, *The G-String Murders* (ghosted by Craig Rice), and peppered her appearances with cultural and political references. Rodgers and Hart wrote into *Pal Joey* (1940) the song "Zip," a newspaperwoman's speculation about what, or who, passed through Gypsy's mind as she stripped, including citations of philosopher Arthur Schopenhauer, political commentator Walter Lippman, Salvador Dalí, and Confucius. She made some minor film appearances, and had an illegitimate child by director Otto Preminger. Her 1957 autobiography, *Gypsy: A Memoir*, with its forgiving portrait of her mother, inspired the musical *Gypsy*.

ALSO

LADY OF BURLESQUE (1943). U.S. film. Directed by William A. Wellman.

Movie of *The G-String Murders,* with Barbara Stanwyck as burlesque star Dixie Daisy, suspected of murdering her competition.

GYPSY (1962). U.S. film. Directed by Mervyn LeRoy. Sugar-coated version of Louise Hovick's life until her escape from burlesque into striptease. A scene-stealing Rosalind Russell puts Natalie Wood's Gypsy in the shade.

LEE, Hyapatia (née Vickie Lynch) (1962–). U.S. adult movie actress.

Hyapatia Lee claimed that one-quarter Cherokee blood accounted for her long dark hair, imperious profile, and coppery skin—assets she used to considerable effect in a thirty-six-film career extending from 1983 to 1993. Beginning as a stripper in her native Indianapolis, Lynch adopted the name Hyapatia to honor, she claimed, her Native American ancestry.

Lee's striking beauty brought a sort of savagery to porn cinema. Her films, mostly co-written and produced by her then-husband, ex-dinner theater actor Bud Lee, exploited her darker skin and exotic features by casting her in tough, assertive roles—typically as a businesswoman who employs sexual gymnastics to save a telephone answering service, dance studio, night club, or model agency—roles rare in a field where the standard female was usually a groveling submissive.

The danger and strangeness of Hyapatia's films emerged in *Saddle Tramp* (1988), a porn Western that was her first film after giving birth to her son, Cochise. Still with clothing draped over her waist to hide the postpartum slackness, she's about to be penetrated by Randy West. As his erection grows, she smilingly squeezes her breast. Milk spurts startlingly over his erection, and she takes his penis in her mouth.

Hyapatia Lee disappeared in the mid-1990s, supposedly dead from diabetes. Subsequently, however, the report proved fake. She'd left porn and was now remarried, living under another name. Her reasons for this dramatic departure were never revealed.

LEGION OF DECENCY. Also CATHOLIC LEGION OF DECENCY (1933–2001).

This archetypal self-appointed religious-based censorship group was founded in response to an appeal by apostolic delegate Amleto Cicognani at the 1933 Catholic Charities Convention in New York. He warned against an incipient "massacre of innocence of youth," and urged a campaign for "the purification of the cinema." Although "National" replaced "Catholic" in 1934, the Legion always reflected Vatican dogma. It wielded particular influence between 1934 and 1954, when Catholic Joseph Breen administered Hollywood's self-censorship PRODUCTION CODE.

Director Busby Berkeley parodied the Legion in his 1934 musical *Dames,* as the Ounce

Foundation for the Elevation of American Morals, founded by bibulous millionaire Hugh Herbert, and MAE WEST attacked it as the Bainbridge Foundation in *The Heat's On* (1943). In 1966, the Legion re-named itself the National Catholic Office for Motion Pictures. Eventually, it was subsumed into the United States Catholic Conference.

LEGMAN, Gershon (né George Alexander Legman) (1917–1999). American folklorist and author.

Uniquely accomplished and unapologetically eccentric, Legman made the study and celebration of sex his life's work. At the age of twenty, he conceived a VIBRATOR, and worked with an inventor to perfect it. A tireless collector, he accumulated a notable archive of erotic folklore, including thousands of LIMERICKS. His expertise made him invaluable to ALFRED KINSEY, for whom he worked for two years as book buyer and bibliographer.

In 1949, he completed *Love & Death: A Study in Censorship*, which attacked our tendency to shun sexual freedom but embrace cruelty and violence, particularly toward women. In this book, Legman coined the later-famous slogan "Make Love, Not War." When no publisher would accept the book, Legman produced it himself, selling copies by mail. Harried by the postal authorities, he abandoned the United States in 1953, and lived the rest of his life in France.

He still traveled widely, however, and in Japan discovered origami, the art of folding paper to create objects and animals, which he did much to popularize in the United States. In 1970, he published *The Limerick*, which contains 1,700 of the more than 4,000 limericks he'd collected, most of them vulgar. He followed this with *The Intimate Kiss*, on techniques of oral sex; *Roll Me in Your Arms and Blow the Candle Out*, a collection of bawdy songs; and the two-volume *Rationale of the Dirty Joke: An Analysis of Sexual Humor*, the standard work on the subject.

LEG OPENER (Australian and British slang, 1950s–1970s). Alcoholic beverage, usually gin, which makes women receptive to sex. See ALCOHOL.

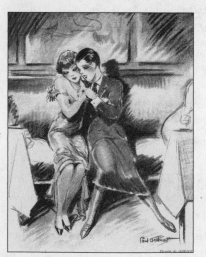

LESBIAN. Female homosexual.

From the Greek island of Lesbos, traditional home of the lesbian poet Sappho, whose poems reflect an admiration and devotion to women over men. *Lesbianism* in the sense of a sexual preference first appears in the 1870 *Oxford English Dictionary*. The adjective *lesbian* appears in the 1890 edition, and was in relatively wide use from 1925 as the preferred alternative to *Sapphist*.

LET MY PEOPLE COME (1974). U.S. stage revue.

Premiered in January 1974 in New York City, and building on the success of *HAIR*, *Let My People Come*, described as "A Sexual Musical," was a plotless revue, with songs by Earl Wilson, Jr., including "I'm Gay," "Come in My Mouth," "Give It to Me," and "The Cunnilingus Champion of Company C." Playing in a basement cabaret, the show attracted a sober collar-and-tie audience, sprinkled with couples. Thirty minutes before curtain, the cast, in a practice borrowed from dinner theater, circulated among them fully dressed, which gave an added frisson to their later appearance nude. The show toured successfully in the United States and had a London season.

LEVENSON, Lawrence (19??-1999). U.S. club owner and entrepreneur.

The self-styled "King of Swing," Levenson, a former fast food and ice-cream vendor at Coney Island, acted as front man for the New York sex club PLATO'S RETREAT. Viewed with equal contempt by the porn community and his backers in organized crime, who twice broke his legs with baseball bats, Levenson could boast only one distinguishing attribute: an ability to ejaculate repeatedly. AL GOLDSTEIN once bet Levenson could not do so fifteen times (in some versions of the story, the figure is eighteen) within twenty-four hours. Ten thousand dollars was wagered, and the process carefully observed by a jury of porn insiders, including BOB GUCCIONE. Levenson won at a walk, ejaculating for the eighteenth time on a photograph of Goldstein's face.

Like many others involved in the sex trade during the 1980s, Levenson was jailed for tax evasion, on $2.3 million skimmed from the club's profits. After serving forty months of his eight-year sentence, he returned in triumph. Wearing a cape and hat of leopard skin, he paraded through Manhattan in the back of a convertible, arriving at Plato's new Midtown premises to be greeted by five hundred enthusiastic supporters. Seven months later, however, on New Year's Eve 1985, Mayor Ed Koch closed Plato's down; it was never to reopen. Levenson ended his days driving a cab.

Richard Dreyfuss, a former resident of the ANSONIA HOTEL and regular patron of PLATO'S RETREAT, was tapped to play Larry Levenson in an unproduced biopic conceived by AL GOLDSTEIN.

LIMERICK. Five-line poem, the first, second, and fifth lines of nine syllables, the third and fourth of six, and rhymed AABBA. The first line traditionally introduces a person and a location, ("There once was a man from East Kent . . .") and ends with a rhyme, usually obscene ("And instead of coming . . . he went"). Credit is given for ingenious concluding rhymes, even if they lack precision, e.g.:

> The jolly old Bishop of Birmingham,
> He buggered three maids while confirming 'em,

As they knelt seeking God,

He excited his rod,

And pumped his Episcopal Sperm in 'em.

The classic collection and study of the limerick was compiled by GERSHON LEG-MAN. The OLYMPIA PRESS published a selection of these in 1956 as *Count Palmiro Vicarion's Book of Limericks*, "Vicarion" being the British poet Christopher Logue. Tom Stoppard performed a prodigy of invention in his play *Travesties* (1974), by writing an entire scene of dialogue, between James Joyce and Tristan Tzara, in limericks.

LIPSTICK LESBIAN (U.S. slang, 1960s–present). Female homosexual who maintains conventionally feminine behavior and wardrobe. See DYKE.

"LITTLE EGYPT" (1893–1910). Stage name of various dancers.

According to legend, "Little Egypt," performed the "belly dance" or *danse du ventre* at the 1893 World's Columbian Exposition in Chicago, so exciting the spectators that one of them, author Mark Twain, suffered a heart attack. In fact, no "Little Egypt" appeared at the 1893 fair. Two exotic dancers of the period, Farida Mazar Spyropoulos and Ashea Wabe, did use "Little Egypt" as a stage name, but while Wabe appeared at the "Street in Cairo" concession in 1893, she did so as "Fatima," and there's no evidence that Twain saw her. In 1897, Mutoscope released a short film of a scantily clad and impressively undulating exotic dancer said to be "Little Egypt," but her identity is unclear. See SHIMMY.

ALSO
LITTLE EGYPT (1951). U.S. film. Directed by Frederick de Cordoba.

Rhonda Fleming poses as Izora, an Egyptian princess, dances at the 1893 fair as part of a confidence trick, and is arrested for indecent exposure.

LIVER.

Popularized as an aid to masturbation in Philip Roth's *PORTNOY'S COMPLAINT*. Its compulsively onanistic hero jerks off into the uncooked liver intended as the family dinner. Parties thrown by Freddie Mercury, gay lead singer of the rock group Queen, sometimes featured a naked youth lying in a dish of raw liver.

LOLITA (1955). Novel by Russian writer Vladimir Nabokov.

Possibly the most famous, but probably least read and understood work of modern erotic fiction, *Lolita* derived from Nabokov's adolescent infatuation with a cousin who died young, and from the contradictory feelings engendered by the birth of his son, Dmitri. Its theme is the obsession of an overeducated and world-weary European intellectual, Humbert Humbert, with a specialized class of underage girl, gawky, infantile, but preternaturally cunning and carnal, whom Humbert and his fellow enthusiasts call "nymphets."

Nabokov was irked intensely by the widespread co-opting of "nymphet"—by Simone de Beauvoir, for instance, in her 1962 essay *Brigitte Bardot and the Lolita Syndrome*—to signify any hot young chick. Taking a cue from his love of butterflies, he had meant "nymph" in the sense of an insect in its unformed state, alien and larval. The mutual lust between nympholepts and nymphets has little in common with a seducer's lip-smacking taste for hard-bodied teenagers, but is closer to the fetishistic need of some men to fuck CHICKENS or paving stones. Asked by Stanley Kubrick to suggest who might play Lolita in the film version, Nabokov unhelpfully proposed a "dwarfess." One uneasy U.S. editor to whom Nabokov initially submitted the book clearly sensed something off-center about its eroticism, and suggested the author change the object of Humbert's affections to a boy.

MAURICE GIRODIAS published *Lolita* from his Paris-based OLYMPIA PRESS, less out of any admiration for its muted eroticism than in appreciation of its complex literary references, word games, and pervasive weltschmerz. While *littérateurs* were grateful for his foresight, the clientele who hoped for the sort of fun and games found in other Girodias productions such as *Sex for Breakfast*, *Until She Screams*, and *The Wisdom of the Lash* must have been sorely peeved.

ALSO

LOLITA (1962). U.S./UK film. Directed by Stanley Kubrick.

Courageous attempt to film Nabokov's novel, but doomed from the start by the LEAGUE OF DECENCY, to which Kubrick was forced to lie that he intended a comedy of an older man tied to a teenager, taking place in one of the southern states where marriage was legal at age fourteen. Sue Lyon's Lolita is sophisticated beyond her years.

LONDON.

The capital not only of the British Commonwealth but of the British Way of Sex, with a thriving but covert erotica industry centered in the SOHO district. Cards in tobacconists' windows advertised "French lessons" and "Correction" by "Young MODELS," or more deviously, "rubber goods." Some prostitutes used antique furniture as a cover ("forty-inch chest, in fine condition"). Nude photographs, suitably AIRBRUSHED, were published as "art studies" or in NATURIST magazines such as *HEALTH AND EFFICIENCY*. Folies Bergère imitators such as the WINDMILL THEATRE, which, by defying the Blitz ("We Never Closed"), had been adopted as a national institution, remained acceptable so long as their nudes posed in goose-fleshed immobility.

Although films were rigorously censored, British actors and filmmakers enjoyed a vigorous sex life in the 1960s. JOHN PROFUMO, implicated in the period's greatest political scandal, was married to actress Valerie Hobson. Both Mandy Rice-Davies and Christine Keeler named movie star Douglas Fairbanks, Jr., as a client. Actress DIANA DORS led a varied sex life. Barbara Windsor, busty star of *Carry On* films, married Ronnie Knight, a henchman for the gangster Kray brothers.

Filmmakers such as Harry Alan Towers featured in testimony during the Keeler affair. Other witnesses recalled a 1961 London party at which a man, naked and masked, was tied between two wooden pillars. Each guest struck him with a whip as they arrived, and he spent dinner cowering under the table. He was Anthony "Puffin" Asquith, director of *The Winslow Boy* and *The Yellow Rolls-Royce*. Asquith, who shared with T. E. LAWRENCE a taste for flagellation and working-class ROUGH TRADE with a military flavor, could be found on many weekends serving behind the counter of a tea stall near the military base at Catterick.

LONGFORD, Lord (né Francis Aungier Pakenham, 7th Earl of Longford) (1905–2001). Politician, author, and social reformer.

As part of a campaign to improve prison conditions, Lord Longford met Myra Hindley, one of the MOORS MURDERERS. The fact that both she and partner Ian Brady acknowledged the role of pornography in their crimes led Longford in the early 1970s to form the Longford Committee Investigating Pornography.

In 1971 the earl, christened by the tabloids "Lord Porn," led a fact-finding trip to DENMARK, then Europe's primary source of erotica. The Danish embassy arranged conferences with bishops, diplomats, academics, and officials from the Ministry of Foreign Affairs, but, ironically, nobody from the porn business.

This proved a grievous mistake. "Two visits were paid to so-called live shows," notes the committee's deadpan report, "from both of which the Chairman felt compelled to walk out after brief encounters, in the second case with a 'lady' who appeared afterwards to have been a man. In his own words, he had 'seen enough for science and more than enough for enjoyment.' When asked whether he had not expected to meet these phenomena, he replied that he had not foreseen the audience participation required of him."

Some committee members thought Longford narrow-minded. One noted, "Lord L's sole reaction is disgust, no more, no less. . . . He sees the problem in black and white, while I think the rest of us can detect a certain amount of shading." Reflecting their doubts, the five-hundred-page *Pornography: The Longford Report* (1972) was relatively subdued. It acknowledged that while pornography may have driven people such as Hindley and Brady to violence, others were unaffected, and it recommended research into the reasons for this.

LOOP (porn slang, 1950s–1970s). Short pornographic film.

From the end of World War II to the production of *DEEP THROAT*, the loop was the standard porn product. Running nine minutes, the length of a single reel of thirty-five-millimeter film, and generally unedited, it was intended for continuous screening in PEEP SHOW booths, where patrons paid by the minute.

In New York, production was controlled by the PARAINO crime family. In Los Angeles, the leading producer was BILL OSCO, and in San Francisco JIM AND ARTIE

MITCHELL and ALEX DE RENZY. Loop production was lucrative. Having paid a model between fifteen and thirty dollars and spent an additional thirty on film stock and processing, a filmmaker had a product that would sell at seventy-five or a hundred dollars a copy to hundreds of sex shops and peep-show arcades across the country. "It's a very hard business to lose money in," confirmed producer-exhibitor Bob Sumner.

Most loops simply showed a lone woman stripping and masturbating. JIM MITCHELL believed "the purest form of titillation is the single girl 'auto-masturbation' film . . . and the BEAVER film was a lot truer form for getting off on some kind of autoerotic fantasy." He felt the introduction of male partners ruined the 'purity' of the loop form. "When you added fucking, you had to show the man, and you covered up the girl. It disrupted the autoerotic trend of sex films. It was boring, because all anyone really wanted to see was the close-up penetration shots."

Once the 1957 Supreme Court decision of ROTH V. UNITED STATES OF AMERICA allowed the law to take existing COMMUNITY STANDARDS into account, loop producers constantly tested the degree of acceptance. "We started with single girls," said Jim Mitchell. "Then there were scenes with two girls (who were not yet allowed to touch each other), and when the competition imitated us, we went to three."

Shooting loops in California was luxurious compared to the conditions in New York. "Imagine a huge loft," said one performer, "where ten different sets are built in a circle with three walls and one open side—all cubicles, with different kinds of bedroom set-ups, baby cribs, walls with harnesses, high school locker rooms, dungeons. Chip [the producer] put a crew on a 24 hour day. While one scene is being shot in a bedroom, people are warming up with whips for the dungeon scene. At the end of five days Chip has eight films in the can. Scripts are written on the way over in a cab, but most of them are improvised."

Another actress evoked an atmosphere even more distasteful. "A filthy loft in Manhattan, sheets draped over the furniture, floors that had never been mopped, a bathroom sink that had never been scrubbed. Two other actors waiting there, a young man named Rob and his wife, Cathy. The director giving us the story line. 'All right, Rob, you lie down on that rubber sheet and Cathy, you and Linda come over and piss on him.' Not believing my ears, watching Cathy try to do it in vain, her saying finally, 'I just can't.' The director announcing, 'Well, fine, if you can't be the pisser, you can be the pissee. Cathy, you lie down and Rob, you and Linda piss on her.' " "Linda" was Linda Boreman, a pale-skinned, dark-haired prostitute of average prettiness, soon to become a household name as LINDA LOVELACE.

LORD CHAMBERLAIN'S OFFICE. Department of the British royal household charged with licensing and, if necessary, censoring theatrical performances.

In the film *Shakespeare in Love*, Queen Elizabeth I's Lord Chamberlain is shown closing London's theaters because of the risk of plague, then because Shakespeare's company has allowed a woman rather than a boy to play a female role. After 1737, however, his office spent most of its time reading every play performed in Britain. Those deemed "acceptable" were licensed. The rest could be presented only privately, or in designated "theatre clubs." Among the plays deemed "unacceptable" were Arthur Miller's *View from the Bridge*, Tennessee Williams's *Cat on a Hot Tin Roof*, and Robert Anderson's *TEA AND SYMPATHY*. Increasing liberalism forced the closure of the Lord Chamberlain's office in 1968.

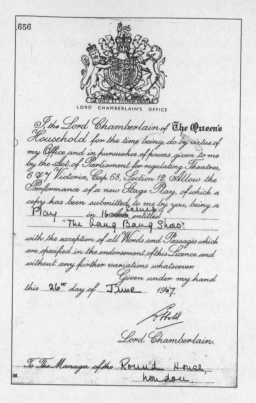

LORDS, Traci (née Nora Kuzma) (1968–). U.S. adult film actress.

The only emblem of 1980s porn comparable in popularity to MARILYN CHAMBERS in the 1970s, Lords lacked Chambers's humor or personality. A parody sex queen, she embodied mindless carnality. Her unblinking stare, toneless voice, and heavily lipsticked mouth, the lower lip swollen as if repeatedly bitten, suggested the infantile greed of a baby for the teat.

In September 1984, *PENTHOUSE* featured Lords as its centerfold, claiming she "spent her 22 formative years in . . . Nevada, Florida, South Carolina, and now Redondo Beach, California." In fact she had actually been born Nora Kuzma in Steubenville, Ohio, on May 7, 1968, and was only sixteen when she posed for the pictures. Having run away from home at thirteen, she made her first porn film a year later, by which time she was freebasing cocaine so lavishly that, as she says, "I lost three years of my life." During those three years, Lords made about eighty porn films, and participated in numerous erotic photo shoots.

Her career might have petered out there, had she not revealed her real age to the FBI. All her films and photos automatically became child pornography—which, charged a lawyer for one producer, "eliminated from the marketplace all the films where she had no royalty interest." The IRS and FBI reduced charges against her in return for testimony against her former associates, some of whom, such as GINGER LYNN, were offered leniency in return for corroboration. (Lynn refused, and was jailed.)

On her eighteenth birthday, Lords, able for the first time to appear in porn legally, flew to France to make *Traci, I Love You* (1987), the distribution rights to which she controlled. Rich on her profits, Lords left porn for a straight career, playing in the horror film *Out of This World*, and John Waters's spoof 1960s teen musical *Cry Baby* (1990). *Vanity Fair* published a charitable estimate of her chances in the mainstream. "No actress," it said, "has successfully crossed over from hard-core to Hollywood films before, but in Lords' favor are her age . . . and the fact that the stigmata aren't quite what they used to be." To date, however, the hopes have not been fullfilled.

LOVE HOTEL (*Rabu Hoteru*). Japanese hotel that offers discreet short-term accommodation for couples wishing to have sex.

In a country where space is limited and some couples still live with their parents, the clients of love hotels can include married people, though more commonly they are partronized by illicit lovers, who take a room for one to three hours for what is technically called a *kyûkei*, or "rest." Most love hotels have vibrating or undulating beds, pornographic videos, and a selection of oils, condoms, and sex aids. Some offer theme rooms, set up for S&M, bondage, and so on.

Discretion is paramount. Entrances and exits are obscured. Check-in is computerized. At most, new arrivals may see only a pair of hands accepting their credit cards and handing over a key. All hotels have automated and untraceable payment systems. Staff even shield the license plates of clients' cars.

LOVELACE, Linda (née Linda Susan Boreman), aka Linda Marchiano (1949–2002). U.S. actress.

Linda Lovelace was an improbable candidate for porn movie stardom. If she is assessed on looks alone, her dreamy demeanor and almost ghostly pallor suggest a natural ascetic, even a nun. "The most amazing thing about Linda," said *DEEP THROAT* director GERARD DAMIANO, "is that she looks so sweet and innocent." High school friends nicknamed her "Miss Holy Holy," for her withholding sexual favors from her dates.

A policeman's daughter from the Bronx, Linda reacted against an overbearing Catholic mother by becoming pregnant at twenty. When the family moved to Florida, she married bar-owner CHUCK TRAYNOR, who, in her version, forced her into prostitution and the Mafia-dominated world of New York porn. She appeared in numerous LOOPS, in one of which she had intercourse with a dog (see *DOG FUCK*). Her claim that Traynor stood off camera with a loaded gun is not supported by either her collaborators or the films themselves, in which she performs with casual expertise.

Like most hookers, Lovelace treated a sex movie as just one part of her working week, which might include turning tricks in a hotel, stripping at a "smoker" or STAG NIGHT, and satisfying any or all the guests who could pay. The only skill that set her apart was the ability to take, sword-swallower style, the whole length of a penis into her mouth. In 1972, seeing her demonstrate the talent at a New York party, Gerard Damiano recognized a gimmick on which he might build a feature. At the same time as he hired her for the role, he proposed a new name—Linda Lovelace.

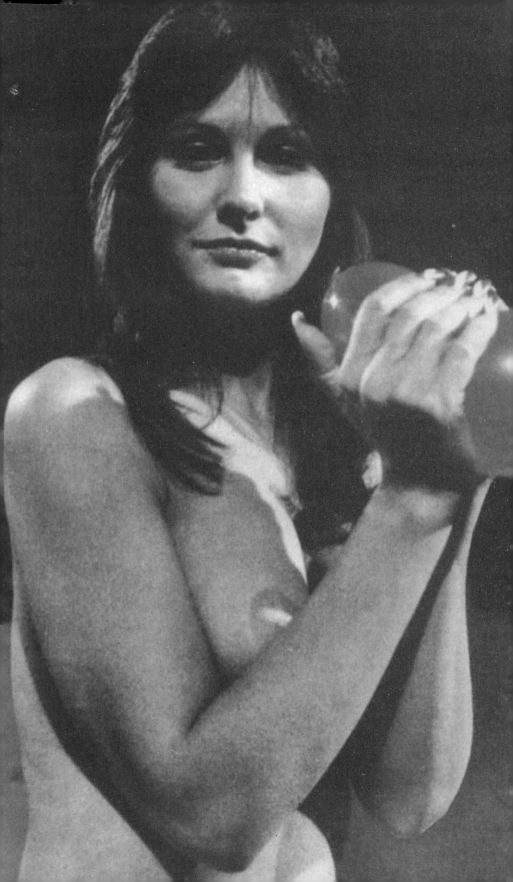

Deep Throat made Lovelace the preferred trophy of every bedroom athlete. Spotting her on a London street, an aged Rex Harrison piled out of his car so hurriedly that he sprained his ankle. Traynor handed her around like candy among those who could further their joint careers. When director Milos Forman and writer Buck Henry proposed featuring Lovelace in Forman's first U.S. production, *Taking Off*, Traynor responded, "If you guys really want to make a movie with Linda, you can have her for a week." They declined.

Fame swept the couple to Hollywood, where sex partner SAMMY DAVIS, JR., offered to include her in his Las Vegas stage act, although after a few maladroit rehearsals, the idea soured. Breaking with Traynor, Lovelace became a house guest at the PLAYBOY mansion. She put her name to a ghosted memoir, *Inside Linda Lovelace*, and stumbled through acting roles in films such as *Linda Lovelace for President* (1975), but it was clear that once her notoriety had faded, her career was over.

The federal crackdown on porn came almost as a relief for Lovelace. She avoided prosecution by insisting that Traynor had forced her into making the film, a claim she pressed in two highly unreliable ghosted memoirs, *Ordeal* and *Out of Bondage*. Having remarried, she rejected the "Lovelace" name and campaigned against her former career with Andrea Dworkin, Gloria Steinem, and the group Women Against Pornography. After surviving a liver transplant, she died in 2002 from injuries sustained in an auto accident.

LYNN, Ginger (née Ginger Lynn Allen) (1962–). U.S. adult film actress.

Many X-rated stars are ex-strippers or beauty queens who share a physical type: tall, slim, languid, with a stripper's haughty stare. In this company, Ginger Lynn stood out. Less than five feet two, she was giggly, bubbling, blond, and bisexual.

Born in Rockford, Illinois, Ginger went to California in 1982. After a year, she answered a WORLD MODELING newspaper advertisement for figure models. She was soon earning $1,500 a day posing for *PENTHOUSE* and erotic photographers Suze Randall, Stephen Hicks, and Ed Holzman, who became her lover.

Lynn shot her first porn movie, *Surrender in Paradise* (1984), in Hawaii; her debut sex scene was a disconcerting beach encounter with the rotund, hirsute RON JEREMY, who appears to be devouring the petite Ginger. For the scenes where she's clothed, she wore the same dress in which she'd graduated from high school four years earlier. In the following two years, she made sixty-nine films, always trading on her pert blond prettiness and California-style freshness.

In 1986, the FBI asked Lynn to testify in the case of underage performer TRACI LORDS. She refused, and was jailed for tax evasion, after which she abandoned porn to become a trophy date among the wilder Hollywood stars, in particular Charlie Sheen (who had also dated Lords). At the same time, she pursued an unsuccessful career in "legit" films, including *Hollywood Boulevard II* (1989) and the *Vice Academy* series. In the first of these, she plays an undercover policewoman exposing a porn filmmaker who directs with a series of placards reading "Fall on Bed," "Moan Louder," and "Degrade Her More"—not far from real-life adult movies. In 1999, having recovered from cancer and given birth to a son, Ginger, now old enough for MILF roles, signed a deal to return to adult films.

L WORD, THE (2004–). U.S. TV series.

Innovative series for U.S. cable channel Showtime, created by Ilene Chaiken and written by Rose Troche and others, which built on the success of *SEX AND THE CITY* (its promotional line was "Same Sex, Different City") by tracing the intertwined lives of glamorous lesbians living in Los Angeles. They included Jennifer Beals as Bette, director of an art gallery; her docile partner, Tina (Laurel Hollomon), whose character is transformed when they decide to have a child; and Jenny (Mia Kirshner), a young writer who discovers she's a lesbian, to the horror of her boyfriend, Tim (Eric Mabius). The series unrepentantly represents most men as dopes, dupes, liars, and bigots, with the occasional dispensation for a character who claims to be an "honorary lesbian" and for the macho star who admits to being a closet homosexual. See LESBIAN.

MACHO (Spanish). Adjective signifying exaggerated masculinity, and its related male pride, *machismo*. Although *macha*, *femacha*, *femacho*, and *feminisma* are sometimes suggested as the female equivalent, the correct term is *hembra*.

MADONNA (née Madonna Louise Veronica Ciccone) (1958–). Singer, actress.

Struggling to make a name as a singer in New York City in the 1970s, Madonna posed for nude shots and starred in the shoestring SOFT-CORE feature *A Certain Sacrifice*, in which she played a tough Manhattanite living with three "sex slaves" who, when she's raped in a restaurant toilet, take revenge on her attacker. Madonna tried strenuously to keep the film out of circulation during the 1980s, even taking director Stephen Lewicki to court. The judge declined to intervene.

Madonna could hardly claim innocence, since her performances as singer and actress were calculatedly erotic. In September 1992, she released *Sex*, a book of photographs by Steven Meisel, for which she and friends modeled in various degrees of nudity, often in public, and in overtly fetishistic settings. The book, spiral-bound in metal covers, and sealed in a metalized bag, debuted at number one on *The New York Times* bestseller list and sold 1.4 million copies in six months.

Accompanying the book was a CD of the song *Erotica*, used in Madonna's album of the same name, which was issued the following day. The inventive video for the song, directed by Fabien Baron (who also shot some of the images used in *Sex*), employs a variety of porn iconography, including jittery hand-held Super-8 film in the style of STAG MOVIES; tableaux resembling the bondage scenarios of HELMUT NEWTON; LEATHER and flagellation images reminiscent of S&M clubs such as THE MINE SHAFT; 1940s amateur CHEESECAKE; shots of a blonde resembling MARILYN MONROE; and MAN RAY's lesbian portraits of Meret Oppenheim and Nusch Eluard, all linked by Madonna wielding a riding crop and wearing a domino mask, black suit, and white collar, recalling BERLIN in the 1920s. MTV ran the clip only three times, then withdrew it permanently.

For the Girlie Show World Tour in 1993, she reprised her *Erotica* performance as a whip-cracking dominatrix, surrounded by topless dancers. The same year, she starred in *Body of Evidence*, a drama in which her elderly millionaire lover is found dead of heart failure, handcuffed to the bed. The presence of cocaine and a pornographic home video leads to her trial for "fornicating" him to death—assault with a friendly weapon? Willem Dafoe is hired to defend her, and the two become lovers, coupling in various uncomfortable locations, e.g., on top of a car in an underground parking garage. Following this flop, Madonna closed the erotic chapter of her career and reincarnated herself yet again, as a wife, mother, and adherent of the Kabbalah creed.

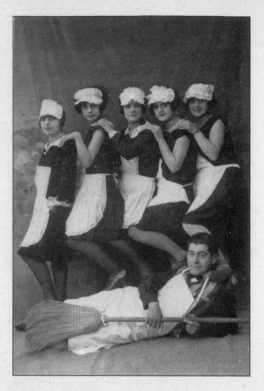

MAID. Female domestic.

A popular figure of twentieth-century erotica, the maid often appears as a frank and uninhibited working girl, sexually initiating her naïve but wealthy young charges, e.g., Jane Fonda in ROGER VADIM's remake of *La Ronde*, and SYLVIA KRISTEL in *Private Lessons*. For the elderly, the maid is represented as a troubling sexual object, tantalizingly omnipresent but not necessarily accessible, as in Stephen Sondheim's gleeful lyrics for "Everybody Ought to Have a Maid" in *A Funny Thing Happened on the Way to the Forum*, and the two film versions by Jean Renoir and Luis Buñuel of Octave Mirbeau's *Diary of a Chambermaid*. An exception to the rule of inaccessibility was Richard Dreyfuss's affair with his Cuban maid, played by Elizabeth Peña, in *Down and Out in Beverly Hills*. JEAN GENET saw a darker side of service in his play *The Maids*, where two sisters murder their employer.

In British and American literature, maids are more commonly middle-aged and frumpish or, if young, terrified or arrogant, but almost always cowed by their employers, e.g., Julia Roberts in Stephen Frears's *Mary Reilly*, about the girl unlucky enough to have to "do" for both Dr. Jekyll and Mr. Hyde, and Kelly Macdonald, hapless helper to the vicious Maggie Smith in Robert Altman's *Gosford Park*. However, Emily Watson's maid in the same film is sufficiently familiar with her master to have slept with him. A rare English-language example of maid erotica is the 1981 novel *Spanking the Maid*, a metafiction in which Robert Coover rehearses in finally ridiculously repetitive detail the numerous permutations of a maid being punished by her master.

***MAÎTRESSE* (1975).** French film. Directed by Barbet Schroeder.

During the 1960s, Dutch-born dominatrix "Baroness" Monique M. K. Von Cleef turned her New York penthouse into a "pain parlor." Closed down in 1967 when the FBI suspected some clients might be members of the Pentagon brass, and as such, vulnerable to blackmail, the business was relocated in Amsterdam, then Paris, where as a *sadotherapiste*, Von Cleef attracted the attention of director Schroeder.

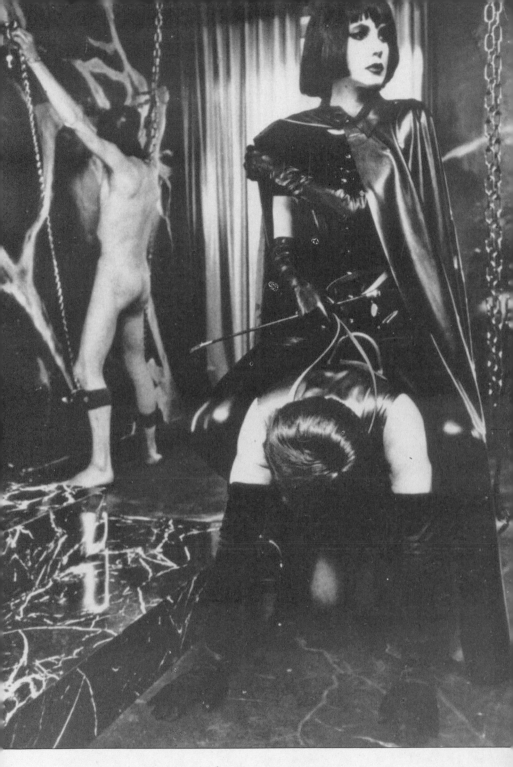

BULLE OGIER AS THE DOMINATRIX IN *MAÎTRESSE*

Maîtresse renders the S&M world in all its eerie fascination and seedy glamour, with costumes by Karl Lagerfeld and a poster by pop artist Allen Jones of Bulle Ogier, in full leather, trailing a whip. Gerard Depardieu plays Olivier, a naïve drifter, new in Paris, who's tempted into some light burglary by a friend. They break into an apparently empty apartment, to find it filled with whips, chains, and bondage costumes. In the bathroom, covered by a tarpaulin, is a cage containing a naked man. "She sent you, didn't she?" he murmurs in pleasure in the beam of Olivier's flashlight. "She's so cruel."

Before they can escape, a metal staircase unrolls from the floor above and the dominatrix Ariane descends, in black wig, full leather, stilettos, and leading a Doberman. She releases the friend but keeps Olivier, initially as assistant (his first job is to piss on one of her clients, then to let himself be fellated, for which the man tips him handsomely) but soon as lover.

Nestor Almendros shot in fluorescent light, giving the images a bilious tone. For smaller roles, Schroeder recruited actual masochists, one of whom has his scrotum pinned out on a wooden board, like a bat awaiting dissection. The beatings are real— strikingly so in a sequence where Ariane takes Olivier to a chateau for what he assumes will be a quiet weekend. They're greeted by the "butler," actually the chateau's owner, who gets off on acting the servant. That night, he hosts an S&M orgy, in which Olivier vigorously involves himself.

"MAKE LOVE, NOT WAR." See LEGMAN, Gershon.

MAKING LOVE (1800s-present). Until the early 1930s, "to make love" meant simply to express admiring or seductive sentiments. Subsequently, however, it became a synonym for sexual intercourse, not necessarily loving.

ALSO
MAKING LOVE (1982). U.S. film. Directed by Arthur Hiller.

Early mainstream Hollywood movie about a wife coming to terms with her husband's bisexuality. The film broke with the tradition of depicting the gay culture as furtive and effeminate, cf., Don Murray's decent but conflicted bisexual senator in *Advise and Consent* or Shelley Berman's creepy snitch in *The Best Man* (1964). Male lovers Harry Hamlin and Michael Ontkean are handsome, masculine, and queer. It would be another twenty-four years before Hollywood had the courage to present a similar pair of homophile hunks, in *Brokeback Mountain*.

MANGA. Japanese comic strips, mostly of an erotic and sadomasochistic nature. See ANIME.

MAN RAY (né Emmanuel Radnitzsky) (1890-1976). American photographer and artist.

Abandoning his American roots and changing his name, Man Ray moved to Paris in 1921 and, with the help of his friend Marcel Duchamp, became photographer by appointment to the SURREALISTS.

If, as Christopher Isherwood confessed, "BERLIN meant boys," for Man Ray, Paris meant pussy. KIKI OF MONTPARNASSE became his model and lover, as well as an enthusiastic collaborator in his more profitable sideline of shooting erotic photographs for magazines that catered to the tourist trade. Images of a naked Ray sodomizing Kiki and being fellated by her appeared in the suppressed book *1929*. His photographs of Meret Oppenheim and Paul Eluard's wife, Nusch, entwined nude, so impressed Henry-Pierre Roche, author of *Jules et Jim*, that he commissioned more of the same. William Seabrook, diabolist, fetishist, and recreational cannibal, invited Ray to photograph the naked girls he kept chained to his stairs.

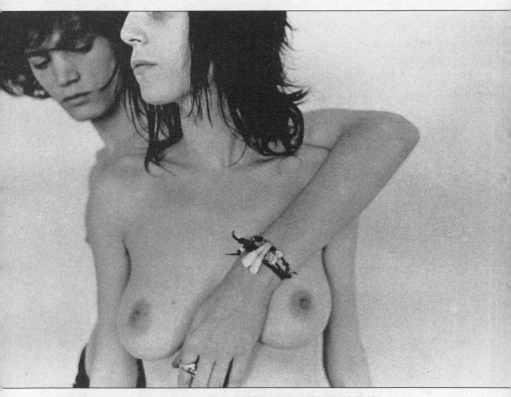

ROBERT MAPPLETHORPE AND PATTI SMITH IN *ROBERT HAVING HIS NIPPLE PIERCED*

MAPPLETHORPE, Robert (1946–1989). American photographer.

Born in Long Island, New York, and raised as a Catholic, Mapplethorpe became the archetype of the outrageous Manhattan photographer, the gay equivalent of Diane Arbus who, in both his work and private life, aimed to shock, although, unlike Arbus, he chose to exercise his imagination not on the marginal and maimed but on the beautiful.

He first attracted attention with portraits of celebrities such as rock singers Grace Jones, Debbie Harry, and longtime friend Patti Smith, who appeared with him in Sandy Daley's 1971 film *Robert Having His Nipple Pierced*, in which Mapplethorpe is pierced while Smith provides a commentary.

ANDY WARHOL made him staff photographer for *Interview* magazine. Meanwhile, Mapplethorpe broke new ground with erotic images of bodybuilder Lisa Lyon, and of male models, mostly black, who were shown urinating through enormous penises into the mouths of others, or being penetrated anally with the handle of a bullwhip. Sexually involved with Warhol and members of The Factory, Mapplethorpe participated in his notorious "Piss Paintings." At the same time, he became fascinated by flowers, which he shot in a meticulous style that puzzled admirers of his erotic work.

Once diagnosed HIV-positive, Mapplethorpe seemed more emblematic than ever of the self-destructive New York arts culture. This made him a target for conservative politicians such as Congressman Jesse Helms, who used the artist's work as a pretext to attack the National Endowment for the Arts, which funded Mapplethorpe's exhibitions. A year before his death at forty-two, Mapplethorpe was unrepentant. "I'm looking for the unexpected," he said. "I'm looking for things I've never seen before . . . I was in a position to take those pictures. I felt an obligation to do them."

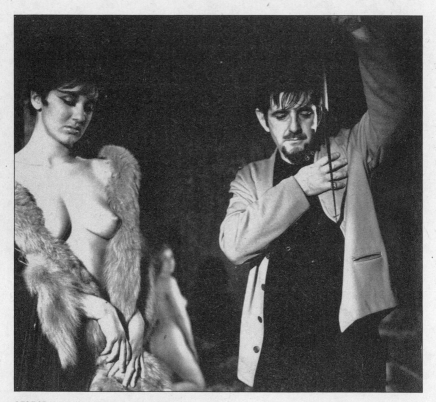

GEORGE HARRISON MARKS AND MODELS

MARKS, George Harrison (1926–1997). UK photographer and film producer.

If HARD-CORE was rare in Britain throughout the 1950s, there was more than enough SOFT-CORE to go around. Its king was George Harrison Marks, a stand-up comedian who developed into a publicity photographer. When a few coffee table books of discreet nudes attracted the attention of a publisher from DENMARK, Marks became a producer-publisher in the IRVING KLAW mold, churning out photos of pale, breasty young women bathing, posing, and frolicking. He used the same girls in ten-minute movies, often shot in his own kitchen and bathroom. People without projectors bought hand-held viewers and wound the films through while holding them up to a light. Since this impeded masturbation, many preferred stills of the same models featured in Marks's magazines such as *Kamera*.

Marks enshrined the prevailing British ideal of sexuality. Milkmaids and farm girls, wide-hipped and bovine, with soft white breasts, his models seem kidnapped from eighteenth-century Flanders. Their Junoesque proportions were replicated in a platoon of husky colleagues in modeling and the cinema: Sabrina, Liz Fraser, Marks's wife, Pamela Green (who, as an art-student-turned-nude-model, knew how to retouch photographs, and found herself blanking out the pubic hair from Marks's photos, including her own), and DIANA DORS, whose charms were emphasized even further by a booklet of "views" employing the prevailing fad, 3-D.

Despite lamenting that "sex bores the arse off me," Marks helped instigate the boom in NUDIE movies by directing *Naked as Nature Intended* (1961) and *The Naked World of Harrison Marks* (1965). By then, alcoholism had almost ruined him. Green left him in 1961, and in 1971 he was prosecuted for selling pornography through the post. Fortunately for him, entrepreneur DAVID SULLIVAN hired him to make *Come Play with Me*, a vehicle for his protegée MARY MILLINGTON. Released in 1977, the film was screened for two years (albeit in a Sullivan-owned theater), a British record.

When video took over the porn market, an increasingly drunk and eccentric Marks turned to S&M films such as *Stinging Tails*, *Flogged Fannies*, and *The Spanking Academy of Dr. Blunt*, and published a magazine called *Kane*. U.S. porn star Richard Pacheco praised Marks's films, particularly *Thrashed by the Brits*, in which a monk spanks a nun who, as he does so, sings "Do-Re-Mi," from *The Sound of Music*. "Done without apology," he wrote, "and produced and acted with a truly European *joie de vivre*, the spanking tapes from Kane are the best the world has to offer."

MARX BROTHERS, THE. Leonard ("Chico") (1887–1961), Adolph ("Harpo") (1888–1964), Julius ("Groucho") (1890–1977), Milton ("Gummo") (1892–1977), and Herbert ("Zeppo") (1901–1970). U.S. vaudeville entertainers and comic film actors.

Although it was Zeppo, with his patent-leather hair and sub–RUDOLPH VALENTINO good looks, who played any romantic roles demanded by their movies, and Chico

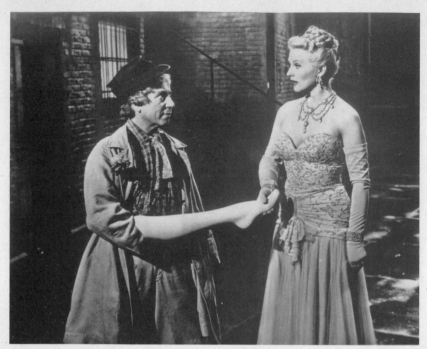

HARPO MARX

who, in real life, was the most priapic of the team—he owed his nickname to his interest in "chicks"—the sexually suggestive material of the Marx Brothers was assigned almost entirely to Harpo and Groucho.

Harpo, a mute, infantile satyr, rolling his eyes and honking on a rubber-bulbed horn, pursued blondes in and out of the ramshackle plots. By contrast, Groucho was almost too vocal, babbling ambiguous verbal woo ("I could dance with you till the cows come home. . . . But I would rather dance with the cows till *you* come home") at the lumbering Margaret Dumont, his one-size-fits-all comic foil.

Intelligent enough to know he needed good scripts, Groucho, albeit grudgingly, accepted the lines written by George S. Kaufman and S. J. Perelman, and remained reliant on writers through his second career, as a TV personality on the quiz show *You Bet Your Life*.

Paradoxically, his best-known quip from this period, as well as the most lubricious, is one he never delivered. In 1947, interviewing a contestant with a large family, he is supposed to have asked him why he had so many children. When the man responded, "I love my wife," Marx, according to legend, said, "I love my cigar, too, but I take it out occasionally." Though it was quoted repeatedly, sometimes by the Marxes themselves, the line is one Groucho never uttered. The closest he came was a tepid "I like pancakes, but I haven't got closetsful of them."

MASSAGE PARLOR. Establishment offering sexual services under the guise of physical therapy.

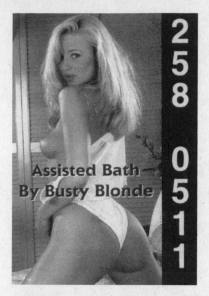

Massage parlors conventionally offer non-penetrative sex acts such as "hand relief" (masturbation) and "assisted showers," usually guaranteeing a "release" or a "happy ending." Girls wear high-heeled shoes, panties, and "happi coats," any or all of which can be shed for an additional payment. In Thailand, the term "full body massage" sometimes indicates that the masseuse uses her nude body to massage the client.

MASTURBATION.

Except for the invention of the VIBRATOR, the last century didn't add substantially to the theory of self-satisfaction, although it did widen the terminology. Euphemisms in use at various times included *self-sexuality*, *self-pleasuring*, *autoeroticism*, *sex without a partner*, *whacking off*, *jerking off*, *pulling your wire*, *beating your meat*, *diddling*, *fiddling*, *frigging*, *twiddling yourself*, *jacking* . . . and . . . *jilling off*, and *visiting the widow Palm and her five daughters*. One of the most elaborate literary celebrations of masturbation was Brian Aldiss's trilogy *The Hand Reared Boy*, *A Soldier Erect* (both 1970), and *A Rude Awakening* (1978). His hero, Horatio Stubbs, practices masturbation solo and with his brother and sister, then with classmates at boarding school, his fellow recruits on military service in Malaya, and on into adulthood. See VIBRATOR.

MAT. Russian slang, obscene and sexual, taking its name from the common obscenity *yob tvo yu mat* ("Fuck your mother"). Mat contains many thousands of words and phrases, but relies almost entirely on reiterations and variations on the words *khuy* (prick), *pizda* (cunt), *blyad* (whore), and *ebat* (to fuck).

MATA HARI (née Margaretha Geertruida Zelle) (1876–1917). Dutch exotic dancer and alleged spy.

Originally a circus horsewoman under the name Lady MacLeod, Zelle moved to Paris and, after working as an artist's MODEL, developed in 1905 a provocative Oriental dance act, which she presented in Paris under the name Mata Hari—Indonesian for "Eye of the Day," conventionally meaning "the sun."

Claiming to be a Javanese princess trained in secret temple dances, she was an instant success, both onstage and off, where she enjoyed relationships with a series of wealthy and influential men across Europe. Since the Netherlands was neutral, these continued even when World War I broke out.

After the war, the chief of French intelligence would claim in a dubious memoir that he had recruited Zelle as a spy, but actual evidence is sketchy. (His claims about another of his "agents," MARTHE RICHARD, were so inaccurate that he even misspelled her name.) In January 1917, French intelligence intercepted German messages from Madrid that mentioned a double agent, code-named H-21. The transmissions were in code that the Germans knew the French could read, which should have aroused suspicion of an exercise in disinformation, but France was smarting from war reverses, and anxious to find a scapegoat.

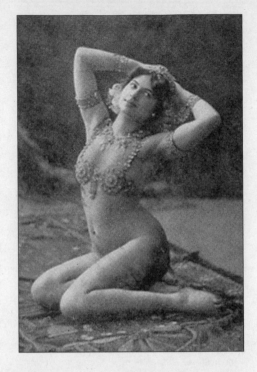

Zelle was arrested in her Paris hotel on February 13, 1917, tried, found guilty on little or no evidence, and shot by a firing squad on October 15.

Hardly was she dead before the legends began; some claimed she had blown a kiss at her executioners; others, that their guns had fired blanks and she was spirited away to fool the Germans one more time. Both Marlene Dietrich and Greta Garbo would incarnate her on-screen, in *Dishonored* and *Mata Hari* respectively. Ironically, the most accurate portrayal may have been in Curtis Harrington's SOFT-CORE *Mata Hari*, made in Budapest and starring SYLVIA KRISTEL—who was, of course, also Dutch, and, also like the forty-two-year-old Zelle when she died, aging and overweight.

MATTACHINE SOCIETY (1954–present). Association pledged to encourage wider public acceptance of male homosexuals and their lifestyle.

Founded by Harry Hay, with early involvement by designer RUDI GERNREICH, Bob Hull, Chuck Rowland, Dale Jennings, and others, the organization was named for a masked jester character in medieval theater whom Hay saw as leading a "hidden" life analogous to that of modern gays. For a decade, the Society was the public face of gay activism in the United States, publishing the *Mattachine Review* and lobbying for repeal of the sodomy laws and other restrictive legislation. It was supplanted by the more militant GAY LIBERATION FRONT, which emerged following the STONEWALL RIOTS.

"MAYFLOWER MADAM." See BARROWS, Sydney Biddle.

MEAT RACK (slang, UK and U.S., 1940s–present). A public place to pick up sex partners.

Applied in particular to covered spaces or colonnades, e.g., the arches at the foot of London's Regent Street, adjacent to Piccadilly Circus, though during the 1930s the whole of Piccadilly was a meat rack, cruised by, among others, Graham Greene. See also CRUISING.

MEESE COMMISSION, THE. This nine-person panel was set up by President Ronald Reagan in 1985, under chairman Henry E. Hudson, to report to U.S. attorney general Edwin Meese on the prevalence of pornography. Its covert aim was to reverse the findings of a 1970 commission convened by Richard Nixon, which had discovered little causal connection between pornography and violence.

The Meese Commission took less time and spent less money than its predecessor, and did no original research. Instead, it held public hearings. These became platforms for such polemicists as Andrea Dworkin, and for LINDA LOVELACE, who offered a revised story of her porn career, claiming she had acted entirely under coercion.

The few pro-porn witnesses, seeing that the commission intended to demonize the industry, were hostile. Producer and critic Bill Margold asserted that, while U.S. society "is drug-infested, violence-racked and polluted by chemical greed, no one has ever died of an overdose of pornography. . . . We are a nation of hypocrites who jerk ourselves off with the left hand and deny the X-rated industry with the right hand."

The commission's 1,960-page report, published in July 1986, was as bad as the industry feared. It advised local and state police not to waste time dragging wealthy publishers and film producers through the courts in the hope of winning convictions under the hazy obscenity laws. Instead, they should target individuals too poor to fight, and do so for old-fashioned offenses such as prostitution and pimping.

As a first step, the commission announced that shops stocking *PLAYBOY* and *PENTHOUSE* risked prosecution. Ten thousand of them withdrew those magazines. New York BDSM clubs such as THE MINE SHAFT were closed for offenses against the health and liquor regulations. The owner of PLATO'S RETREAT was jailed for tax evasion. Porn cinemas and sex shops found themselves cited for infractions of fire regulations, or accusations that prostitutes solicited on or near their premises.

In California, where selling and renting porn was legal, police targeted performers. A porn performer arrested for drug possession would be offered immunity in return for testimony against producers. Though it worked in the short term, the policy did nothing to slow the expansion of the porn industry, and may even have hastened it by driving away the small fry, leaving the market to the larger and better-financed producers and distributors, who were immune to such piecemeal attacks.

MEMORIES WITHIN MISS AGGIE (1974). U.S. film. Directed by Gerard Damiano.

In a secluded farmhouse in snowbound Pennsylvania sometime in the 1930s, an aging Miss Aggie (Deborah Ashira) describes to a companion Richard (Patrick L. Farrelly) a series of youthful sensual experiences, with her character played in each case by a different actress. A young blond Kim Pope chooses to lose her virginity with Eric Edwards in a sequence notable for its extended, carefully observed foreplay. Edwards then visits a whore (Darby Lloyd Raines), who inflames him with a long episode of masturbation. And finally a girl (Mary Stuart), having excited herself by masturbating with a small doll, seduces a delivery man (HARRY REEMS).

After each recollection, Richard casts doubt on Aggie's veracity. It's finally revealed that she is insane and the Richard to whom she speaks is the ghost of her first and only lover. She murdered him when he threatened to leave her. Now, *PSYCHO*-like, his corpse shares the lonely house with her, a truly captive audience for her erotic ramblings.

Miss Aggie was screened at that year's Cannes Film Festival and became the most widely circulated of all Damiano's early films. It decisively dispels LINDA LOVELACE's picture of him as a hack. The shooting is atmospheric, the direction of actors, both in the erotic scenes and the framing story, skillful, the music unassertive and atmospheric. It, in what must surely be its only use in a porn film, includes a few bars of the hymn "Amazing Grace."

MERKIN (1600s–present). Pubic wig, originally worn by prostitutes who had shaved to eradicate vermin, but during the twentieth century developed for decorative purposes. Also, less commonly, a man who dates or marries a gay or bisexual woman so that the woman can pretend to be heterosexual. See BEARD; LAVENDER MARRIAGE.

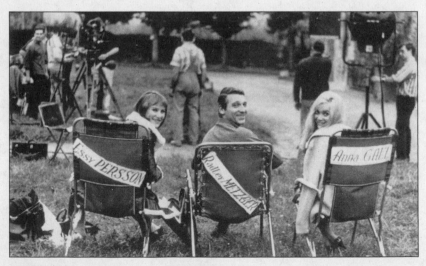

RADLEY METZGER ON THE SET OF *THERESE ET ISABELLE*

METZGER, Radley (aka Henry Paris) (1921-). U.S. film director.

Metzger entered movies as editor of trailers for Janus Films, a U.S. distributor of foreign films. Having failed with his first feature as director, a conventional drama, *Dark Odyssey* (1961), he began buying European movies and "editing" them for the United States. His first success was Mac Ahlberg's *I, a Woman*, which he shortened, and released with subtitles rather than dubbed—proof it was art, not porn. Having paid only $20,000 for the rights, he made $4 million. For the lesbian drama *Les Collegiennes*, he changed its title to *The Twilight Girls* and shot additional nude scenes—some with GEORGINA SPELVIN.

Metzger became a fixture on the European adult movie scene, making *Therese et Isabelle* (1968) in Germany, *The Lickerish Quartet* (1970) in Italy, and *Camille 2000* (1973) and *L'Image* (1976) in France. Always happy to "tweak" his films to avoid CENSOR-SHIP, he screened the lesbian *Therese et Isabelle* to both French and British censors, and amended it in line with their comments. For Britain, he removed the subtitles for two minutes while Essy Persson described her reactions to sex. "The theory here," said one critic, "is that if you don't know French, you won't be depraved or corrupted by it. It follows, I assume, that if your French is up to standard, you'll have the wit and intelligence to resist depravity and corruption."

The Punishment of Anne (1976) was adapted from *L'Image*, a 1956 novel by "Jean de Berg," alias Catherine Robbe-Grillet, in which a jaded Parisienne and her ex-lover collaborate on tormenting her beautiful young sex slave. Indignities escalate from the trivial (being forced to visit restaurants without underwear; urinating in a semi-public garden) through the piquant (a lesbian changing-room encounter with a sexy *vendeuse*) to a perverse conclusion involving whips, chains, and red-hot needles in the nipples.

THE OPENING OF MISTY BEETHOVEN (1976), Metzger's most ambitious film, was emblematic of his hope to bring porn into the mainstream. Like *The Lickerish Quartet*, in which a family is encouraged to experiment sexually after watching an erotic film, the film has the implied lesson "in porno veritas." In a technically impressive but unintentionally hilarious *Quartet* sequence, a couple copulate on giant pages of a dictionary, humping vigorously across definitions of *masturbate* and *fornicate*; Hugh Hefner's *PLAY-BOY* philosophy literally writ large.

Metzger continued to make ambitious porn features, notably *Barbara Broadcast* (1977), with ANNETTE HAVEN, an attempt at a New York–oriented psychedelic erotic film, but in 1979 returned to the mainstream with a non-porn version of the 1920s thriller *The Cat and the Canary*. He retired in 1984. He's the most likely of many filmmakers to have inspired the character of the idealistic porn producer Jack Horner in the film *BOOGIE NIGHTS*.

MEYER, Russ (né Russell Albion Meyer) (1922–2004). U.S. film director.

A World War II combat cameraman, Meyer was a virgin until his company commander, Ernest Hemingway, persuaded a brothel just outside Paris to open

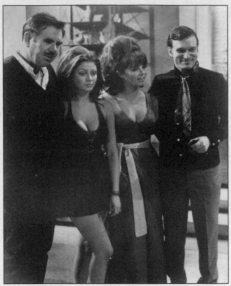

HUGH HEFNER (RIGHT) AND FILMMAKER RUSS MEYER, WITH COMPANIONS

up for his men in 1944. From among the fifteen girls, Meyer, exhibiting a lifetime preference, chose the one with the biggest breasts.

After the war, he took up still photography, specializing in PINUPS. One of the six centerfolds he shot for *PLAYBOY* was the busty ex–Miss Sweden ANITA EKBERG. In 1959, he graduated to movies with *THE IMMORAL MR. TEAS*. When he retired in 1979, he had produced, directed, written, and shot twenty films. In most of them, heavy-breasted heroines—e.g., Candy Samples, Edy Williams, Uschi Digard, and Francesca "Kitten" Natividad—were grossly imposed upon by a succession of villains, only to surge back triumphantly and knee their traducers in the groin.

Little about Meyer was subtle. His characters employed pickaxes, chainsaws, and dynamite as weapons. Names were as broad as the fake casts of stag films: "Mr. Peterbilt" and "Semper Fidelis" in *Beneath the Valley of the Ultravixens*; "Babette Bardot" in *Common Law Cabin*; "Martin Bormann" in *Supervixens*. Relentlessly emphatic, Meyer punched home his scenes with zooms, pans, and fast cuts, jumping from long shot to close-up.

Mayer shared the stag film's fondness for outdoor locations, but photographed his lake, forest, and mountain settings with as much glamour as a 1960s backwoods melodrama. He was also adept at avoiding the "porn" label by introducing a political or social subtext. *Vixen*, a romp in the Canadian woods, with the buxom Erica Gavin pleasuring almost all the male cast, ends with a twenty-minute discussion of draft-dodging, plane hijacking, and civil rights.

The French enjoyed the connections to pinups and comic strips, and hailed Meyer as an auteur for controlling every aspect of his films. Richard Zanuck of 20th Century Fox invited him to make a sequel to Jacqueline Susann's *Valley of the Dolls*. Cheekily hiring film critic Roger Ebert as writer, Meyer made *Beyond the Valley of the Dolls* (1970), for $2 million. Zanuck wanted to commission three more such films from Meyer, but his father, Darryl, called back from Europe by an irate board, cancelled the deal.

Meyer made millions when VIDEO transmogrified the sex film. Rated X in the days when even a whiff of sex was enough to win condemnation, his films shared the adult shelves next to much harder material, and benefited accordingly. He spent his retirement with a succession of busty actresses, including "Kitten" Natividad, star of his last production, *Beneath the Valley of the Ultravixens*, and stripper Melissa Mounds, forty years his junior. Of his declining years, Meyer, always in character, said, "I get up, I sit around, I write, I fuck."

> *"I'd rather play cards if I can't have a lady with big tits."*
>
> —RUSS MEYER

MIDNIGHT COWBOY (1965). U.S. novel, by James Leo Herlihy.

Unsparing picture of the life of a bisexual GIGOLO in New York City, and his friendship with a dying derelict.

ALSO

MIDNIGHT COWBOY (1969). U.S. film. Directed by John Schlesinger.

Newcomer Jon Voight starred as GIGOLO Joe Buck in this adaptation, with Dustin Hoffman as his tubercular companion "Ratso" Rizzo. Schlesinger, who was gay, is said to have been inspired to make the film by seeing *MY HUSTLER*, by ANDY WARHOL. Warhol, invited to appear in the film, declined, but screenwriter Waldo Salt added a party scene in which Warhol regulars Viva, Ultra Violet, International Velvet, Taylor Mead, and Paul Morrissey appear.

> *"Uh, well, sir, I ain't af'real cowboy. But I am one helluva stud!"*
>
> —JON VOIGHT AS JOE BUCK IN *MIDNIGHT COWBOY*

MILE-HIGH CLUB (U.S. slang, 1960s–present).

Members must have achieved sexual intercourse in an aircraft, as demonstrated by SYLVIA KRISTEL in *EMMANUELLE*. By the early 2000s, aerial sex was so common that designer Fcuk produced the Mile-High-Club Pack, a pink toilet bag "ideal for playful nights, flights and weekends away." Contents were "Love knickers, mini body spray, mini massage oil, lip gloss, feather tickler, eye mask, mirror, stayfresh wipes, and toothbrush and toothpaste set." See AVIATION.

MILF (U.S. slang, 1990s–present). Acronym for "Moms I'd Like to Fuck," signifying a mature woman who remains sexually attractive.

Taken to its extreme by *The Mother* (UK film, 2003), in which the unglamorous Anne Reid has a sexual relationship with Daniel Craig, her daughter's lover, a man half her age.

MILLER, Henry Valentine (1891-1980). U.S. writer, painter.

A ramshackle literary stylist and indifferent artist, Henry Miller made up for his deficiencies with heaping servings of the Life Force. Prolific, outspoken, visible, audible, he installed himself as the great unignorable presence of the twentieth century's bohemian literature. Compared to his bawl, Jack Kerouac is a whisper.

In Paris in 1930, on the run from American provincialism, Miller became a proofreader on the same paper as his friend Alfred

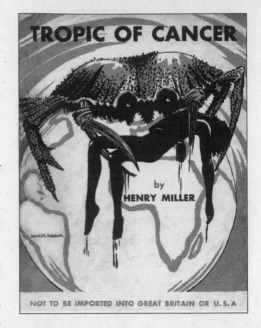

Perles, with whom he haunted the bars and brothels, writing copy for the brochures issued by one of the latter, *LE SPHINX*, in return for his choice of its girls. In even thinner times, he taught English at a regional college.

In between, he wrote feverish books that depicted him as merely one more upwardly mobile spermatozoid in the flood of fecundity he called "the ovarian trolley." To fornicate was, for Miller, not only a pleasure but an affirmation of his role in life—though he was offended when an illustrator for a French *de luxe* edition of *Tropic of Cancer* depicted him with a penis for a nose.

Miller never met a free meal he didn't like. Attaching himself to wealthy expatriate Hugh Guiler, he seduced Guiler's bored, self-regarding wife, ANAÏS NIN, who in 1934 underwrote Jack Kahane's OBELISK PRESS to produce a thousand copies of Miller's first autobiographical outpourings, *Tropic of Cancer*. Banned in the United States and the UK, it sold briskly in the cafés of Paris, becoming one of the most famous and profitable of dirty books.

The same fountain of prose produced *Tropic of Capricorn, Black Spring, The Rosy Crucifixion, Max and the White Phagocytes*, and scores more. In 1940, George Orwell praised Miller. "Here in my opinion is the only imaginative prose-writer of the slightest value who has appeared among the English-speaking races for some years past." The same year, Miller returned to the United States and gravitated to Northern California, where he evolved over the next four decades into the world's favorite Dirty Old Man, enjoying a crapulous and prolonged retirement in the prelapsarian paradise of Big Sur, his physical and social needs catered to by idolatrous acolytes and a succession of ravishing young women.

MILLET, Catherine (1948–). French art historian and author.

Millet, who edited the monthly magazine *Art Press* and wrote the definitive guide to French contemporary art, became a sexual heroine overnight upon the 2001 publication of *La Vie Sexuelle de Catherine M.*, her memoir of thirty years devoted to *LA PARTOUZE*, or group sex. She described enjoying sex in private clubs, apartments, rural chateaux, and, at the other end of the spectrum, parking garage, workmen's huts, or the Bois de Boulogne, the wooded park long a popular hangout of prostitutes, voyeurs, and exhibitionists. She admitted to sex with her dentist and his nurse in the chair, and with moving men in their van as they shifted paintings from airport to gallery, the driver watching in the rearview mirror.

Le Monde, France's leading daily, called *Catherine M.* "an excellent book, very well written, and absolutely staggering." This might have been the general opinion had publication not coincided with the launch of *Loft Story*, France's version of *Big Brother*. Overnight, 21 percent of the TV audience became absorbed in the doings of a dozen unemployed young Parisians locked in a suburban penthouse. *L'Express* yoked *Loft Story* and *Catherine M.* together under the headline "The Triumph of Voyeurism."

Auchan, one of France's biggest supermarket chains, suddenly decided not to stock Millet's book. Bernard Pivot's highbrow TV show *Bouillon de Culture* spotlighted the phenomenon. JEAN-JACQUES PAUVERT called her book "the end of eroticism." The left-wing *Liberation* found her "clinical, an entomologist with the style of Robbe-Grillet, scrutinising with a magnifying glass these specimens of licentiousness." But sales increased, particularly after Millet's husband, novelist Jacques Henric, published *Legendes de Catherine M.*, which documented another of her sexual tastes, to be photographed naked in public places.

MILLINGTON, Mary (née Mary Quilter) (1945–1979). British model and porn star.

In Robert Hamer's 1949 film *Kind Hearts and Coronets*, the charming serial killer hero describes his mistress Sibella (Joan Greenwood) as "the perfect combination of imperfections. I'd say that your nose was just a little too short; your mouth just a little too wide. But that yours was a face a man could see in his dreams for the whole of his life. I'd say you were vain, selfish, cruel, deceitful . . . I'd say you were adorable."

Mary Millington fitted this profile almost exactly. Sibella is cunning enough to blackmail her lover into rescuing her from suburban tedium, a move for which Mary lacked the smarts. "I haven't got much upstairs," she confessed ruefully. Too short at four feet, eleven inches to model clothes, she became a nude photo model, actress in porn shorts, and an expensive prostitute; clients included the Shah of Iran, with whom she spent a weekend in Switzerland. He gave her a diamond-and-gold bracelet, which she promptly sold. Like most successful sex performers, she was bisexual. Her partners included DIANA DORS.

Drifting into the orbit of porn entrepreneur DAVID SULLIVAN, she became his lover. He featured her in the sex comedies *Come Play with Me* (1977), *The Playbirds* (1978), and *Queen of the Blues* and *Confessions from the David Galaxy Affair* (both 1979). *Come Play with Me*, advertised by a poster of Millington in nurse's uniform, stockings, and suspenders, ran for two years, a British record.

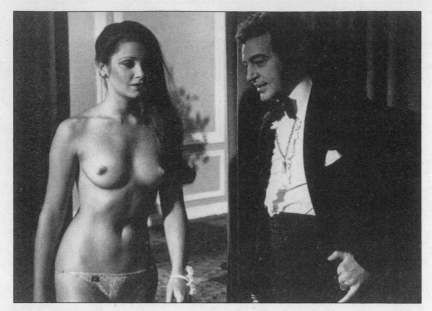

MARY MILLINGTON IN *CONFESSIONS FROM THE DAVID GALAXY AFFAIR* (1979)

Realizing that the confident beauties of *PENTHOUSE* and *PLAYBOY* could daunt the average patron, Sullivan made Millington his emblem, an ordinary girl whom any man could imagine possessing. He opened a sex shop in her name, where she invited patrons to write to her. She put her name to a ghosted "diary" of sexual exploits, and provoked officialdom with stunts such as appearing nude in front of 10 Downing Street, arm in arm with the prime minister's police guard.

In 1977, Millington was investigated for tax evasion, and arrested for shoplifting. In August 1979, she committed suicide. She was thirty-three. She'd written Sullivan a long letter before her death. "I can't face the thought of prison," she confessed. "Please put in your magazine how much I wanted porn legalized, but the police have beaten me. I do hope you are luckier."

Sullivan traded on Millington's death, using portions of her suicide note in his magazines and later in *The Naked Truth*, a documentary "tribute." As "a mark of respect," London's sex cinemas closed for the day of her funeral, but neither Sullivan nor any of her former clients attended the funeral. The only mourners of note were DIANA DORS and her husband, Alan Lake.

MINE SHAFT, THE (1970s–80s). Gay male S&M New York nightclub situated in New York's meatpacking district, at 835 Washington Street, near Little West Twelfth Street.

Along with The Spike, The Anvil, The Ramrod, The Tambourlaine, The Hellfire Club, and The Eagle's Nest, The Mine Shaft offered FISTING, flagellation, UROLAGNIA, and other violent sexual pursuits in an atmosphere of High Grunge and Biker

Chic. A strict dress code applied: "No Cologne or Perfume. No Suits or Ties. No Lacoste or rugby shirts. No (Designer) sweaters. No 'Disco' or other drag. No sandals or Guccis. No ruffled shirts. . . . We welcome jockstraps, T-shirts and *sweat*."

These clubs enjoyed a vogue among the international intellectual glitterati. When visiting New York, German gay film director Rainer Werner Fassbinder liked to convene meetings with his financiers at The Mine Shaft. In 1977, ANDY WARHOL visited The Eagle's Nest and watched fascinated as a man urinated into a beer bottle and left it on the bar for someone to drink. "They were all fighting over it," he told his colleagues at The Factory the next day. "It was so abstract." Inspired, Warhol, in December 1977, began his "Oxidation" or "Piss" Paintings.

The Tambourlaine closed in the early 1970s after a Cuban drug dealer castrated a Puerto Rican drag queen in the club's washroom, but The Mine Shaft survived until 1985, when it was shut down by the city—ostensibly for an unhygienic kitchen. By then, the ambiance and wardrobe, thanks in some part to Warhol, had been enshrined in the work of gay filmmakers and photographers such as ROBERT MAPPLETHORPE, whose shots of well-hung models shoving whips and, occasionally, their arms up the anuses of their friends were usually taken after all-night sex sessions, which often began in clubs such as The Anvil.

The S&M chic of those pre-AIDS days became celebrated in gay porn as a vision of prelapsarian delight. *Nighthawks* (1987), a gay *BEHIND THE GREEN DOOR*, takes place in a club called Paradise, a visit to which is like a tour through a lost world. Every door opens on hard, oiled, hairless, healthy bodies, lounging, fondling, or, in one case, dangling in straps while a brute in a leather harness and biker's cap languidly greases a brawny forearm to the elbow.

MINSKY'S. New York BURLESQUE house, 1912–1937.

Regarded as the ne plus ultra of burlesque houses, Minsky's remained independent of the three major "wheels," or booking circuits. Owner Billy Minsky pioneered the Parisian idea, soon standard, of a runway extending into the audience, and presented lavish themed shows that attracted a more discriminating audience. Most had faux-intellectual titles, e.g., *Panties Inferno*, *The Sway of All Flesh*, and frequently featured stripper GYPSY ROSE LEE. Despite its high tone, Minsky's was regularly raided by the police—an event featured in numerous films, including *Applause*; *Gold Diggers of 1933*; *Dancing Lady* (1933), which starred JOAN CRAWFORD as a reluctant burlesque dancer and marked the screen debut of Fred Astaire; and *The Night They Raided Minsky's*. Minsky's closed in 1937, a victim of the campaign of New York mayor Fiorello LaGuardia.

MIPORN (for "Miami Porn"). Code name for the FBI investigation, begun in 1980, which indicted such porn film figures as ANTHONY PARAINO and HARRY REEMS.

Supposedly aimed at eradicating porn production in the United States, MIPORN's primary target was a much more important part of the illegal industry, the bootlegging of mainstream feature films. Responding to Hollywood pressure, the police, unable to pinpoint the organized crime figures in charge, harried performers. A porn actor arrested for a drug or prostitution offense would be offered immunity in return for testifying against producers. In 1985, in such a case, producer Harold Freedman was given a three-year jail sentence. The charge wasn't obscene publishing, notoriously difficult to prove, but "pandering," procuring a woman for an immoral act—i.e., making a porn film.

"They arrest you, cost you a lot of lawyers' fees," complained WILLIAM ROTSLER, "and then you're never convicted. They try a lot of things they know are not going to work. And they *know* it's not going to work. But what they're trying to do is make it so difficult for you, and so costly to stay in operation, that a lot of people—actors and producers—go out of the business."

Legal or not, it worked. By 1987, the number of Manhattan porn theaters, bookstores, peep shows, and strip joints had fallen to 42, from the 1977 high of 121, while porn cinemas across the country had dwindled from 600 to 300. Persuaded that its money would be better invested elsewhere, East Coast organized crime moved out of porn, which continued to flourish in the more relaxed moral climate of California. By 1995, the San Fernando Valley was producing 70 percent of the world's X-rated product.

Effective in the short term, Miporn proved finally futile. VIDEO and DVD technology had arrived, rocketing the porn industry to new heights and also, ironically, simplifying the bootlegging of mainstream Hollywood films.

MITCHELL, James Lowell (1943–2007) and Artie Jay (1945 –1991). American porn-film producers.

Sons of a small-time gambler, the Mitchells were raised in San Francisco, and inherited its laid-back style. In the late 1960s, watching STAG FILMS, both were struck by the idea that someone who improved on these joyless efforts might make money. Jim took courses in film at San Francisco State University. Once he'd mastered the basics, the two bought a sixteen-millimeter camera and advertised for talent.

There was no shortage. The runaway teenagers or young wives who arrived in California by the hundreds preferred posing for porn to waiting tables. "You could make $45 for half an hour of filming for a peep show," said one. "I remember feeling nudity was okay and natural, so photos of it must be okay too."

With their profits from the sale of LOOPS, the Mitchells turned their garage studio on Polk and O'Farrell Streets into the O'Farrell Theatre, painting the exterior sky blue with giant floating multicolored flowers. Later, they renamed it The Eros Center, and gave it a new decorative motif of rain forest and aquaria, embedding it even deeper into the Californian ethos.

Through the 1980s the Mitchells remained loyal to the values of the SUMMER OF LOVE. When HARRY REEMS, harried by vice charges, tax problems, and alcohol and cocaine dependency, was reduced to anonymous guest shots, the Mitchells starred him in 1985 with the equally discredited JOHN HOLMES, in *The Grafenberg Spot*. They were also the first producers to campaign against AIDS. Every man in their 1986 *Behind the Green Door: The Sequel* wears condoms and there are frequent and visible displays of safe sex propaganda.

Those who attacked the Mitchells, such as San Francisco assistant district attorney Bernard Waller, a longtime adversary, often unwittingly augmented their luster. "The First Amendment," Waller complained, "was the Mitchells' license to make millions selling oral copulation and digital intercourse to thousands of tourists"—a statement not likely to offend anyone, least of all the Mitchells' happy customers.

"I ask those who say flattering things about the Mitchells," Waller continued. "Would you say the same about two brothers from Sicily or two handsome black pimps?" Given the racial diversity of San Francisco, this argument was hardly designed to win friends, especially since the Mitchells were, in the best tradition of the 1970s, scrupulous in distributing work in their films among ethnic and cultural subgroups.

Waller dubbed the O'Farrell "a Cadillac of whorehouses," but this didn't deter tour buses from depositing passengers for an hour's browsing in its Kopenhagen strip theater, cinemas, and X-rated video store. It may even have encouraged them. Nor was his final accusation likely to sway their supporters. "The Mitchells had the money to hire the same legal talent that defended Huey Newton, the Weather Underground, IRA gunrunners, and other First Amendment Communist front organisations," he protested. To which the citizens of California, the most litigious state in the union and home to 11 percent of its lawyers, would generally have responded, "Right on!"

The Mitchells relished their image as renegades. "We were raised to be torpedoes against the state," said Artie. They proudly displayed a framed letter from Yippie leader Abbie Hoffman on their office wall. For a time, Gonzo journalist Hunter S. Thompson acted, inadequately, as the O'Farrell Theatre's night manager. And the brothers could bite back if provoked. To counter attacks from Mayor Dianne Feinstein, they displayed her unlisted home phone number on the O'Farrell marquee, inviting people to express their resentment in person. After a New York judge compared the activities in the Mitchells' films to those of Sodom and Gomorrah, the brothers announced a new production: *Sodom and Gomorrah: The Final Days* (1977). At $350,000, it became the most expensive porn film to that time.

What their detractors had not been able to do, the brothers did themselves. Artie, a heavy drinker and drug user, known to his friends as "Party Artie," became increasingly unstable. "I always thought the Mitchell brothers were immortal," MARILYN CHAMBERS said, "but Artie lived on the screaming edge of insanity, and that can never last forever." In May 1991, Jim Mitchell shot his brother dead. With both a bang and a whimper, the SUMMER OF LOVE came decisively to a close.

MODEL.

Like *actress* during the eighteenth century, *model* during the twentieth was, in sexual terms, an ambiguous label. Depending on context, it could indicate someone who represents a social, cultural, or moral idea ("a model child"), a man or woman who hires out as a living clotheshorse for the creations of designers ("a fashion model"), a person who poses, fully clothed or in various stages of undress, for artists or photographers ("an artists' model"), as well as a prostitute, and even a dummy of wax or plaster.

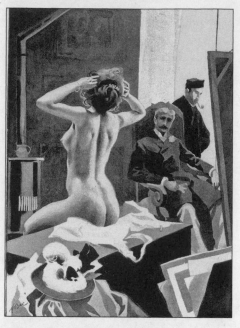

MODEL WITH ARTIST AND "PATRON"

The aristocrats who modeled for John Singer Sargent had little in common with models such as KIKI OF MONTPARNASSE, who posed nude for painters and photographers such as Jules Pascin and MAN RAY, who in turn were not the same models who paraded in the *defilés* of dress designers such as Paul Poiret. These women were more properly called *mannequins*, which, to confuse matters still further, was the name also given to the plaster and wax DOLLS on which the same clothes were displayed in shop windows.

Between the wars, the term *artist's model* called up instantly a vision of beautiful naked women reclining in Paris studios, then slipping into bed with either the young artist or, more likely, a wealthy older patron. Most belonged to the families of the Italian sculptors who gravitated to Montparnasse to produce stonework for the city's burgeoning art nouveau architecture. Montparnasse become synonymous with a society of free-living artists and accommodating models. Once a year, they celebrated their libertarian lifestyle in the BAL DES QUATZ'ARTS, an event notorious in sexual mythology for the fact that almost everyone, but particularly the models, attended near-naked. Soon, the terms *photographic model* or *figure model* became synonymous with *whore*. Throughout London's SOHO, the hand-lettered sign NEW MODEL UPSTAIRS appeared on invitingly open doors.

Many actors and actresses spent some time as models, though usually of the more inhibited kind. Humphrey Bogart modeled for the soap ads drawn by his mother. Lauren Bacall first attracted attention when she posed for the cover of *Harper's Bazaar* (March 1943). MARILYN MONROE famously modeled for a nude calendar. HELMUT NEWTON was the first photographer to coax mannequins into stripping and posing for his S&M fantasy tableaux.

Movies love models. Statuesquely posed seminude models appear in numerous 1920s films inspired by the stage revues of Florenz Ziegfeld and his many imitators. After the establishment of the PRODUCTION CODE, Hollywood used the convention of the fashion show to sneak parades of lightly draped girls into films such as *Fashions of 1934*, inspiring a parody in *Singin' in the Rain*. *The Powers Girl* (1943) celebrated the New York City agency that launched Grace Kelly, Lee Remick, and Jennifer Jones. BETTIE PAGE both drew attention to the ambiguous role of the photographic model and gave the job the glamour it didn't always possess. The seamier side was explored by Jacques Demy in *Model Shop*, where Lola (Anouk Aimee), heroine of his earlier film of the same name, is forced, after being abandoned by her American lover, to pose seminude for photographers in the suburbs of Los Angeles.

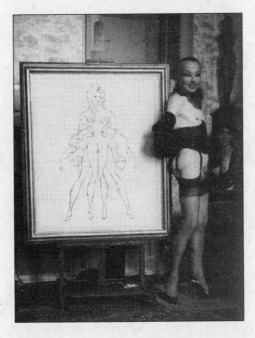

MOLINIER, Pierre (1900–1976). French fetishist photographer and artist.

Molinier lived in the regional city of Bordeaux, and developed his personal brand of fetish art entirely independent of the art world. At eighteen, he learned photography, and for the next thirty years pursued a sex life that involved CROSS-DRESSING, PORNOGRAPHY, and AUTOFELLATIO. At fifty, he started photographing himself dressed in women's LINGERIE and STILETTOS, often also incorporating artificial limbs and DOLLS, and with DILDOS and, occasionally, flowers anally inserted. André Breton, to whom he sent some of his elaborately symmetrical photomontages and paintings, accepted him as a genuine SURREALIST and arranged his first exhibition in 1956.

Following the publication of *EMMANUELLE* in 1957, Molinier, excited by a woman apparently able to gratify her desires with the confidence and independence of a man, sent ARSAN a portfolio of his work. After a long and torrid correspondence, he visited the couple in Paris. He photographed Emmanuelle nude in front of one of his paintings and, upon leaving, presented the couple with a selection of exotic dildos. In May 1967, they repaid the visit, during which the sixty-seven-year-old Molinier, according to Emmanuelle's husband, "did what he had already done hundreds of time in imagination; that is, he made love with her." Arsan's husband photographed the encounter, but they and Molinier never met again. At seventy-six, Molinier calmly committed suicide, leaving a note on his door indicating the fact, and explaining where the keys of his apartment could be found. See ARSAN, Emmanuelle; SURREALISM.

MOM AND DAD (1942). U.S. film. Directed by William Beaudine. *THE FAMILY STORY* in UK.

Shot in six days for $62,000 by veteran Beaudine, this sex-education feature served primarily as a platform for the merchandising skills of producer-distributor KROGER BABB, a leading member of THE FORTY THIEVES. Ignoring conventional distribution, Babb hired independent theaters across the country to screen it, and made enormous profits.

Mom and Dad tells the wartime story of a young American innocent who, kept in ignorance about sex by her parents, sleeps with her pilot lover, later killed in action. Finding herself pregnant, she approaches a teacher who's been fired by his school for answering his students' questions about sex. Together they confront her mother, with the teacher accusing her of "neglect[ing] the sacred duty of telling their children the real truth."

At this point, the lights went up, and audiences, which were segregated sexually, either with men and women on separate floors, or by showing the film on consecutive nights, were lectured from the stage by an actor posing as a sex-education campaigner. He urged the purchase of two books, written and published by Babb and his wife, and on sale in the cinema. The film then continued, with diagrams of the reproductive system and scenes of the baby being born.

"This fucking MOM AND DAD was everywhere. There ain't a theatre in America that didn't play this picture. They had a show for women at two o'clock in the afternoon, another show for women at seven o'clock, and then a show for men at nine, and everybody had to listen to the lecture, and everybody bought the book—no, two books—how to do it, how not to do it, when to do it, why to do it, how not to get the clap, how to get the clap..."
—DAVID F. FRIEDMAN,
LATER DISTRIBUTOR
OF *MOM AND DAD*

The form in which *Mom and Dad* was screened depended on the region. In some versions, the baby was born dead; in others it was handed to a loving couple for adoption. Elsewhere, a documentary warning against sexually transmitted diseases accompanied the film. Babb presented *Mom and Dad* for decades across the United States, then sold the rights to Britain and Australasia. Estimates of its total profits, mostly from the books, range from $40 million to $100 million. See BABB, Howard W. "Kroger."

MONEY SHOT. Also COME or CUM SHOT, PROOF SHOT (1960s–present). Cinematic image showing a male ejaculating.

British critic Alexander Walker wrote in 1977 that "sexual ejaculation [was] now visibly portrayed and indeed regarded as an earnest of authenticity ... Where pelvic thrusts and erect members were deemed sufficient only a few years ago, visceral evidence is now wanted as a guarantee that the act is not being simulated."

Far from being a phenomenon of the 1970s, however, the money shot features in the earliest porn films. Its justification isn't as "an earnest of authenticity"—the actors' erections supply that—but rather a need to satisfy those viewers to whom the emission of SEMEN has become fetishized.

San Francisco producer-director Lowell Pickett tried in films such as the 1973 *Rendezvous with Annie* to show sex more realistically, and omit the money shot. However, the films failed; audiences demanded a visible ejaculation. So crucial is the cum shot that films go to extraordinary lengths to include it. If an actor can't produce a sufficiently photogenic emission, a grip will fake one with dishwashing detergent, shampoo, or egg white. Credit for the most spectacular cum shot in porn history belongs to *BEHIND THE GREEN DOOR*, which features a flamboyant and extended ejaculation, filmed in vivid color and slow motion, and multi-imaged with an optical printer. See SEMEN.

MONKEYS. See ZOOPHILIA.

MONROE, Marilyn (née Norma Jean Mortensen) (1926–1962). Actress.

It's debatable whether Monroe ever actually enjoyed sex, although she became an expert in using it. As a starlet in Hollywood, she was famed for her fellatio skill. Executives sent her to colleagues with a note that simply said, "This kid just loves to give head." She even agreed to be filmed on her knees fellating an unknown man. The fifteen-minute film, shot on sixteen-millimeter and long regarded as another improbable Hollywood legend, surfaced in 2008, to be snapped up by a Manhattan businessman for $1.5 million.

Like GYPSY ROSE LEE, Monroe strove to be taken seriously. Yet the more she struggled to become a serious actress and to mix with intellectuals and men of power and influence, the more her admirers demanded to see her wriggling nude and pouting. Watching her on the arm of George Sanders as the acerbic critic in *All About Eve*; breathily singing, "Happy Birthday, Mr. President," to her secret lover JOHN F. KENNEDY; or clinging to her ill-matched husbands, sportsman Joe Di Maggio and playwright Arthur Miller, simply made her audience hungrier to possess her.

A more stable person might have reconciled the rival impulses in her character, but Monroe was ill-equipped psychologically to juggle the demands of her admirers and her own confused sexuality. Director George Cukor, who endured her erratic behavior on her last, uncompleted film, *Something's Got to Give*, dismissed all elaborate depictions of Monroe as tragic heroine. "If you ask me," he said, "I think she was crazy. Her mother was crazy, and so was she." See ST. CYR, Lili.

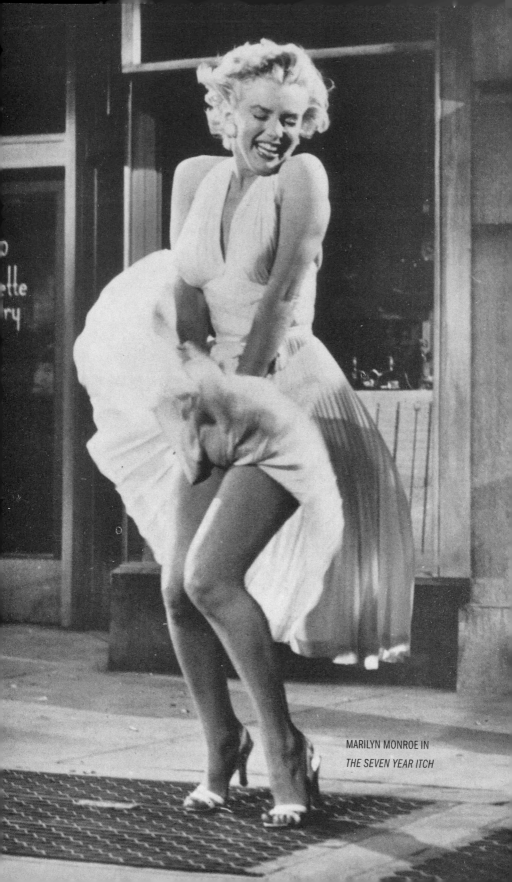

MARILYN MONROE IN
THE SEVEN YEAR ITCH

MOORS MURDERS, THE. Five sadistic child sex murders committed in 1963-1965 near the city of Manchester, and so named because the killers, Ian Brady and Myra Hindley, buried some of their victims on nearby moorland.

Brady, a seductive psychopath, dominated the impressionable Hindley, introducing her to pornography and recruiting her in the killings, some of which they photographed and recorded. The sexual theatricality of their relationship made them among the first serial murderers to attract media attention, and because Britain had abolished the death penalty, both were jailed for life in 1966, which meant they lived on as sources of attention. They inspired various books, including *Beyond Belief*, by Emlyn Williams, Edward Gorey's *The Loathsome Couple*, and films such as *Longford*, which dramatizes the efforts of LORD LONGFORD to befriend and arrange the release of Hindley.

MORGAN, "Chesty" (née Liliana Wilczkowska) (aka Zsa-Zsa) (1928–). Actress.

Polish-born Morgan possessed only one talent—or, more correctly, two, since she measured 73-32-36. Her enormous breasts were shown off in *Deadly Weapons* (1974), in which she revenges her gangster boyfriend by suffocating the killers (one played by HARRY REEMS). FEDERICO FELLINI hoped to lure her into his film *Fellini Casanova*, as the whore Astrodi, but compromised with Marika Rivera.

MUFF DIVER (U.S. slang, 1950-1980s). Person who enjoys cunnilingus.

MUSICAL (British slang, 1890s-1910s). Adjective once used euphemistically to identify homosexuality.

[His elder uncle] Henry was delighted to find a blood relative who shared his [homosexual] tastes—using the slang expression of his generation, he referred to himself as being "musical" or "so" (Christopher Isherwood, in *Christopher and His Kind*)

MY HUSTLER (1965). U.S. film. Directed by Charles Wein. Photographed by Andy Warhol.

Shot on Fire Island beach over a Labor Day weekend, this seventy-minute film consists of two largely unedited conversations about male prostitutes. Ed Hood has called "Dial-a-Hustler" and been sent Paul America, who lies on the beach sunning himself while Hood discusses him with two companions, Joe Campbell (the "Sugar Plum Fairy" of Lou Reed's song "Walk on the Wild Side") and Geneviève Charbon. In the second part, two hustlers dressing in front of a mirror debate the problems and rewards of life as a GIGOLO. According to Warhol, "It's about an aging queen trying to hold on to a young hustler, and his two rivals—another hustler and a girl. The actors were doing what they did in real life; they followed their own professions on the screen." *My Hustler* succeeded on the underground circuit, but Warhol suppressed it once he set his sights on Hollywood-style films. *My Hustler* inspired John Schlesinger to film James Leo Herlihy's novel *MIDNIGHT COWBOY.*

MY LIFE AND LOVES. See HARRIS, Frank.

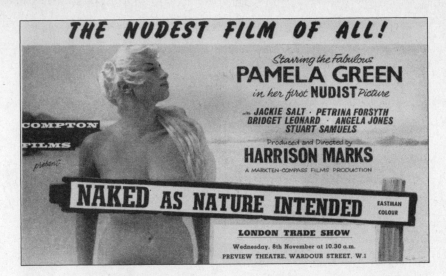

THE NUDEST FILM OF ALL!

Starring the Fabulous
PAMELA GREEN
in her first NUDIST Picture

with JACKIE SALT · PETRINA FORSYTH
BRIDGET LEONARD · ANGELA JONES
STUART SAMUELS

Produced and Directed by
HARRISON MARKS
A MARKTEN-COMPASS FILMS PRODUCTION

COMPTON
FILMS
present

NAKED AS NATURE INTENDED   EASTMAN COLOUR

LONDON TRADE SHOW
Wednesday, 8th November at 10.30 a.m.
PREVIEW THEATRE, WARDOUR STREET, W.1

NAKED AS NATURE INTENDED (1961). UK film. Directed by George Harrison Marks.

A secretary, a dancer, and a sales girl visit a Cornish nudist camp in their holidays and, after initial nervousness, learn to revel in the experience. The British Board of Film Censors required that such films be shot in actual "sun clubs," which Pamela Green, the star (and the director's wife) described as "grotty and unsuitable." The amateur performers were clumsy, and uncomfortable with their nudity, while a male who consistently forgot to cover his "dangly bits" with a towel had to be posed behind hedges and pieces of furniture. None of this deterred London audiences, which queued on both sides of the street in the rain on opening night. Some were back again at 11:00 a.m. next day. Within a few months, the avalanche of NUDIES began.

NECK BRACES.

An obscure FETISH. Proponents are attracted to surgical apparatus such as orthopedic corsets and supports. In the "Princess with the Golden Hair" episode of Edmund Wilson's 1946 *Memoirs of Hecate County*, the narrator articulated his sexual attraction to a girl who, because of a childhood riding accident, wore "a harness of leather thongs, steel uprights and rubber pads [with] a collar round her neck, and two straps that came down over her shoulders and held up a small band of steel which stretched across her chest and two pads which went under her arms, rather like a decolleté, below which her lovely bare white breasts emerged in a perverse and provocative way." A British Neck Brace Association claimed fifteen thousand members—85 percent male—in 2007.

NEWTON, Helmut (né Helmut Neustädter) (1920–2004). German-born erotic photographer.

As a boy in BERLIN, Newton encountered fetishism and prostitution, which left an indelible mark on him. Fleeing Germany in 1938, he worked in Singapore, then settled in Australia as a photographer for *Vogue*, before moving to Paris in 1961, where he won a reputation for innovative fashion and portrait photography, generally with erotic or violent elements.

High-fashion models, tall, unsmiling, and imperious—"glaciers with breasts," in the words of critic Anthony Lane—were his favorite subjects. His signature work, *Sie kommen!* (*Here They Come!*), shows a group of such women first strolling toward the cameras fully clothed, then nude except for high-heeled shoes. In similarly startling celebrity portraits, actress Charlotte Rampling perched nude on the corner of a table, and jewelry designer Elsa Peretti strutted in a PLAYBOY BUNNY costume.

Newton's trademark was the elaborate staged erotic tableau, often set in luxurious private homes or hotel suites, with nude or seminude models acting out fetishist scenarios.

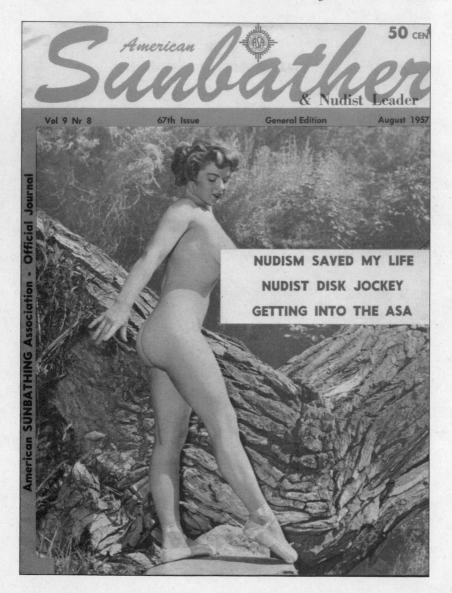

American *Sunbather* & Nudist Leader

50 CENT

Vol 9 Nr 8   67th Issue   General Edition   August 1957

American SUNBATHING Association · Official Journal

NUDISM SAVED MY LIFE

NUDIST DISK JOCKEY

GETTING INTO THE ASA

(He claimed dryly that his work documented "the harshness of everyday life amongst the rich."). His first book, *White Women* (1976), influenced Irvin Kershner's film *The Eyes of Laura Mars* (1978), in which Faye Dunaway plays a Newton-like fashion photographer who can foresee murders. The producers commissioned Newton to stage the erotic tableaux that Dunaway photographs, but rejected them as insufficiently violent.

NATURISM. Belief in the health and moral values of socializing while naked.

The first naturist club was the *Freilichtpark* (Free-Light Park), opened near Hamburg in 1903. In 1906, Heinrich Pudor's *Nackt-cultur* (*The Cult of the Nude*) and Heinrich Ungewitter's *Die Nacktheit* (*Nakedness*) extolled the benefits of nudity in everything from education and health to sports and sex.

In the 1920s, the cult spread to Britain, where in 1924, a group calling itself the New Gymnosophy Society opened the UK's first private club, at Wickford in Essex, known simply as The Camp. Membership was strictly controlled, and members identified only by pseudonyms; the donor of the land chose "Moonella," and the club became known as the Moonella Group.

Naturism arrived in the United States in 1929, when German national Kurt Barthel organized an event in the woods just outside New York City. He later founded the American League for Physical Culture. Private clubs soon sprang up in many states. Like their German and British equivalents, they exhibited a high moral tone; the first director of the national movement was a Baptist minister. Sex was discouraged, alcohol forbidden, and families preferred to individuals.

Although Leni Riefenstahl's film of the 1936 Olympics opened with an ecstatic celebration of the naked body, the Nazis suppressed naturism, mainly at the instigation of the obese Hermann Goering. It was revived in the late 1940s, when the wave of new liberalism, the leisure society, and the beginning of mass tourism encouraged the setting up of "sun clubs" and naturist colonies in warmer regions of Europe and the United States. The wave of NUDIE movies followed inevitably.

9 1/2 WEEKS (1986). U.S. film. Directed by Adrian Lyne.

Nine and a Half Weeks: Memoir of a Love Affair, by the pseudonymous "Elizabeth McNeill," was the supposedly true account of a sadomasochistic relationship. After failing to finance the film version as director, co-scenarist Zalman King sold the project to Lyne, who changed the female character from a business executive to the manager of a SoHo art gallery, and cast little-known Kim Basinger and Mickey Rourke as the curator and her manipulative arbitrageur lover.

By shuttling between Rourke's minimalist all-black apartment and the clutter of SoHo, Lyne played on the exoticism of New York life and the imagined corruption just under its surface. In the process, *9 1/2 Weeks* became a Manhattan *EMMANUELLE*. Some scenes were imaginatively erotic, such as Basinger masturbating while watching slides of classic paintings in her empty gallery or stripping for Rourke to Joe Cocker's grating

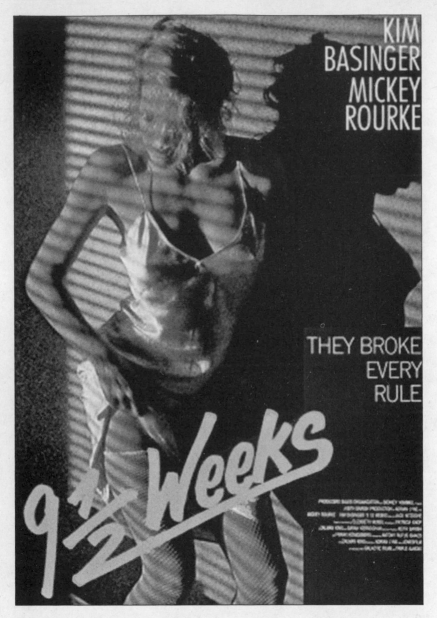

KIM
BASINGER
MICKEY
ROURKE

THEY BROKE
EVERY
RULE

9 1/2 Weeks

version of Randy Newman's fetishist "You Can Leave Your Hat On." Too often, however, the film tipped into the absurd, as in Basinger's unconvincing attempt at cross-dressing, complete with cigar and false moustache, and a sex scene in an alley during a rainstorm, with photogenic rats watching from the shadows.

Lyne extracted performances by extreme means, fomenting tension between his stars, and shooting in sequence, to graph Basinger's real-life emotional deterioration. As a result, Basinger refused to appear in a proposed sequel, *Four Days in February*, or in *Another 9½ Weeks*, starring Rourke. A further spin-off, *The First 9½ Weeks*, featured neither.

1929. Book by Louis Aragon, Benjamin Péret, and MAN RAY.

In October 1929, it was no surprise to the SURREALISTS, gathered for their daily séance at the Café Radio on Place Blanche, to hear that the Brussels-based surrealist group was bankrupt. Its leader, Edouard Mesens, later the doyen of London's surrealists, was, and remained, as hopeless in business as he was charming in person.

To raise money, it was decided to publish a special issue of the Belgian group's magazine *Varieties*. To guarantee success, its theme would be erotica. With Benjamin Péret, Louis Aragon, the lieutenant of the group's founder André Breton, created a number of lubricious poems. One of Aragon's began, "Ah the little girls who lift their skirts / and diddle themselves in the bushes / or in museums / behind the plaster Apollos / while their mother compares the statue's rod / to her husband's / and sighs. . ." For illustrations, Aragon approached MAN RAY, who offered four pornographic photographs of himself having sex with his model and companion KIKI OF MONTPARNASSE.

Breton edited the production, calling it arbitrarily *1929* as a gibe at the almanacs produced by the Post Office and Fire Brigade, members of which distributed them door to door as a means of extorting their annual bonus. Dividing the poetry into four sections, he named them for the seasons, with a Ray photograph prefacing each one. Mesens printed five hundred copies and shipped them to Paris, only to have Customs seize and destroy the entire printing at the frontier.

1929 remained one of the better-kept surrealist secrets until 1996, when the first English-language edition was published in Paris, with translations by "Zoltan Lizot-Picon," i.e., Christopher Sawyer-Laucanno and André Breton's biographer Mark Polizotti.

NOONER (U.S. slang, 1920s-present). Sexual encounter during the lunch hour. See also HOT LUNCH.

> *Your daddy was a real ladies' man, now there was a man who knew his way to the bedroom . . . Back in his bachelor days, you never saw anybody could rustle up a nooner like Benny could. He had a cock like a ballpeen hammer. We used to go round north Minneapolis, we knew where all the hot babes were. He was a pistol, your old man.*
>
> —Garrison Keillor, *WLT: A Radio Romance*

NO SEX, PLEASE—WE'RE BRITISH (1971). UK stage farce by Alistair Foot and Anthony Marriott.

The wife of a provincial bank manager orders some Scandinavian glassware but receives pornography by mistake. As erotic photographs, books, films, and finally girls pour in to their home, she and her husband try frantically to hide them from neighbors and colleagues. A classically British response to the unexpected emergence of SWEDEN and DENMARK as sources of pornography, this play ran for ten years in London, but flopped in the United States.

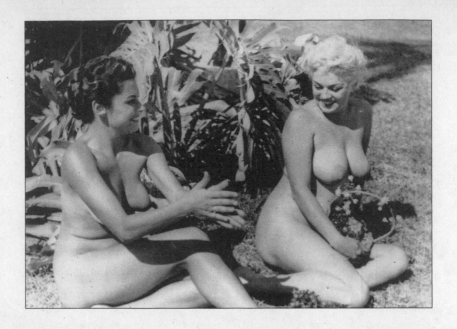

NUDIE (1960s–1980s). Cinema film that exploits NATURISM for salacious effect.

In the wake of the 1957 Supreme Court decision in *Roth v. United States of America*, progress in porn became a question of inching forward, testing the limits of COMMUNITY STANDARDS. The requirement that any film featuring nudity should exhibit "redeeming social merit" produced a plethora of quasi-documentaries about naturism, beginning in Britain with *NAKED AS NATURE INTENDED*. It was followed by *World Without Shame*, *The Isle of Levant* (set on that French naturist resort), *The Reluctant Nudist*, *It's a Bare, Bare World*, and *Some Like It Cool* (written and directed by Michael Winner).

While the vogue lasted, a handful of U.S. producers cranked out a nudie every ten or twelve weeks for the fifty or sixty theaters nationwide that dared to show them. *Nudes Around the World*, *The Bare Hunt*, *The Nude and the Prude*, *Hollywood Nudes Report*, *My Bare Lady*, and *Career Girls on a Naked Holiday* were as ritualized as their British equivalents. Attractive girls, initially skeptical, encounter naturism while taking a holiday, pursuing a boyfriend, looking for a job, or, in one extreme case, searching for buried treasure (*Take Off Your Clothes and Live*). Since the average nudist was dismally unattractive, most of the performers were professional models. Even then, nudity was confined to rear views and the occasional breast shot, low in what prime-time U.S. TV in the seventies would christen "jiggle quotient."

Once naturism palled as a subject, nudie producers looked elsewhere for a pretext to show naked bodies. Barry Mahon made twenty nudies a year in New York during the early 1960s, all involving painting or photography. The film *1000 Shapes of a Female* showed an artist at work, college art classes featured in *Naughty, Naughty Nudes*, and glamour photographer BUNNY YAEGER in *Nude Las Vegas*.

Producers impatient with the legal restrictions tried vainly to stretch the limits. Mahon's nudie comedy *She Should Have Stayed in Bed* was banned everywhere. In 1965, however, *The Raw Ones* broke the rules by showing frontal nudity in a naturist film. Ingeniously, producer-director John Lamb packed the commentary with libertarian quotes from such impeccable sources as Bertrand Russell and Thomas Jefferson. This disarmed his opponents, and though the law took Lamb to court, he won every case. His success led inevitably to the production of the first major sex features *DEEP THROAT* and *BEHIND THE GREEN DOOR*.

ALSO

NUDIE, BOBBIE (NÉE HELEN BARBARA KRUGER) (1913-2006). Costume designer.

Kruger gained her name from her husband Nuta Kotlyarenko, who was rechristened "Nudie Cohen" by an impatient immigration officer. Together they ran Nudies for the Ladies, which manufactured G-STRINGS and lingerie for BURLESQUE dancers, with the insignia of a nude cowgirl. The Nudies also designed stage outfits for Elvis Presley and Johnny Cash.

NUDISM. See NATURISM.

NUTRIX (1947-1966). Company name under which New York pornographer IRVING KLAW produced his books and films.

Klaw's pocket-size booklets, sold mainly by mail, contained BONDAGE and spanking fantasies, either in text form or as comic books, many drawn by ERIC STANTON. The action was ritualized, with men and women willingly bound, often by stiletto-wearing dominatrices, in belts, chains, and rubber suits; in one, a victim is embedded in an inflated rubber sphere and bounced.

Even those not excited by the content conceded the expertise

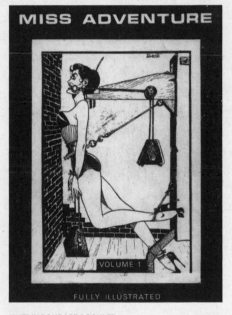

NUTRIX BONDAGE BOOKLET

of the Nutrix productions. "*Slave Mistress* is to be commended for its variation and style," wrote Gillian Freeman in *The Undergrowth of Literature*. She also acknowledged the merit of *Bondage Enthusiasts Bound in Leather*, *Bondage Devotees Tied, Gagged and Disciplined*, *Initiated and Spanked by Satin-Clad Bondage Fans*, and *Holiday in Fetterland*,

and complimented works such as *Dominating Tame-zons Shame Men into Subjection* for their "novel devices."

The "devices"—wooden racks or frames equipped with ropes, straps, and belts— were conceived by Irving's sister PAULA KLAW, who supervised their construction and oversaw their use in photo sessions featuring BETTIE PAGE and other models. Along with other Klaw enterprises, Nutrix was put out of business by the KEFAUVER COMMISSION.

NYMPHET (diminutive of nymph). Sexually active underage girl, not necessarily beautiful, but possessing a preternatural allure to a member of the opposite sex attuned to such attraction. Invented by Vladimir Nabokov for his novel *LOLITA*. Nabokov argues that nymphets are aware of their effect on the susceptible, and use their skill calculatedly.

NYMPHOMANIA. Psychological state that induces excessive sexual desire in women.

A popular diagnosis in the late nineteenth century, nymphomania, sometimes called "sexual catarrh," was supposedly marked by physical as well as psychological symptoms, including swollen genitals and enlarged clitorises. Most noticeable, however, was a tendency toward erotic fantasy, profanity, and immoderate sexual desire. Treatment involved cooling baths and compresses, soporifics, and bleeding.

Nymphomania came into its own when discovered by popular novelists, who decided, paradoxically, that their readers preferred nymphomaniacs not as feverish victims of sexual distress but as chilly sexual athletes, tireless and unemotional. In antiquity, Messalina, wife of the aging Claudius, and Poppaea, empress to Nero, are cited as examples. In modern times, real-life porn star NINA HARTLEY played the nymphomaniac wife of director William H. Macy in *BOOGIE NIGHTS*, ready to have unemotional sex with anyone anytime anywhere. A similar promiscuous urge in men is known as SATYRIASIS.

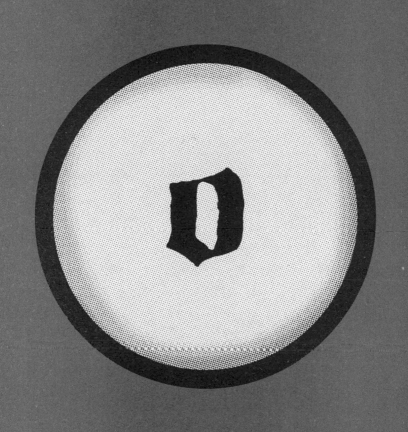

OEDIPUS COMPLEX. Psychological state, first proposed by SIGMUND FREUD, in which the subject subconsciously desires to monopolize the attention of the mother by murdering the father.

Named for the myth of Oedipus, prince of Thebes, whose father, Laius, is told by a sibyl that his infant son will kill him. Laius pierces the child's feet, giving him a permanent limp, and leaves him to die, but Oedipus is rescued, grows up knowing nothing of his ancestry and, as foretold, kills a man he does not realize is Laius. He then marries the widow, Jocasta, and becomes king of Thebes, unaware that Jocasta is his mother until a plague is traced to a curse placed on the city by the gods. Jocasta hangs herself, their sons kill each other, and Oedipus, after blinding himself, becomes a wanderer.

This myth attracts artists preoccupied with their sexuality. Oedipus appears as a character in various works by JEAN COCTEAU, and WOODY ALLEN evokes him in *Oedipus Wrecks*, his episode in *New York Stories*, in which the spirit of his meddling mother, separated from her body, continues to interfere in his intended marriage to a shiksa, and relents only when he dumps her for a nice Jewish girl. The title implies that the Woody character lusts after his mother, a grisly thought, since she's played by the tiny, querulous, and unattractive Mae Questel, one-time voice of the comic strip character Betty Boop and of Olive Oyl in the Popeye cartoons. However, the relationship may have had some basis in real life, since Allen's actual mother acquired in old age a disturbing resemblance to GROUCHO MARX.

OH! CALCUTTA! (1966).

Revue conceived by KENNETH TYNAN. An enthusiastic eroticist, Tynan regretted that "there was no place for a civilized man to take a civilized woman to spend an evening of civilized erotic stimulation. At one end, there's BURLESQUE, at the other, an expensive night club, but no place in between."

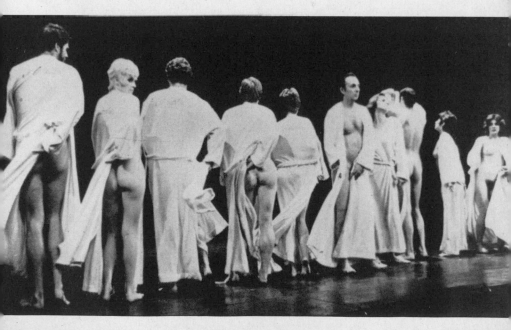

In 1965, he invited film directors, playwrights, novelists, and musicians to contribute an erotic sketch, film, or song to such an entertainment. He aimed initially to satirize national tastes in sex, and suggested sketches of "a nun being raped by her confessor (Italy), a middle-aged bank manager bound hand and foot by a superwoman (U.S.A.) and a St. Trinian's sixth-former being birched (Great Britain)." His model was Paris's CRAZY HORSE SALOON. As an emblem, he took a painting by SURREALIST Clovis Trouille of a girl draped in black silk showing her ample backside, which Trouille, punning on a friend's response to the picture—"*O quel cul t'as*" ("O what an ass you have")—called *OH! CALCUTTA!*

OH! CALCUTTA! made it to Broadway in 1966, with contributions by Samuel Beckett, Edna O'Brien, Jules Feiffer, Kurt Vonnegut, John Lennon, and Tynan, among others. Trotting onstage in white bathrobes, the ten-person cast dropped the robes to reveal themselves totally naked, then, for two hours, mimed, talked, or sang about sex in bed and in a bath, in Edwardian England and contemporary Manhattan, between couples, in groups, and with a man wielding a cane while a naked girl hung, bound and gagged, in a net.

Reviews were almost universally negative. Intellectuals who welcomed novels such as *LOLITA* were hostile to erotica in the glare of the footlights. Nor was the show prosecuted (to Tynan's disappointment), although a British bookseller was fined £150 for importing a U.S. book about it. The public, however, loved *OH! CALCUTTA!*, which ran for more than 1,300 performances in New York and 2,400 in London. It also spawned imitators, such as *The Dirtiest Show in Town* and *LET MY PEOPLE COME*. A 1971 film directed by co-producer Jacques Levy sparked a revival, and Tynan later produced an unsuccessful imitation, *Carte Blanche*.

OLYMPIA PRESS.

In 1953, the year HUGH HEFNER launched *PLAYBOY*, MAURICE GIRODIAS inaugurated the Olympia Press, with the aim of publishing a better class of pornography.

Having lost his first publishing business through mismanagement, Girodias, adopting his mother's maiden name to distance himself from the bad reputation of his father, JACK KAHANE, founder of the OBELISK PRESS, was rootless in Paris when, in his version of events, a doctor, applying the theories of SERGE VORONOFF, gave him ten injections of monkey testicles. Rejuvenated, he conceived The Olympia Press. HENRY MILLER, an old friend from the Obelisk days—Girodias drew the cover design for the first edition of *TROPIC OF CANCER*—offered him *Plexus*, which became the press's first book.

Beginning under the imprint Atlantic Library, with yellow paperback bindings imitating the popular but unerotic Albatross imprint, Girodias soon adopted the title Traveller's Companion, which became his trademark, and the uniform binding in the same establishment green card used by auctioneers Sotheby's for catalogues of objets d'art.

Olympia's run-of-the-mill dirty books were often composed, tongue-in-cheek, by moonlighting novelists and expatriate intellectuals such as Alexander Trocchi (writing as "Frances Lengel"), Christopher Logue ("Count Palmiro Vicarion"), and Terry Southern, who, with Mason Hoffenberg (as "Maxwell Kenton"), wrote *Candy*, a parody of the pornographic novel, distantly derived from Voltaire's *Candide*. The Olympia editorial policy was simple: "Three sex scenes per chapter," decreed Girodias. "Anything less and you're fired."

From the start, Olympia mixed flagrant erotica with serious literature. The pseudonymous works of "Marcus Van Heller" (John Stevenson) and "Akbar del Piombo" (Norman Rubington) appeared alongside Samuel Beckett's *Watt* and *Molloy*, Nabokov's *LOLITA*, J. P. Donleavy's *The Ginger Man*, and William Burroughs's *The Naked Lunch*.

To satisfy the market for unrepentant porn, Olympia launched cadet imprints such as Ophelia and Ophir. Bound in pink or white, they concentrated on flagellation and BONDAGE, with the indefatigable Van Heller/Stevenson turning out titles such as *The Whipping Post*, *The Whipping Club*, *The Whip Mistress*, and *Terror*.

Even more strenuously than his father, Girodias resisted censorship. "What probably offended the authorities," writes Olympia Press bibliographer Patrick Kearney, "was the fact that Girodias . . . stubbornly refused to give up. Whereas most publishers in his line of business would simply stop selling a book if it were banned, Girodias would fight the ban to the highest court, organize support from notable literary figures, and even bring lawsuits against the French government. Worst of all, he often won."

The 1955 publication of *LOLITA* made Girodias briefly solvent, but he rashly invested his profits in La Grande Severine, a nightclub-theater-restaurant in Paris's Latin Quarter. In 1964, having been convicted of selling obscene literature and sentenced to a year in jail and fined $20,000, he prudently fled to New York, where he relaunched the Olympia Press with titles such as *Bondage Trash*, by "Jon Horn," and *The Sexual Life of Robinson Crusoe*.

In 1967, Valerie Solanas, mentally disturbed founder of SCUM, the Society For Cutting Up Men, who had been carrying on a sulphurous correspondence with Girodias as publisher of its manifesto, arrived at his Gramercy Park offices carrying a gun. Finding him absent, she went on to shoot the unlucky ANDY WARHOL. She was far from the only writer furious at Girodias, whose business methods were cavalier. He and Nabokov warred endlessly over *Lolita*, as did Donleavy, over *The Ginger Man*. To retrieve the rights, Donleavy finally purchased the bankrupt company when it was sold to satisfy its debts.

In 1974, Girodias disastrously published *President Kissinger: A Political Fiction*, an erotic fantasy based on Henry Kissinger. Not only did Girodias lose the subsequent libel case; he was also deported. He spent the remainder of his life composing an extensive but fanciful memoir, *The Frog Prince*, and attempting, unsuccessfully, to find a publisher for his one work of fiction, a science fiction novel. Called *Atlantis*, it was, ironically, totally free of all erotic content. See GIRODIAS, Maurice; KAHANE, Jack; OBELISK PRESS; D.B.

A four-letter word never killed a reader.
—MAURICE GIRODIAS

OMORASHI. See UROLAGNIA.

ONE-NIGHT STAND (U.S. slang, 1900s–present). A sexual encounter that lasts a single night. Adapted from the show-business term for a single performance by a traveling show.

OPENING OF MISTY BEETHOVEN, THE (1975). French film. Directed by "Henry Paris," i.e., Radley Metzger.

A porn variation on *My Fair Lady*, in which wealthy sex writer Seymour Love (JAMIE GILLIS) meets Dolores Beethoven, alias "Misty" (Constance Money) in Paris's Pigalle, where she administers HAND JOBS to men watching Claude Mulot's erotic feature *Le Sexe Qui Parle* (*Pussy Talk*). Misty takes a no-nonsense attitude to paid sex, similar to Melanie Griffith's in *BODY DOUBLE*. "I do a straight fuck," she tells Love. "I don't take it in the mouth. I don't take it in the ass. I don't take it in the bed." This both disconcerts and delights him. When Misty says later, "I think men stink," he responds, "They think *you* stink. It's one of the most perfectly balanced equations in nature."

Love recruits Misty, intending to turn her into the most desirable of all sexual partners. After high-tech training, she's unleashed on the jaded and undersexed editor of *Goldenrod* magazine, Larry Layman, based on HUGH HEFNER. Sensing Layman's secret desire, Misty dons a STRAP-ON and sodomizes him while he's fucking his mistress—the first screen depiction of PEGGING.

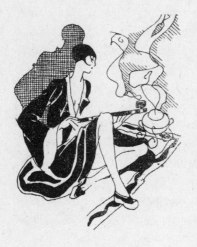

OPIUM. Gum of the opium poppy, from which morphine is derived.

In the nineteenth century, the British cultivated opium in India, then forced it on China as a substitute currency for buying expensive tea. Though the Chinese resisted, opium soon became a major recreational drug, so firmly associated with China that most people believe it emerged there.

Dissolved in alcohol to make laudanum, opium was a much-abused medication in Victorian Europe. Legends grew of female addicts driven to nymphomaniac frenzy by the drug. The paperback edition of *Black Opium*, the English translation of Claude Farrere's *Fumée d'Opium*, shows a nude woman emerging from the smoke of an opium pipe, with the advertising line "The Shocking Ecstasy of the Forbidden." In fact, opium suppressed sexual desire, and was much less addictive than its derivative, morphine.

Imported into France by civil servants returning from its Indochinese colonies, opium developed an enthusiastic following. Regular users included JEAN

COCTEAU and Pablo Picasso, who called the odor of opium smoke "the least stupid smell in the world, after that of the sea." A pea-size ball of opium gum, heated over a flame and placed in a special pipe, gave an hour of smoking, during which the smoker drifted in a timeless haze. Users customarily spent whole evenings in opium "dens" (in France *fumeries*), which provided beds, and a staff to replenish the pipes. In 1922, the Folies-Bergère featured a sequence in which three seminude women in gorgeous costumes played "Opium," "Morphine," and "Ether."

ORGASM ACTIVISM (1960s-present). The belief that the coordinated mass expenditure of sexual energy can influence events.

Orgasm activity was prefigured by the Bed-Ins for Peace held in March 1969 by John Lennon and Yoko Ono, who stayed in bed for a week on two occasions to protest the Vietnam War. In October 2006, London HIV/AIDS charities held a Masturbate-a-Thon in which participants indulged in sponsored masturbation, one of them continuing for seven and a half hours and raising £500. On December 22, 2006, Donna Sheehan and Paula Reffell, San Francisco organizers of the Baring Witness protests, in which supporters undressed for peace, launched Synchronized Global Orgasm with Global Orgasm Day, which urged people all over the world to induce an orgasm for peace.

ORGY. Originally a secret religious rite. In contemporary usage, any unrestrained activity, normally but not exclusively sexual, and involving a group.

"Home is heaven, and orgies are vile," wrote Ogden Nash. "But you need an orgy, once in a while." Some argue that the true orgy is indiscriminate, embracing the gratification of all the senses and the participation of all interested beings. Hence the donkeys, bunches of grapes, and so on that feature in classical depiction. Given the shortage of obliging quadrapeds in modern suburbia, it's not surprising that the twentieth-century orgy was usually 100 percent human, and on a modest scale, so that the point at which group sex becomes an orgy has never been adequately defined. In *MORE JOY OF SEX*, ALEX COMFORT suggested abandoning the term altogether in favor of "Sharing," but insisted on the therapeutic effect of the orgy's mass outpouring of sexual energy, which, he insisted, left participants "breathless, guiltless and ready to return to propriety."

ORTON, Joe. (né John Kingsley Orton) (1933-1967). British playwright.

Orton incorporated elements of his promiscuous homosexuality into plays such as *Loot*, *Entertaining Mr. Sloane*, and *What the Butler Saw*. Surfing the new climate of sexual acceptance in 1960s Britain typified by the Beatles (for whom he wrote a screenplay, never filmed), Orton embodied the cheeky, cheap street boy. His plays, as he boldly explained at an awards ceremony, "were about getting away with it."

Before he became famous, Orton and his older lover Kenneth Halliwell were jailed for six months for "defacing" library books with scatalogical collages (subsequently the most treasured holdings of that institution). In 1967, a jealous Halliwell battered Orton to death with a hammer, then committed suicide. Orton's life and the efforts of biographer John Lahr to document it were described by Lahr in *Prick Up Your Ears* (1978) (the title a coded reference to sodomy, as in "Prick Up Your Arse"), and in a 1987 film with screenplay by Alan Bennett, with Gary Oldman as Orton and Alfred Molina as Halliwell.

OSCO, William (194?-). (also Rexx Coltrane, Johnny Commander). Film producer and actor.

Self-styled "Boy King of L.A. Porn," Osco belonged to the Osco drugstore dynasty. Affecting a full-length fur coat over jeans and boots, and cruising Los Angeles in a $35,000 Rolls-Royce, he inhabited a walled mansion in Encino, where he emulated the lavish lifestyle of HUGH HEFNER on the other side of the Hollywood Hills.

In 1967, still in his mid-twenties, Osco formed Graffity Productions, with Howard Ziehm, to make porn LOOPS. Within a year, they were turning out fifteen or twenty a week. Unusual among loop makers, Osco signed his films, and soon established a following among the cognoscenti who learned to look out for Graffity's logo, a parody of Universal's opening credits from the 1930s, showing the earth encircled by a tiny plane that, unlike the original, jerks and sputters.

Osco varied the camera's unblinking stare of the MITCHELL BROTHERS' films, changing angles to show off the models, many of whom were young, attractive wannabe starlets. He graduated to longer films in 1967–1968, plunging $7,000 on the forty-minute *Whatever Happened to Stud Flame?*, directed by Ziehm and Michael Beneviste (as "Mike Light"). *Mona, The Virgin Nymph* was more ambitious. Shot largely outdoors, a characteristic of Osco's productions, it starred Fifi Watson, who performs oral sex on a man in the middle of a field, and with a woman in a sunlit domestic interior.

Osco followed *Mona* with another film by Ziehm and Beneviste, *Harlot*, about Melody and Mary, students at Hollywood High who take the day off to go TRICKING on the streets of L.A. In slow motion, Melody (Patty Alexon) runs naked with her overweight biker boyfriend through a shopping center—watched in obvious astonishment by passersby—and a scene on top of the Federal Bank Building ends in a helicopter shot pulling away from the writhing bodies on the roof. Taking a cue from the FORTY THIEVES, Osco hired small cinemas in cities such as Denver and Phoenix and presented the films himself. In some locations, they took in as much as $25,000, unheard-of figures for porn.

When VIDEO arrived, Osco tried to crash the big time with the science fiction spoof *FLESH GORDON* and a 1976 porn musical version of *Alice in Wonderland*, then drifted into the fringes of "legit" production with the horror film *The Being* and the 1983 comedy *Night Patrol*. In 1991, he directed and produced *Gross-Out*, a comedy that lived up to its name with liberal helpings of defecation. The same year, he, his mother, and a business partner were convicted on eighteen counts of illegal money transfers, bank fraud, false accounting, and tax evasion.

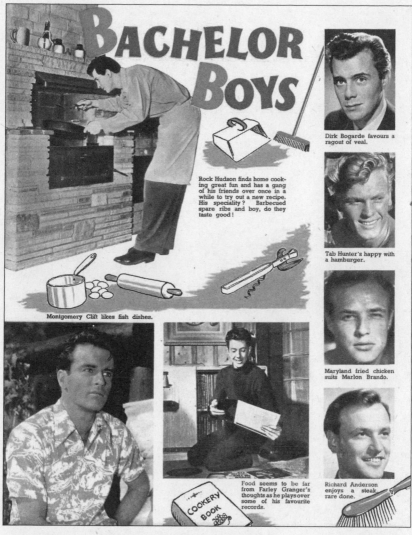

THIS HOLLYWOOD GOSSIP MAGAZINE NOT VERY SUBTLY "OUTED" A NUMBER OF MOVIE GAYS, AND THE BISEXUAL BRANDO

OUTED (1980s–present). To have one's true nature, usually sexual, publicly revealed, as in "out of the closet."

Popularly used to describe the hostile exposure of a celebrity's homosexuality. In a 1982 issue of *Harper's* magazine, Taylor Branch predicted that "outage" would become a political tactic. In *Time* (January 29, 1990), "Forcing Gays Like Mike Howes Out of the Closet," by William A. Henry III, introduced the term to the general public.

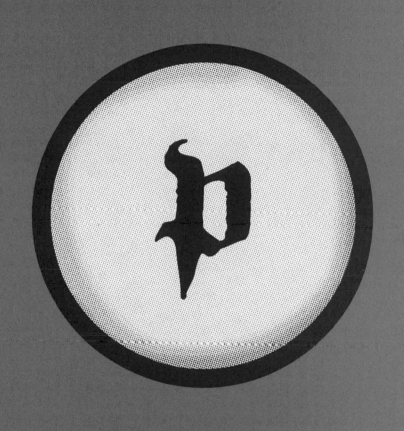

PAEDOPHILIA, also PEDOPHILIA. From the Greek *pais* (child) and *philia* (love or friendship). The tendency of a person, usually male, to be sexually attracted to children. See *LOLITA*, NYMPHET.

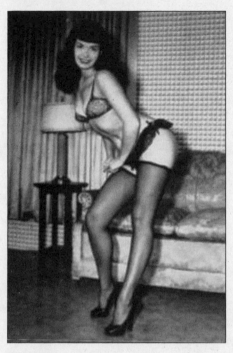

BETTIE PAGE

PAGE, Bettie (sometimes Betty) (née Betty Mae Page) (1923–). Model.

During the early 1940s, a new image of the U.S. male's sexual ideal emerged from the collective unconscious of men drawn to the sleek woman of movies and advertising but desiring at the same time a simple woman who might accept them without resistance: "the girl next door," as a later porn star, GINGER LYNN, put it, "who did the things the girl next door would never do."

This ideal had the perfect body, legs, and hair of a movie star, combined with a farm girl look, humorous and unsophisticated. She first appeared in the work of PINUP artists such as Hugh Petty and Alberto Vargas. She decorated the sides of Flying Fortresses during World War II, and was recycled in comic strips as the "Dragon Lady" of Milton Caniff's *Terry and the Pirates* and "Sand Serif" of Will Eisner's *The Spirit*.

Bettie Page embodied this vision to perfection. She was born with a body made for the airbrush and a face as gleaming and open as the chromed grille of a Detroit gas guzzler; David Denby was right to call her "a Buick that smiles." More important than her proportions was the pleasure she obviously took in them. No matter what contortion or costume her job demanded, she retained her good humor.

Page was born in Tennessee to parents who divorced when she was ten. For a year, she and her sister lived in an orphanage, which left her with a desperate desire to be liked. In high school, she was date-raped by fellow students. Moving to New York, she worked as a secretary while looking for stage roles. Amateur photographer Jerry Tibbs spotted her at Jones Beach on Long Island in 1952 and sent his pictures to Robert Harrison, publisher of the magazines *Wink, Titter, Eyeful*, and the notorious *Confidential*.

Tibbs refined Page's image, suggesting her trademark pageboy hairdo. Page launched herself as a model for photographs and glamour LOOPS produced by IRVING KLAW. In 1950 and 1951, she made more than fifty such films. They include BOND-

AGE and CAT FIGHT films, and a number of STRIPTEASES. The five-minute reels sold for twelve dollars each in sixteen-millimeter and eight dollars in eight-millimeter. At such low prices, they quickly found their way into thousands of surreptitious basement screenings and stag nights.

Page's career was transformed by model and figure photographer BUNNY YAEGER, whom she met on a Florida holiday. Yaeger's pictures emphasized her girl-next-door quality. One showing her as Santa Claus became *PLAYBOY*'s centerfold for January 1955. HUGH HEFNER later took Page under his wing, and helped rescue her financially when she faced bankruptcy.

Periodically, Page tried to abandon porn for acting but could score only bit roles in TV dramas. Pressured to return to modeling, she compromised by hiring out to camera clubs for "glamour weekends," where she posed for scores of admirers, not all of them entirely serious photographers. One who attended such events was Buck Henry, actor-screenwriter (*The Graduate*, *What's Up, Doc?*), who remained an unashamed Page admirer.

Four unhappy marriages drove Page from modeling to religion. During the sixties, she worked behind the scenes for Christian organizations, including the crusades of evangelist Billy Graham, but also spent time in prison and in mental hospitals.

Page was unaware that she was becoming the object of international and discerning admiration. Bernardino Zapponi, screenwriter for FEDERICO FELLINI's films *Fellini Satyricon* and *Fellini Casanova*, wrote an enthusiastic appreciation. Her image permeated the work of illustrator Frank Frazetta and British artist Allen Jones, who incorporated her figure into paintings after seeing her in a mail-order catalogue.

Bettie herself was a character in Dave Stevens's comic strip *The Rocketeer*, and the feature film based on it. Stevens was so fascinated with Page that he made over his wife, Brinke, into a Page lookalike. In 2005, Page was the subject of a feature film, *The Notorious Bettie Page*, with Gretchen Mol. The best evidence of her appeal remains, however, her own films. That they exist today almost entirely in prints so battered, scratched, and recopied they are often barely visible is an index of Page's popularity. Yet through the grain and the flare, beyond their blankly utilitarian photography, and irrespective of the naïve sets—couch, carpet, curtain, and lamp, if that much—something is communicated by this girl in the black underwear, undulating and smiling through the debris of half a century: an innocence and sensual pleasure that's archetypally American.

PAGE-THREE GIRL (1969–present). British tabloid newspaper pinup.

Though the tradition of the PINUPs in newspapers was long and venerable, the British tabloid *The Sun* was the first to include a nude or seminude photograph of a girl on its page three as a regular feature. After Stephanie Rahn, the first such model to pose TOPLESS, appeared in the issue of November 17, 1970, sales rose 40 percent.

PAN'S PEOPLE (1968–1976). British dance group.

Prototype of the scantily dressed, leggy, and provocative TV female dance group, Pan's People was formed to provide interludes for the BBC's *Top of the Pops*. Its original members were Babs Lord, Ruth Pearson, Dee Dee Wilde, Louise Clarke, Andi Rutherford, and Flick Colby, who created the choreography. Pan's People were replaced on *TOTP* by Legs and Co., and in the United States quickly imitated by the Solid Gold Dancers and by numerous "girl bands" more adept at shaking their BOOTY than singing.

PARAINO, LOUIS "Butchie" (aka Lou Parish, Lou Perino, Lou Perry, Stanley Stevens) (1940–1999). Film financier.

Son of Anthony "Big Tony" Paraino, a member of the "family" of Mafia don Joseph Colombo, Paraino, described by LINDA LOVELACE as "a 250 pound hulk" but by others as "a fun guy" with "a Lou Costello quality," was active in porn distribution before borrowing $25,000 from his father to finance *DEEP THROAT* on which, as "Lou Perry," he is credited as producer. After *DEEP THROAT*, the Parainos were rich enough to diversify into non-porn films. Butchie produced *Flesh for Frankenstein: Andy Warhol's Frankenstein* (1973) and *The Texas Chain Saw Massacre* (1974). Following the MIPORN investigation, he was jailed from 1976 to 1982, which terminated his film career.

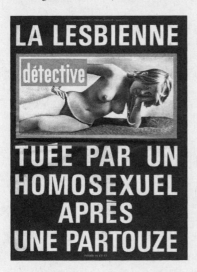

PARTOUZE (French slang, 1922–present). Wife-swapping. Probably invented by the novelist Victor Margueritte in his novel *LA GARÇONNE*.

PARTY (1960s–present). Prostitute term for sexual act, e.g., "Do you want to party?" "What sort of party did you have in mind?" In WOODY ALLEN's *Celebrity*, Leonardo DeCaprio signals that an incipient incident of GROUP SEX should move into the bedroom by saying, "Let's take this party indoors."

PARTY GIRL (1920s–1960s). Semi-professional prostitute.

Often a showgirl or minor actress, the party girl makes herself available mainly as ARM CANDY, and expects no more than a fun night out, a meal, and incidental "expenses." In real life, party girls have, as Sky Masterson says in *Guys and Dolls*, "nice teeth and no last names." Sex is optional, and normally raises the relationship to a new, and more expensive, level. Speaking of the practice in Paris earlier in the twentieth century, Mavis Gallant writes about the "mute invitation [that] used to be known as '*Suivez-moi, jeune homme*' ("Follow me, young man."). It was the prerogative of married women. The unmarried were chaperoned, or didn't dare, or were semi-professional—which means to say, just now and then, hoping just for a good dinner in a decent restaurant, a cab home, a bit of cash. A new hat was a lot to hope for."

Movies of the 1920s and 1930s show actresses routinely moonlighting as party girls, accepting free meals, entertainment, and sometimes cars, jewels, and apartments from wealthy men. In *Stage Door* (1937), young tenants of a theatrical boarding house spend nights on the town with visiting businessmen in return for a good meal. In the 1920s, it was usual for a party girl to extract money from her escort, ostensibly for other purposes, e.g., to tip the ladies' room attendant. See ARBUCKLE, Fatty; ESCORT.

ALSO
PARTY GIRL (U.S. MOVIE, 1958). Directed by Nicholas Ray.

Cyd Charisse and fellow chorus girls in 1930s Chicago are offered $100 each to decorate a party at the home of gangster Lee J. Cobb, who is throwing it to assuage his misery at the marriage of his sexual ideal JEAN HARLOW. Perversely, she elects to go home with Cobb's embittered and crippled but brilliant lawyer, Robert Taylor.

> *"Just about a year ago this time I was on my way to Havana—and I said to the big mug in the next pew, 'I need a coupla hundred dollars, big boy,' and he said, 'In my pants pocket.' I reached over and took $500 out of the back pants pocket, just like that. Now all I've got left is his pajamas."*
>
> —ALINE MacMAHON, LAMENTING THE ONSET OF HARD TIMES IN
> *GOLDDIGGERS OF 1933*

PASTIES. Adhesive nipple shields worn by STRIPTEASERS.

PEEPING TOM (1960). UK film. Directed by Michael Powell.

Assured and eerie, *Peeping Tom* depicts the mid-twentieth century's clandestine LONDON, where pornography and prostitution flourished behind a screen of evasion and circumlocution. Karl Boehm plays a camera assistant in a London film studio. Nights, he photographs porn, or roams SOHO stalking women, whom he impales on a spike attached to one leg of his tripod, filming them as they watch themselves die in a mirror attached to the lens.

Powell catches this furtive world precisely. Pamela Green, then Britain's most popular nude model and wife of GEORGE HARRISON MARKS, has a featured role. Venerable character actor Miles Malleson, a specialist in vicars and literary eccentrics, plays a patron smacking his lips over an album of erotic "views." Upstairs, where the murderer shoots his pictures, the women wear the "exotic" outfits—Spanish hats, net stockings, fringed shawls—typical of British pinups of the time, but pose against

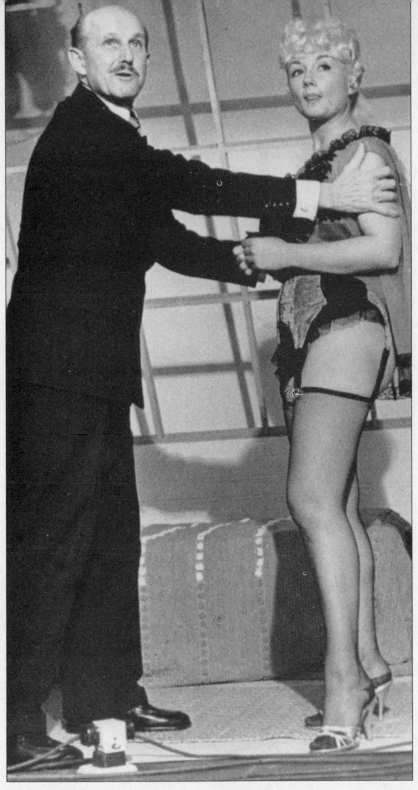

MICHAEL POWELL DIRECTING PAMELA GREEN IN *PEEPING TOM*

mocked-up Paris street backgrounds. Revealingly, director Powell, in private an enthusiast for flagellation and sadism, appears as the psychologist father whose experiments drive Boehm to homicide. Contemporary reaction was uniformly hostile, and effectively ended Powell's career. Only after his death did *Peeping Tom* win acceptance for its macabre sexual satire.

PEEP SHOW. Originally a show or illusion manipulated by levers or strings while viewers watched through individual peepholes. A corruption of the old Scots *keek*, meaning to watch furtively, *peep* always implied secrecy and the forbidden, and was soon attached to the voyeur FETISH.

The first twentieth-century peep shows were WHAT THE BUTLER SAW Kinetoscopes or Mutoscopes in penny arcades. After World War II, adult bookstores began providing booths where clients viewed porn LOOPS, masturbating with one hand while feeding coins to the voracious machine with the other. These developed into live peep shows where "private dancers" performed on a circular stage, watched by patrons in booths set around the periphery. As with film peep shows, a shutter cut off one's view unless one fed it coins. Tina Turner's 1984 hit "Private Dancer" was a scornful lament for the lives of such women, well depicted by Season Hubley in the film *HARDCORE*.

> The video booths are small spaces where 25c in the slot will buy one and a half minutes of video porn. In this particular place there is a row of ten brown cubicles, like confessionals. . . . I locked the door behind me and in the unfamiliar blackness was assailed with the strong smell of semen . . . My eyes adjusted to the light. I put the coin in the slot and the space filled with flickering electric color. . . . In one of the cubicle walls, at about hip level, there was a roughly scratched hole in the plywood, straight into the next cubicle. My feet were sticking to the floor. The space was filled with a blur of groans as the horny, naked stud started coming into the rear of one of the accommodating models. Then it went black, needing more coins. In the quiet I heard a door bang in the next cubicle. Someone shuffled and unzipped and a coin clonked into place.
>
> —GAEL KNEPPER, *Sex in Australia*

PEGGING (U.S. slang, 2001–present). Sexual act in which a woman wearing a STRAP-ON anally penetrates a man while he's copulating with a woman.

The practice appeared in *THE OPENING OF MISTY BEETHOVEN*, less flagrantly in *Myra Breckenridge*, but wasn't named until sex columnist Dan Savage invited suggestions for a title in 2001. In a variation, Atom Egoyan's *Where the Truth Lies* (2005) showed the comedy team of Peter Firth and Kevin Bacon breaking up when the former tries to sodomize the latter while Bacon is having sex with a girl. See also BOB.

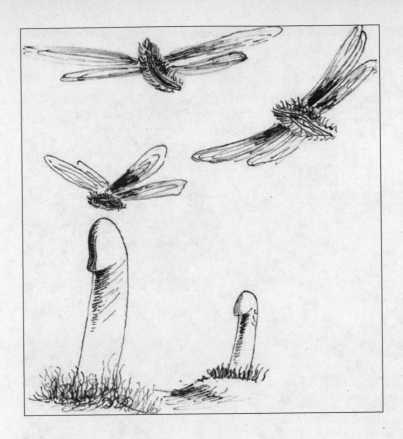

PENIS.

Notwithstanding a "Size Doesn't Matter" campaign, a big penis remains among the most seductive of all fetishes. A writer to the feminist magazine *Cosmopolitan* in the 1990s said dismissively, "I don't date hamsters."

PENTHOUSE (1956–present). Monthly magazine.

BOB GUCCIONE launched *Penthouse* initially in Britain in 1956 and in the United States in 1958. It quickly became the most effective of the monthlies to compete with *PLAYBOY.* Guccione had worked as an artist, was a collector of art, and a sufficiently expert photographer to shoot the nudes for the first issues of the magazine. In place of HUGH HEFNER's Californian cheerleader freshness, Guccione offered an Italianate soft focus that echoed the style of films such as *EMMANUELLE*, and immediately won a following.

Penthouse surfed the wave of the permissive 1970s, wherever possible testing the prevailing COMMUNITY STANDARDS. "We began to show pubic hair," boasted Guccione. . . . "We introduced lesbian pictorials. . . . We were the first to show full frontal nudity. The first to expose the clitoris completely."

Soon a multimillionaire, Guccione accumulated a museum-quality art collection, and knocked together 14 and 16 East Sixty-seventh Street to create Manhattan's larg-

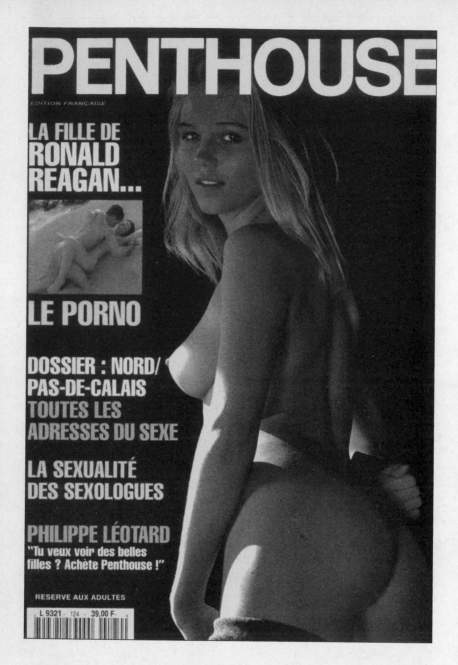

est private residence to house it. Confident in his mastery of his brave new world, he launched the glossy science monthly *Omni*, another called *Longevity*, the women's magazine *Viva*, and *Spin*, intended to eclipse *Rolling Stone*. He also financed the soft-core porn feature *CALIGULA* and a scientific project to perfect the dubious "cold fusion" process.

But the flair that fired his earlier innovation had deserted him, and all these ventures failed spectacularly. Hoping boldness would again be his salvation, Guccione decreed a change in direction for *Penthouse*, typified by *HUSTLER*-style photo features depicting urination, fetish wear, humiliation, and "FACIALS." Both readers and advertisers fled, and the magazine was even banned from U.S. military bases. Guccione filed for bankruptcy and, in 2004, was evicted from his home, which realtors diplomatically rechristened "Milbank Mansion," to remove the stigma of Guccione's name. Ironically, the new owners of the *Penthouse* franchise have responded to dwindling newsstand sales by diversifying into the INTERNET dating sector, specifically the overtly Christian www .BigChurch.com, committed to "Bringing people together in love and faith."

PERCY. Euphemism for penis, probably coined by Australian comedian Barry Humphries, who described urination as "pointing Percy at the porcelain."

ALSO
PERCY (1971). UK film. Directed by Ralph Thomas.

Sex comedy in which Hywel Bennett, emasculated in the same car accident that kills a well-known playboy, receives the dead man's penis as a transplant, and sets out to learn something of its previous owner.

PETTING (U.S., 1910s–1960s). When more strenuous, HEAVY PETTING.

Sexual foreplay, usually in public, e.g., AUTOMOBILES. Celebrated in the film *42nd Street* with an elaborate production number called *Pettin' in the Park*, featuring Ruby Keeler, Dick Powell, midget Billy Barty, and a corps of half-nude showgirls.

> *"As far back as 1915 the unchaperoned young people of the smaller cities had discovered the mobile privacy of that automobile given to young Bill at sixteen to make him 'self-reliant.' At first petting was a desperate adventure even under such favorable conditions, but presently confidences were exchanged and the old commandment broke down.... But petting in its more audacious manifestations was confined to the wealthier classes—among other young people the old standard prevailed until after the War, and a kiss meant that a proposal was expected, as other young officers in strange cities sometimes discovered to their dismay."*
>
> —F. SCOTT FITZGERALD, *Echoes of the Jazz Age*

PHONE SEX. Telephone conversation on a sexual topic during which one or both of the speakers masturbate or are aroused.

In some services, the recipient of the call assumes a character and purports to be performing a sexual act as demanded by the caller. Alternatively, the caller can "listen in" on a supposedly private sexual conversation. Such services were known as 900 or 976 numbers, a reference to the premium-rate telephone code, but following widespread fraud and unauthorized use by children, the regulations were tightened in 1996.

Private phone sex was celebrated in Nicholson Baker's *Vox: A Novel* (1992), which depicts a sexual relationship carried on almost entirely by phone. The stage and screen musical *Bells Are Ringing* (1955) flirted with the potential risks, legal and emotional, of a telephone answering girl becoming involved with her clients. In *Hustle* (1975), Catherine Deneuve as a French prostitute in Los Angeles provides phone sex, to the chagrin of her cop lover Burt Reynolds; Jennifer Jason Leigh in *Short Cuts* (1993) delivers phone sex from the family home while managing husband and children. *Girl 6* (Spike Lee, 1996) is set in a phone sex office.

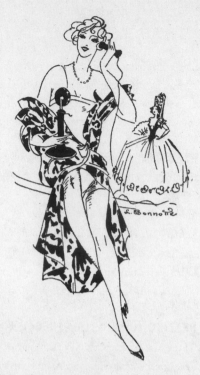

In France during the last decades of the twentieth century, the *Minitel Rose*, a text-only telephone link (originally launched to replace printed telephone directories) allowed clients and sex workers to communicate in typed conversations. Such services, like much professional phone sex, have been supplanted by the Internet.

Celebrity enthusiasts for phone sex include Prince Charles, who was overheard telling mistress Camilla Parker-Bowles that he wished to be reincarnated in her trousers, perhaps as a pair of knickers, but, if he had bad luck, as her tampon, and ANDY WARHOL, who preferred "sex-phone" with lovers such as Truman Capote because "I don't like my hair messed up." Warhol also fantasized an elaborate phone sex enterprise in which clients could talk to operators pretending to be celebrities, alive or dead. "You can believe you're making it with anyone, or having an orgy with Elsa Maxwell, Cleopatra, James Dean, Queen Elizabeth, anyone."

PICKLE (1950s–1960s). Movie shorthand for penis.

In NUDIE movies, if a performer inadvertently showed his penis, the cameraman yelled, "Pickle," and stopped shooting. See also BEAVER; FRANKS AND BEANS.

PIERCING. Puncturing or cutting the body in order to attach or insert an object for decorative or ritual reasons.

Ear piercing in particular dates back to prehistoric time. Nose and earrings are mentioned in the Bible, and earrings were worn by women throughout the Middle Ages, as well as men in marginal occupations, e.g., the merchant marine; hence the association of earrings with piracy. The practice was revived as a FETISH in the 1960s, along with TATTOOING, particularly among American homosexuals and enthusiasts of bondage and sadomasochism. Male and female nipple rings were adopted by celebrities such as rock stars Madonna and Axl Rose, and photographer ROBERT MAPPLETHORPE, who had his fitting of a nipple ring documented in the 1971 film *Robert Having His Nipple Pierced*. With the revival of interest in bondage and BDSM in the 1960s, multiple ear piercings and piercings of the nostrils, eyelids, navel, and tongue became common.

Genital piercing flourished after the publication of *HISTOIRE D'O*, in which the heroine has her labia pierced and a ring inserted. Such rings were popularized by porn stars such as MARILYN CHAMBERS. Clitoral and penile piercing enjoyed a vogue among the group calling themselves Modern Primitives. Penile piercing in particular became extremely elaborate, ranging from the insertion of an ALBERT, a metal bar attached to an Edwardian watch chain, to the opening of the urethra and its refastening with a series of metal rings. Metal beads are also inserted under the skin to give the penis a textured surface, and supposedly increase sexual pleasure.

Records for the greatest number of piercings are regularly broken, but permanent piercings in excess of one thousand are not uncommon. See ALBERT; AMPALLANG.

PIG FOOT (U.S. slang, 1900s–1920s). Jazz and blues euphemism for *penis*, cf., the Bessie Smith blues "Gimme a pig foot and a bottle of beer." See also JAZZ; JELLY ROLL.

PILL, The. All-purpose term for oral contraceptives.

No scientific advance of the twentieth century had such a far-reaching influence on sexual behavior as the introduction in the early 1960s of oral contraception for women in the form of a pill that, if taken regularly each day, offered more than 90 percent protection against unwanted pregnancy. It had been known from the 1930s that disturbing the hormone balance affected birth patterns in rabbits by preventing them from ovulating, but human application had to wait for the synthesis of the two hormones, estrogen and progesterone, which regulate the process.

No one scientist invented the Pill. Margaret Sanger, a lifelong proponent of birth control, raised the necessary $150,000 for the research conducted by Gregory Pincus of the Worcester Foundation for Experimental Biology. In 1952, Pincus and gynecologist John Rock began testing a pill that contained synthetic progesterone. Concurrently, Carl Djerassi, working for Syntex in Mexico also synthesized the hormone. Two different companies, Searle and Syntex, started testing pills in 1953. Searle entered the market first with Djerassi's pill, but it was surpassed by Enovid, developed by Frank Colton and launched in 1960, after John Rock—ironically a fervent Catholic—had supervised the clinical trials and presented the Pill to the U.S. Food and Drug Administration for approval in 1960.

Hormone levels in early versions of the Pill were too high, leading to dangerous side effects, but in the half century since its introduction, repeated refinements have drastically reduced the risk to health. Catholic opposition to the Pill remains implacable, and a continuing source of controversy within the Church.

At the time of writing, no reliable contraceptive pill exists for use by men, though a number are in development.

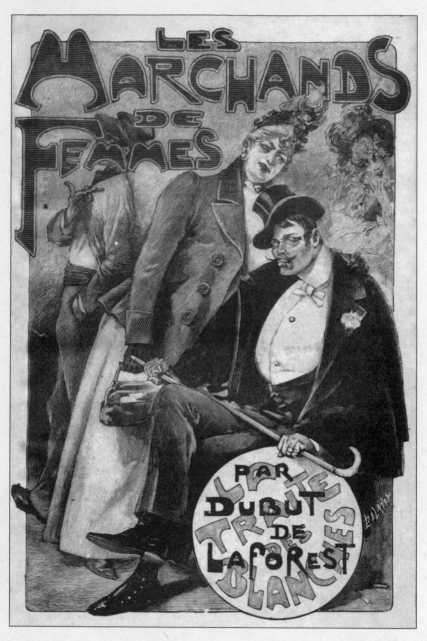

PIMP (also PROCURER, PONCE, PANDER) (1600s–present). Person who manages or controls a prostitute, and lives off "immoral earnings." From Old French *pimper*, "to allure or entice," usually through smart dressing, and *pimpant*, "looking trim and fresh."

Pimping, not prostitution, is "the oldest profession," if one accepts the 1972 claim of a London panderer that "Adam was the first TRICK [and] Snake the first pimp." Pimps occupy an ambiguous position in the moral hierarchy. Though they prey, often violently, on women, both prostitutes and police tolerate them, with the law seeing them as a control on unrestricted prostitution and the women as acting as go-betweens, protecting them from rival pimps, keeping them out of jail, and paying the necessary bribes. In the film of *IRMA LA DOUCE,* a Parisian cop walks into the pimps' bar, puts down his hat, and picks it up a few minutes later filled with banknotes.

Unlikely pimps include black activist Malcolm X and jazz musician Charlie Mingus, who held his fellow procurers in high esteem: "I often see them down at the [Chicago] Art Institute. They are especially fond of the legitimate drama. At the opening night of Eugene O'Neill's *The Hairy Ape* . . . there were twenty-five pimps in the audience, many of them with their girls. A play such as *Frankie and Johnny,* or MAE WEST's *Diamond Lil,* will attract half the pimps and whores in town."

A 1931 study of prostitution in the United States found that "some pimps hold their women by genuine love and devotion, some by lying and bluffing, and others by fear and beating." Many women simply wanted someone with whom they could have sex free of the taint of commerce. A STORYVILLE pimp of the 1910s with a string of eight girls complained, "I have to lay each one of 'em once or twice a month."

Since some prostitutes maintained their pimps in an expensive lifestyle as a sign of professional value, as they might boast a smart car or expensive clothes, the terms *pimp* and *ponce* became associated with a flamboyant style of dressing and living, and with a tendency to pose and preen. Pimp style is typified by the *mecs* of Paris whores, then by the "zoot suits" affected by New York's black pimps in the late 1940s; wide-brimmed felt hats, gaudy clothing with exaggerated lapels and shoulders, and enormous cars ("pimpmobiles"), often in pink and with elaborate interiors. "To pimp" came to mean redecorating a person or thing in a similar extravagant style (cf., MTV's TV series *Pimp My Ride,* in which engineers "pimp" cars with outrageous bodywork and accessories). From this, the word, much used by rappers, became an approving synonym for expertise. Its original meaning forgotten, it's even been adopted for a proprietary "energy drink," Pimpjuice. See also SUITCASE PIMP.

PINK. Adjective with multiple sexual applications:

1. Euphemism, popularized by *HUSTLER* magazine, for porn in which female models displayed the inner "pink" area of the vulva.
2. The color connoting homosexuality, probably because the German government of the 1930s forced homosexuals to identify themselves with a pink triangle on their clothing.
3. In French, as *rose,* an indication of erotic intent, e.g., *GUIDE ROSE* for a book listing brothels, *MINITEL ROSE* for a computer sex chat line.

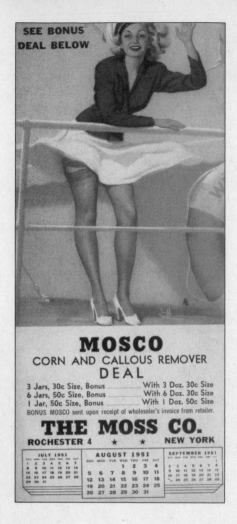

PINUP, sometimes PINUP GIRL (U.S. slang, 1920s–present).

Provocatively posed image, almost always of a lone girl, suitable for semi-public display, as on a calendar.

The term first appears in 1941, but the idea goes back to the 1890s, when magazine printing first produced images sufficiently clear and durable to survive long periods pinned on a wall without fading or yellowing. H. L. Mencken attributed the term to Walter Thornton, self-styled "Merchant of Venus," who ran a large U.S. model agency.

PLATO'S RETREAT (1977–1985). New York sex club.

Opened by entrepreneur LAWRENCE LEVENSON in 1977 on the site of the former CONTINENTAL BATHS, in the basement of the Ansonia Hotel, Plato's Retreat transformed Manhattan's most popular gay hangout into a center for heterosexual SWINGERS. In the club's heyday, 6,500 people a month paid five dollars per couple for a six-week "membership," and twenty-five dollars per visit, or ten dollars for a woman alone. Unattached males were barred, although many hung around outside, soliciting women as they emerged.

By the art deco swimming pool, or in carpeted mirror-walled rooms, with piped music and discreet lighting, visitors could cruise the (usually nude) talent of both sexes, and ogle porn stars such as RON JEREMY and JAMIE GILLIS and low-rent celebrities such as SAMMY DAVIS, JR., Margaux Hemingway, Richard Dreyfuss, Jill St. John, George Hamilton, and scenarist-actor Buck Henry. "We used to wander over there in the *Saturday Night Live* days to take a look," admitted Henry, screenwriter of *The Graduate*, insisting he went mainly for the fine food. Did he also sample the club's other attractions? "Maybe," he replied circumspectly.

The "other attractions" were all that any twentieth-century sensualist could desire. One could slip into one of the alcoves for a semi-private orgy, rent a "mini-swing" room with another couple, take steam in the tiled sauna with its copies of suggestive classical

Greek statues, or catch the action in the Mat Rooms, where couples screwed in crepuscular proximity on pads laid out on the floor of a gymlike space. (Unknown to the management, one of the building's janitors had bored a hole from the adjoining basement, and charged friends two dollars a peek.)

The club, a regular stopover on the Manhattan porn tour, appeared in a number of films, including the SOFT-CORE feature *New York Nights*, and is the setting for a scene in Spike Lee's 1999 *Summer of Sam*. In 1981, Levenson was convicted on charges of tax evasion. Released in 1985, he reopened the club, this time in Midtown Manhattan, but it was not a success. Erstwhile regulars such as Buck Henry found the new premises cavernous and unwelcoming. Even then, it might have survived had Mayor Ed Koch not listened to complaints from the gay community that his crackdown on sex clubs unfairly discriminated against homosexual meeting places such as The Anvil and The Man Hole. On New Year's Eve 1985, patrons arriving at Plato's Retreat found the doors locked, never to reopen.

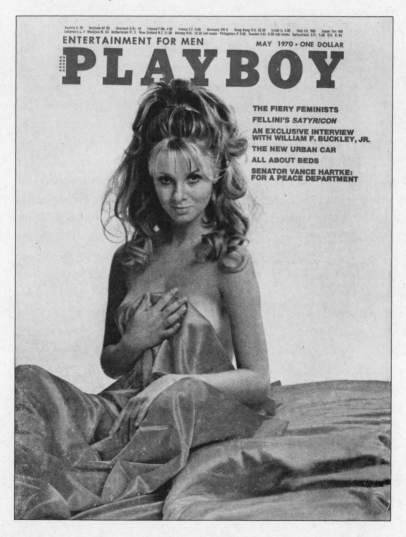

PLAYBOY (1953–present). U.S. men's magazine.

There was little new about *Playboy* when Hugh Hefner assembled the first issue on his living room table, with a nude MARILYN MONROE on the cover. Other magazines had used the same name—Hefner initially preferred "Stag Night" or "The Gentlemens' Club"—and the mix of erotic illustrations with cartoons and stories went back to *La Vie Parisienne* at the end of the nineteenth century. But it's a truism of marketing that "it's not the 'who' or the 'why' but the 'when.' " *Playboy* appeared at a time when COMMUNITY STANDARDS were ready to accept a discreet magazine of erotica, when color printing had improved to the point where flesh tones could be rendered with accuracy, and when the eighteen-to-thirty-five male audience was wealthy enough to buy not only the magazine but the products it advertised.

The first issue of *Playboy* sold fifty-three thousand copies, and circulation continued to climb, peaking in 1972 at just over seven million. Such success allowed the magazine to offer top rates to its contributors, who included Graham Greene, John Updike, Ray Bradbury, Vladimir Nabokov, WOODY ALLEN, Norman Mailer, and IAN FLEMING, and to scores more—significantly predominantly male. It became fashionable to claim one "only bought it for the articles," though the only buyers who could say this with total honesty were the visually impaired, since the Braille edition omitted the pictures.

Playboy's rabbit symbol became the second most familiar emblem in the world, after Coca-Cola's "wave." Foreign editions proliferated, as did Playboy Clubs, where "bunny girls" in abbreviated costumes, complete with ears and tail, served drinks using a backward "Bunny Dip" that didn't expose their décolletage.

Hefner supervised his empire from the Playboy Mansion in Chicago, then from the Playboy Mansion West, in Los Angeles, where he tried to live the high life celebrated in the magazine. Photo spreads showed him as a sober, avuncular pipe-smoking presence, usually in a smoking jacket, surrounded by mid-level celebrities and adoring Playmates of the Month. Every SWINGER aspired to an invitation to the Mansion. Even Elvis Presley succumbed, checking in secretly for one night, and sharing his bed with eight Playmates. Hefner kept the suite locked thereafter, allowing no other person to enjoy the hallowed chamber.

Others were less welcome. Hefner barred SUITCASE PIMP Paul Snider after his protégée, Dorothy Stratten, left him for filmmaker Peter Bogdanovich. Enraged, Snider murdered Stratten, then killed himself, events that inspired the film *Star '80* and Bogdanovich's anguished memoir *The Killing of the Unicorn*.

Tragedies such as the Stratten killing exposed a less idyllic side of both the *Playboy* image and Hefner himself. LINDA LOVELACE, who lived in the Los Angeles mansion during an abortive attempt at Hollywood stardom, claimed that "Hef" was more interested in watching sex than in participating. She described him prowling the overcrowded Jacuzzi, a bottle of baby oil in hand, and finally sodomizing her. Larry Layman in RADLEY METZGER's *THE OPENING OF MISTY BEETHOVEN*, the undersexed publisher of a men's magazine called *Goldenrod* who secretly wants to be PEGGED, seems intended as a parody of Hefner.

The magazine, too, never lived up to its libertarian ideals as expressed in interminable editorials about a *"Playboy* philosophy." Those who did buy it were seldom the sort of people featured in the in-house advertisements that enquired "What sort of man reads *Playboy?"* The ads showed young middle managers being fitted for Savile Row suits or frowning up at the Big Board, when, as the British media critic Raymond Durgnat remarked caustically, the answer was more likely to be "the henpecked, mortgage-harassed, ulcer-ridden, prematurely ejaculating sort."

Playboy's numerous imitators included *PENTHOUSE*, which published more overly erotic photo spreads, and the unabashedly vulgar *HUSTLER*. In France, *Playboy* was shadowed by *Oui*, and in Britain, by *Mayfair*, *Whitehouse*, and many others. As sales fell off, the *Playboy* corporation, now managed by Hefner's daughter, responded by diversifying into video and film production, cable TV, and even, via the purchase of JENNA JAMESON's company, HARD-CORE porn.

PLAYGIRL (1973–present). U.S. erotic lifestyle monthly.

Launched at the height of the feminist movement, *Playgirl* ostensibly catered to liberated women with nude or seminude photographs of men. While it was true, as one staffer contended, that the magazine targeted "young entertainment-starved and sex-starved women in places such as the Midwest, the Deep South, and Texas. Florida and Texas always led the sales," *Playgirl's* slogan, "Entertainment for Women," was ambiguous, since it survived on its gay male audience—estimated at 30 percent by editor Michele Zipp in 2003, but by others as high as 50 percent.

Like *PLAYBOY*, the magazine courted celebrities to pose, even offering Prince Charles $45,000 in 1990, after nude paparazzi shots of him surfaced in a French magazine. For much of its life, it also functioned as a money launderer for organized crime. In 2000, the FCC charged Crescent Publishing, which then produced the magazine (plus much hard-core pornography), with over $180 million in online credit card fraud. Company president Bruce Chew was subsequently indicted, along with members of the Gambino crime family.

POCKET BILLIARDS (UK and Australian slang, 1920s–1960s). Stimulating the testicles via a hand in the pocket, sometimes directly through a convenient hole. Anti-masturbation tracts from the early twentieth century specifically nominate "trouser pockets for boys" as an incitement to self-abuse, on a par with "the *Odes* of Horace . . . ballet . . . phosphorus, cocaine, OPIUM, camphor, and the inhalation of oxygen."

POLAROIDS. Photographs taken with the Land Polaroid camera system, launched publicly by inventor Edwin Land in 1948.

The pornographic possibilities of a system that developed its own prints were immediately obvious, and a Polaroid camera became as common a bedroom accessory as the VIBRATOR, remaining so until superseded by digital technology. Polaroid images featured in numerous scandals, most notably the rift between WOODY ALLEN and Mia Farrow, after she discovered Allen's Polaroids of a nude Soon-Yi Previn, her adopted daughter.

POLE DANCING. Exotic dancing in which the performer, usually in a bar or small club, works in a stationary position, clinging to or hanging from a vertical metal pole extending from bar top to the ceiling.

The introduction in the 1980s of pole dancing to STRIPTEASE considerably increased the variety and range of acrobatic movements, and favored the trained dancers who were finding their way into the now-almost-respectable profession. Following films such as Adrian Lyne's *Flashdance*, which implied that exotic dancing shared skills with modern ballet, pole dancing developed an aesthetic and, like belly dancing, was welcomed by some feminists as a liberating experience. An international school, PoleStars, even offered classes.

PONY PLAY. Fetish in which a participant, sometimes called a Pony Boy or Pony Girl, dresses in a stylized horse costume—commonly a high-cut maillot, stockings, and heels, with the addition of a horse's tail and head plume. In some cases, the "pony" is harnessed to a small sulky and driven in public, often with bridle and bit. See FURVERSION; ZOOPHILIA.

POONTANG (U.S. slang, 1920s-present). Vaginal sex, analogous to PUSSY. Probably of New Orleans origin, a corruption of the French *putain*, "prostitute."

POPPERS. Amyl nitrate capsules. Muscle relaxants, commonly used in FISTING.

PORN CREEP (1990s-present). Psychological condition by which a reliance on pornography renders one impotent with a partner. Also: The process by which sexually explicit content enters popular culture, e.g., via advertising and popular performance. Often cited in relation to the performances of pop star MADONNA, some of whose videos adopt STAG MOVIE iconography.

PORNOGRAPHY. Art intended exclusively to excite sexual desire.

In Roman times, "pornography" applied only to works produced by prostitutes, usually as advertising. Anything else was "erotica." This distinction survived into modern times. Pornography, flagrant, cheap, and readily available, was regarded as a greater threat to the innocent than erotica, which was traditionally produced in editions too expensive for the average reader, or in languages they wouldn't understand. In the 1960 prosecution of *LADY CHATTERLEY'S LOVER*, counsel for the Crown asked the jury, "Is it a book you would wish your wife or servants to read?" The question implied that aristocrats and intellectuals would not be depraved or corrupted by pornography, but that they had a duty to keep it out of the hands of the lower orders.

Mass media and cheap publishing blurred the distinction between pornography and erotica until it became largely a matter of opinion. In 1964, Justice Potter Stewart of the U.S. Supreme Court famously ruled, "I shall not today attempt further to define [pornography] . . . [b]ut I know it when I see it." Described as the "commonsense" approach, this argument faltered once individual states and even towns, given the right to make up their own minds, banned books and films that other, more sophisticated communities accepted.

With the constitutional right to freedom of speech under threat, "commonsense" was abandoned. The new definitions required a work to show "redeeming artistic merit" and prove it did not intend "to corrupt and deprave"—tests that proved difficult, if not impossible, in practice. During the 1970s, the U.S. Supreme Court reluctantly accepted the concept of COMMUNITY STANDARDS, acknowledging that a work that might outrage rural Idaho would raise no eyebrows in Manhattan. Cynics pointed out that, in essence, this was the old "them and us" rule applied on a national basis. Nevertheless, it has survived repeated legal attacks, and looks likely to continue to do so.

"Dirty movies have gotten better, I'm told. Smut and weaponry are the two areas in which we've improved. Everything else has gotten worse."

—JOSEPH HELLER, IN *SOMETHING HAPPENED* (1972)

PORTNOY'S COMPLAINT (1969). U.S. novel, by Philip Roth.

The popularity and social effect of Roth's comic novel equalled that of its contemporaries *LOLITA* and *The Ginger Man*. Alexander Portnoy defines his "complaint" or illness to his psychiatrist as "a disorder in which strongly felt ethical and altruistic impulses are perpetually warring with extreme sexual longings, often of a perverse nature." Portnoy's urges induce him to have sex with FRUIT, to masturbate into a piece of LIVER intended for the family's dinner, and to fornicate indiscriminately with groups and individuals, notably the girlfriend who calls herself "The Monkey," after a sexual variation of her own invention. The memoirs of Roth's ex-wife Claire Bloom suggest that the novel is in part autobiographical. See MASTURBATION.

POSTCARD. Card, normally six inches by four inches, with space for a message on the verso, and designed to be mailed without envelope.

Photographic printing had hardly been invented before small pornographic photographs appeared in France. Though never meant to be mailed, they were of postcard dimensions, and the label stuck. As the trade flourished, the phrase "French postcard" entered the language, along with the cliché of shifty vendors who preyed on the gull-

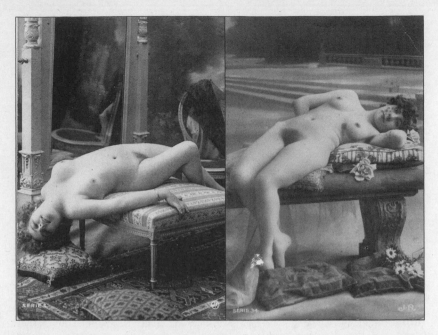

ible tourist, flashing one inflamatory example, then substituting an envelope filled with views of churches and chateaux.

France became the world center for the production both of pornographic post-cards and those that, merely suggestive, could actually be mailed. The latter, featur-ing fully clothed couples flirting or kissing, were often sold in sets of eight, showing the progress of a romance or seduction. Models who appeared nude in photosets were AIRBRUSHED for the postcard market, but there was a busy clandestine market in the unretouched variety. D. H. LAWRENCE attacked these as "of an ugliness to make you cry. The insult to the human body, the insult to a vital human relationship! Ugly and cheap, they make human nudity ugly and degraded; they make the sexual act trivial and cheap and nasty." All the same, British tourists were big customers, although at home they preferred the comic cards of Donald McGill, which parodied cliché British experiences, e.g., overweight men at the seaside ogling scantily clad beauties.

PRIMAL SCENE. In psychoanalysis, the "primal scene" is the actual or imagined observation by a child of sexual intercourse, particularly between parents.

SIGMUND FREUD, using the evidence of THE WOLF MAN case, was the first to propose that such a sight might deeply affect an impressionable mind. Memories of such scenes do appear in many erotic memoirs, most recently those of CATHERINE MIL-LET but also in books by Yukio Mishima and other writers preoccupied with sex.

PRODUCTION CODE. System of internal self-censorship introduced by the U.S. film industry in 1934 after threats of government control.

The Code's first supervisor was ex-Postmaster General Will H. Hays, who headed the Motion Picture Producers and Distributors of America (MPPDA), later Motion Picture Association of America (MPAA). Any film not bearing its seal of approval would be barred from cinemas owned by or contracted to the major studios—which meant almost all of them.

Hays's puritanism permeated what became known as the Hays Office (and subsequently, as its administrators changed, the Breen Office, Johnston Office, etc.). Nudity and suggestive dances were prohibited. So was the ridicule of religion and its ministers. You couldn't illustrate how to crack a safe or smuggle goods through Customs. It was forbidden to show cocaine, opium, or marijuana, and the Code even tried to limit the depiction of alcohol. There could be no overt depiction of "sex perversion" (i.e., homosexuality), sexually transmitted diseases, or childbirth.

Certain words and phrases were proscribed; not simply profanity or references to WHORES, BROTHELS, and so on, but also phrases such as "TRAVELING SALESMAN" and "FARMER'S DAUGHTER," which might evoke the bawdy jokes that employed them. Films were enjoined to uphold the sanctity of marriage and the home. Adultery and illicit sex, however justified—"wife a hopeless invalid," etc.—could not be explicit, or presented as an attractive option. Any pleasure in such situations must be shown to be bitterly regretted afterward.

Racism was implicit in the Code. The only permissible relationship between a white person and an African American, Mexican, or Asian was that of servant and master. As late as 1950, in *Young Man with a Horn*, Juano Hernandez, as the black jazz trumpeter who teaches Kirk Douglas how to play, addresses him throughout a twenty-year friendship as "Mister Rick" and his friend Doris Day as "Miss Jo."

Under Joseph Breen, the tone of restrictions moved from the Protestantism of Hays to an even more restrictive Catholicism. Breen's decisions reflected the views of successive cardinals, notably Joseph Spellman. A body of case law soon spelled out how long a kiss could be, how low-cut a dress, how brutal a beating. Couples had to sleep in twin beds and, if sharing one, keep a foot on the ground at all times. Costumes could not reveal the navel, condemning successive Tarzans to loincloths as high-waisted as miniskirts.

The industry learned to edge past some restrictions. Mercedes McCambridge wasn't necessarily a lesbian just because she dressed mannishly and had a gruff voice, and the fastidious Clifton Webb was never quite homosexual, despite taking prissy roles in *Laura* or *The Razor's Edge*. The proprieties were observed in films such as *Marked Woman* or *From Here to Eternity* by calling a brothel a "club," and its girls "hostesses," or making whore Joan Bennett in *Man Hunt* into a "seamstress."

When the courts forced Hollywood studios to relinquish control of its cinema chains in the 1950s, the MPAA lost the power to enforce censorship. In 1953, Otto

Preminger refused to cut the words *virgin, pregnant, seduction,* and *mistress* from *The Moon Is Blue*, and released it without MPAA authority. As late as 1962, however, Hollywood's self-censorship remained sufficiently powerful that Stanley Kubrick and partner James Harris were forced to promise that they'd make their film of *Lolita* conform by setting it in a southern state where marriage was legal at fourteen. See LEGION OF DECENCY.

PROFUMO AFFAIR, THE. British political scandal.

In 1961, British Minister of War John Profumo was forced to resign after confessing to an affair with PARTY GIRL Christine Keeler, whose other lovers included Yevgeny Ivanov, senior naval attaché at the Soviet embassy.

Keeler had been a showgirl prancing in careful near-nudity round the minuscule stage of the Cabaret Club in SOHO when she and her friend Mandy Rice-Davies were spotted by osteopath Stephen Ward, who acted as PIMP for his aristocratic friends, including William, Third Viscount Astor.

Profumo met Keeler during a nude swimming party at Astor's country mansion, Cliveden. Their affair was soon exposed by the tabloid press, as was Keeler's relationship with Ivanov. Profumo denied the reports, both to Prime Minister Harold Macmillan and, publicly, to the House of Commons. The lie, quickly exposed, ended his political career, and he spent the rest of his life in obscurity, doing charity work in London's East End. The subsequent judicial enquiry by Lord Denning briefly lifted the lid on the world of upper-class vice, only to let it drop back before the public could catch more than a glimpse. Stephen Ward, made the scapegoat, committed suicide.

> *"Well, he would, wouldn't he."*
> —MANDY RICE-DAVIES, ON BEING TOLD THAT LORD ASTOR
> HAD DENIED HAVING AN AFFAIR WITH HER

PROMOTION CANAPÉ. French equivalent of the CASTING COUCH.

PROSAPHISM (French, 1850s-present). The pleasure taken by some men in watching sex acts between women. Credited to the French philosopher Charles Fourier (1772-1837), who also coined the term *feminism*.

PSYCHO (1959). U.S. novel by Robert Bloch.

One of the earliest and most successful attempts to reflect the mind of a sexual psychopath. Inspired in part by the acts of Wisconsin murderer and grave robber Ed Gein (1906–1984), *Psycho* was particularly innovative in its setting, showing the psychopathic killer Norman Bates not as an urban predator but the superficially amiable proprietor of a rural motel.

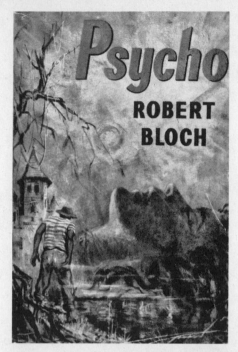

ALSO

PSYCHO (1960). U.S. film. Directed by Alfred Hitchcock.

Psycho was a startling change of pace for Hitchcock, whose well-crafted but old-fashioned adventures had been gradually losing audiences. Based on a raw paperback novel by horror and science fiction author Robert Bloch, and shot in black-and-white, it sent a shock through the cinema. Critics who dismissed it as the cheesiest kind of thriller, an upmarket competitor to William Castle's *Tingler* and *House on Haunted Hill*, recanted to acknowledge it as perhaps his most innovative film, second only to the equally uncommercial *Vertigo* in its acknowledgment of the sexual perversity that lurks behind the most complacent exterior.

From the first shot, a slow crane through the window of a city hotel to a heavy-breasted Janet Leigh enjoying an illicit HOT LUNCH with lover John Gavin, audiences were alerted that this was not another of Hitchcock's bloodless exercises in suspense. Nothing, however, prepared them for Leigh's slaughter a few reels later at the hands of Anthony Perkins in drag. The Shower Scene, a virtuoso exercise in cinematic sleight of hand, depicts the butchering of the nude Leigh without revealing a single nipple or pubic hair, nor one contact between knife and flesh.

PUPPETRY OF THE PENIS. Stage show, 2004, conceived and presented by Australian comics David Friend and Simon Morley, who appeared naked, and manipulated their genitals with a few props to create comic effects.

One admiring review noted that the act "involves the boys contorting their meat marionettes into various shapes from snail and hamburger to Eiffel Tower . . . But the pièce de résistance is when one of them is wafted across the stage on a skateboard using an electric fan and a sail fashioned from his scrotum."

PUSSY (U.S. slang, 1940s–present). Vagina, and by extension, sex in which a vagina is involved.

> *"Pussy rules the world."*
> —MADONNA

PUSSY-WHIPPED (U.S. slang, 1960s-present). To be dominated by a wife or female partner for fear of losing sexual favors.

PUTTING ON AN ONION (Australian slang, 1960s-present). Submitting to serial copulation with a number of partners in succession. Also PULLING A TRAIN.

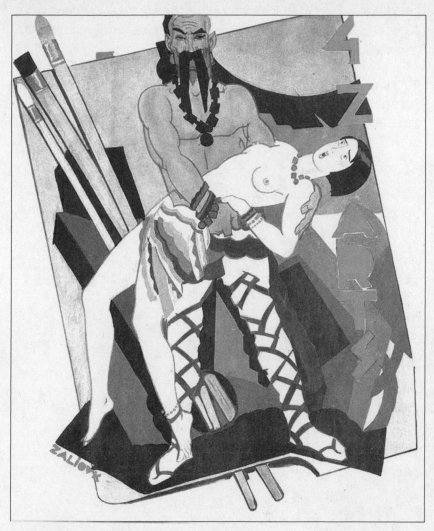

ARTIST'S IMPRESSION OF QUATZ'ARTS BALL, PARIS, 1920s

QUATZ'ARTS, BAL DES (The Ball of the Four Arts). Notorious annual event of Paris in the first half of the twentieth century, traditionally an opportunity for art students and MODELS to behave outrageously, and wear as little clothing as possible. Anything more than a coating of BODY PAINT and a G-STRING was looked on as overdressing.

QUEEN (U.S. slang, 1920s-present). Male homosexual with an effeminate manner, adapted to describe any gay preoccupied with a single sexual aspect. See LEATHER QUEEN; RICE QUEEN.

QUEENING. Bondage position in which a woman squats on the partner's face, anus aligned with his nose, vagina covering his mouth, which places the subject's ability to breathe under her control.

QUEER (noun and adjective) (U.S. slang, 1920s–present). Male homosexual. Originally used in the sense of "odd" or "eccentric." Adapted as a term of abuse, then, defiantly, by the homosexual community as a synonym.

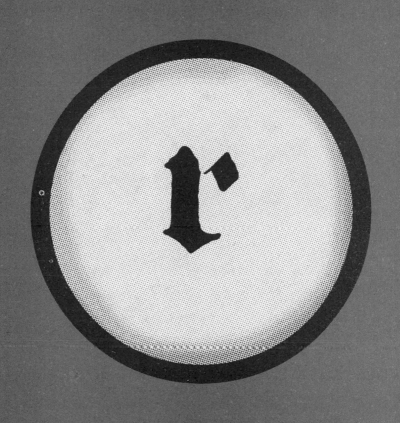

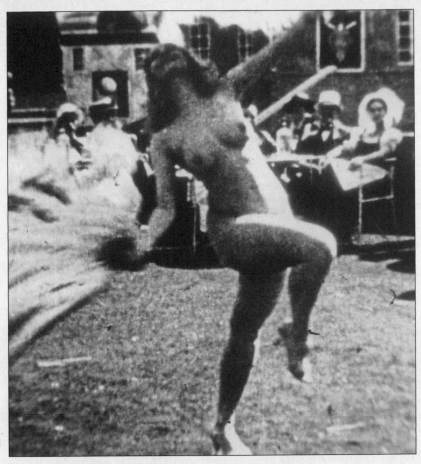

SALLY RAND DOING HER FAN DANCE AT THE 1933-1934 CHICAGO EXPOSITION

RAND, Sally (*née* Harriet Helen Gould Beck) (1904–1979). Exotic dancer.

After a brief acting career from which she emerged only with her stage name, coined by director Cecil B. DeMille, Rand gained notoriety at the 1933–1934 Chicago Century of Progress Exposition, where young entrepreneur Mike Todd presented an attraction called *The Streets of Paris*, as part of which Rand performed her Fan Dance, apparently nude but for two sheaves of ostrich feathers and a pair of high-heeled pumps. Filming the show, Todd sold hundreds of prints as souvenirs. Her performance won Rand a part in the film *Bolero* (1934), opposite George Raft and Carole Lombard, where she danced in a nightclub setting, and even had a minor acting role. First with fans, then with balloons, Rand continued to perform into her sixties, when she appeared at a reception for the astronauts of the Apollo program, an event celebrated in the film *The Right Stuff*.

Rand curtailed her activities during World War II when her body paint, without which she couldn't perform, was reserved for use on fighting ships. College students who sat in the front row of her shows, shooting bent pins from elastic bands, also drove up the cost of her act by forcing her to buy industrial-strength balloons.

REACH-AROUND (U.S. gay slang, current). Masturbating a sex partner with one's hand during sodomy.

RÉAGE, Pauline. See DESCLOS, Anne.

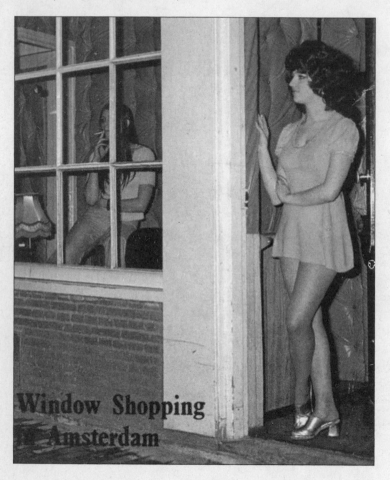

Window Shopping in Amsterdam

RED LIGHT DISTRICT. Brothel quarter, so named because prostitutes customarily displayed a red lamp in their windows.

REEMS, Harry (né Herbert Streicher). Aka Bruce Gilchrist, Charles Lamont, Tim Long, Harry Reams, Harry Reemes, Ned Reems, Harry Rheems, Herb Streecher, Herb Stryker, Bob Walters (1947–). U.S. actor.

Dinner theater, summer stock, Off- and Off-off-Broadway were the nurseries of porn. Actresses with good looks and not much talent could always find work in sex

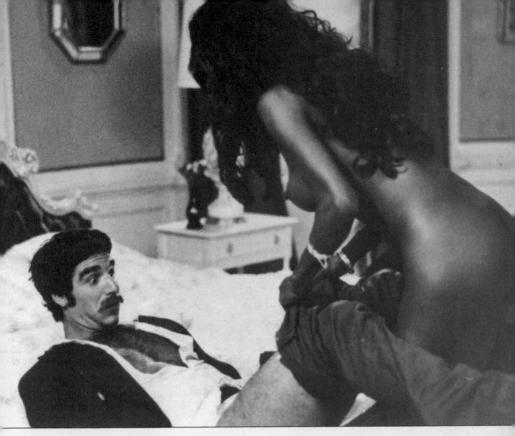

HARRY REEMS IN *BEL-AMI*

films, and actors who were well-built, well-hung, and with an ability to maintain an
erection were equally employable. Reems, a stocky man with a bushy moustache, wasn't
classic leading-man material, but he had worked in New York's Café La Mama and the
National Shakespeare Company, as well as appearing in commercials for products such
as Wheaties breakfast cereal.

At Christmas 1969, he was out of work, with no prospects, when he heard
one could earn seventy-five dollars for a morning's work in porn LOOPS. Over
the next three years, he appeared in more than four hundred, before playing the
doctor in *DEEP THROAT*. "I made little on *Deep Throat*," he says, "but subsequently I was paid thousands of dollars a day just to have my name on the title
credits [in other films]. I'd end up with three teenage girls in a bed and get paid
a thousand dollars to do it. Every week the number of women grew and the number of dollars grew."

Once the FBI launched its MIPORN investigations, Reems was an obvious target—
director GERARD DAMIANO and star LINDA LOVELACE having been granted immunity. Presenting the prosecution as not so much an attack on Reems as on freedom of
speech, lawyer Alan Dershowitz rallied an array of showbiz greats to his defense, including Jack Nicholson, Mike Nichols, Stephen Sondheim, and Gregory Peck. Reems toured

the United States, lecturing on anomalies in the obscenity laws. After an appearance at the Harvard Law School, the president of its organization Forum wrote, "To be honest, you were not at all what we had been expecting, and we were pleasantly surprised not only at your general articulateness, but especially at your knowledge of the legal issues involved in your case and their ramifications."

Despite these efforts, Reems was convicted in 1976 of conspiracy to distribute obscene material across state lines. Though the sentence was overturned, the case left him with massive debts and a dependency on cocaine and alcohol. Unable to work in the United States, he appeared in the German *Young Butterflies* and a 1975 Swedish update of De Maupassant's *Bel-Ami*. As the poet and journalist in the latter, trying to fuck his way into a connection with *Playhouse* magazine, he was less than convincing.

Resurfacing in the United States in 1982, he made several brief pseudonymous or anonymous appearances, becoming an increasingly disagreeable member of the Los Angeles porn community. Jerry Butler, working on *Marilyn Chambers' Private Fantasies #6* in 1985, was distracted in part by CHUCK TRAYNOR's gun-toting presence but more by a furious Reems bursting on the set to demand his pay from the director. Director Harley Cokeliss, visiting an L.A. police station around the same time, encountered Reems manacled to a steel bench in a holding cell, raging, "Don't you know who I *am*?"

After spells in mental institutions, Reems drifted to Utah. In Park City, a tiny ex-silver-mining town of five thousand people mainly known as the site of Robert Redford's Sundance Film Festival, he kicked alcohol, married, moved into real estate, and became a trustee of the local Methodist church.

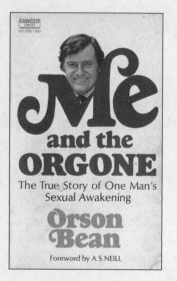

REICH, Wilhelm (1897–1957). Austrian-born psychiatrist whose theories on human sexuality led to imprisonment and death.

Reich's rural childhood fitted him to be more a patient for psychoanalysis than a therapist. At age ten, he was already experimenting with ZOOPHILIA, driving himself to orgasm by masturbating a mare with a whip handle. He spied on the family MAID having sex, and by age eleven was sleeping with the cook. When he was fourteen, his mother, in remorse over her affair with his tutor, killed herself, profoundly affecting Reich.

As a therapist in Vienna, Reich showed a particular interest in adolescent sexuality. Building on the work of SIGMUND FREUD and Karl-Gustav Jung, he proposed the existence of the "orgone," a form of energy that permeated all living things. An inability to conserve orgone energy not only led to psychosis and sexual dysfunction but also accounted for political movements such as communism and fascism.

He tried to measure the energy expended during the male orgasm and, arguing that the force could be conserved and amplified, designed the "orgone accumulator"—a box whose mirrored interior restored the depleted orgone energy of the patient who sat inside. He also, according to 1960s TV personality Orson Bean, a Reich convert, found that "by kneading, pressing or jabbing at certain muscles used to inhibit crying, he could make the patient spontaneously start to sob, and he found that other muscles, when jabbed at or pressed, would cause rage-filled screaming. He encouraged his patients to give in to these natural functions."

Reich's theories were widely disputed, and many in the medical community regarded him as a crank, or even mentally unstable. Resistance hardened with the publication of his books *The Sexual Revolution* and *The Mass Psychology of Fascism*, which argued that both Nazism and COMMUNISM exhibited the effects of sexual repression. Targeted by both the right and left, and ostracized by the medical community, Reich fled to Scandinavia in 1933, then to the United States in 1939.

In the United States, he extended his theories to claim that orgone accumulators could cure cancer. The Food and Drug Administration banned their sale. When Reich persisted, his books were burned, and in 1956 he was sentenced to two years in prison, where he died. Reich's theories have gained support since his death, helped by celebrities such as KENNETH TYNAN, William Burroughs, and Orson Bean, whose book *Me and the Orgone* celebrated his own Reichian therapy. Dusan Makavajev, director of the 1971 film *W. R.: Mystery of the Organism*, was another convert to Reich's ideas.

RENT BOY. Young male prostitute. Also title of novel by Gary Indiana.

RENZY, Alex de (1935–2001). Aka Rex Borski, Rex Borsky. U.S. porn producer and director.

De Renzy entered porn as the proprietor of The Screening Room, a San Francisco cinema that ran a continuous program of LOOPS. He soon started production, turning out five or six loops a week, which, like the MITCHELL BROTHERS, he sold on to other cinemas across the country. The de Renzy loops were distinctive, often using attractive outdoor locations and off-beat sexual imagery.

In 1970, de Renzy directed the more ambitious feature-length *Censorship in Denmark: A New Approach*, for which he covered a Danish porn film in production, interviewed a (nude) porn actress, visited sex shops and a pornographers' trade show, and filmed nightclub acts such as Olga and Her Sex Circus, whose performers prowled among the audience, encouraging them to masturbate or join in the action—the kind of show from which LORD LONGFORD fled during his fact-finding visit with his anti-pornography committee. He also produced the feature-length *A History of the Blue Movie*.

Unfortunately this early enterprise didn't survive the relentless pressures of the market. During the 1990s, de Renzy reverted to the name Rex Borsky, and to anal porn, ending his career with a succession of sodomy titles such as the manic *Anal Booty Burner*, *Anal Cornhole Cuties*, *Borsky's Backdoor Bitches*, the despairing *Another Fuckin' Anal Movie*, and, most intriguing of all, *Anal Crash Test Dummies*.

RICHARD, Marthe (aka Marthe Betenfeld, Martha Crompton, Martha Richer) (1889–1982). French prostitute, spy, and social reformer.

Though she never admitted it, Richard began her career as a prostitute in Bordeaux. Infected with syphilis, she fled to Paris, married a wealthy businessman named Richer, took up aviation, and by faking some epic flights, became a famous aviatrix. During World War I, by then a widow, she spied for France as mistress of Baron Von Krohn, head of the German navy in Madrid. The war won, she again married money, this time the British financial director of the Rockefeller Foundation.

She might have remained an obscure figure had her ex-employer in the Secret Service not mentioned her in his fanciful memoirs (along with his other unsuccessful recruit, MATA HARI). Though he got her name wrong in the process, changing "Richer" to "Richard," she accepted the change, demanded a share of his royalties, then wrote her own even-more-imaginative account. *My Life as a Spy in the Service of France* was filmed in 1937. Glamorous Edwige Feuillere portrayed Richard as a patriot roused to vengeance by German atrocities against her family. Erich von Stroheim played Krohn as a monocled eccentric who so misses the cavalry that rather than sitting in a chair behind his desk, he straddles a saddle.

During World War II, Richard consorted with the Nazi-backed puppet government in Vichy, then moved to Paris, where, while supposedly spying on the Gestapo, she actually arranged sex parties for Nazi officials and collaborators. In 1945, in a wave of national contrition, Paris's 4th Arrondissement elected her to the municipal council.

Desperate for a vote-getter, she proposed turning Paris's 180 brothels into student housing, then in short supply. The crackpot proposition passed, leading in 1946 to the closing of 1,400 *maisons closes* nationwide. Since most students indignantly refused to live in ex-bordellos, the brothels became *HOTELS DE PASSE*, renting rooms by the hour to prostitutes, who, forced back onto the streets, were no longer subject to the obligatory weekly health check. Sexually transmitted diseases proliferated. An unrepentant Richard lived to ninety-three, pontificating on feminism, contraception, and sex in general. Asked for the secret of her longevity, she claimed, "Abstinence has helped me age so well."

RIMMING. Sexual stimulation by licking the anus.

Primarily a gay activity, but also popular with straights, including BILL CLINTON. According to the Starr Report, he and Monica Lewinsky, in addition to FELLATION, "engaged in oral-anal contact." See also TROMBONE.

ROCKEFELLER, Nelson Aldrich (1908–1979). U.S. politician.

A philanthropist and politician who served as New York State governor and vice president of the United States from 1974 to 1977, Rockefeller entered the sexual mythology when he died on January 26, 1979, following a heart attack during sex with his twenty-six-year-old mistress. In the film *Dave* (1993), Kevin Kline plays a presidential lookalike who is called upon to impersonate a president who has suffered a similar fate. The same year, in *Indecent Proposal*, billionaire Robert Redford pays $1 million to spend one night with Woody Harrelson's wife, played by Demi Moore. Lawyer Oliver Platt includes a clause in the agreement to cover the "Rockefeller Scenario."

ROOT, ROOTED (Australian slang, 1900s–present). To indulge in sex. Also, to be exhausted. Source obscure—perhaps from *rut*.

ROTH V. UNITED STATES.

At first glance, this 1957 decision by the U.S. Supreme Court appeared to criminalize erotica by declaring that it wasn't protected by the First Amendment's guarantee of freedom of speech. However, the court also chose to discard the so-called common sense definition of pornography proposed in 1964 by Justice Potter Stewart, who had decreed, "I shall not today attempt further to define the kinds of material I understand to be embraced [i.e., pornography] . . . [b]ut I know it when I see it."

Instead, the court decided that "the standard for judging obscenity . . . is whether, to the average person, applying contemporary COMMUNITY STANDARDS, the dominant theme of the material, taken as a whole, appeals to prurient interest." Under this ruling, lawyers could argue that an item considered obscene in conservative Georgia might be acceptable in more liberal California. Among the far-reaching effects of the decision was the wholesale migration of adult film production from New York to Los Angeles.

ROTSLER, William Charles (1926–1997). (Aka Barney Boone, Shannon Carrse, Shannon Carse, W. A. Chrisfield, Clay McCord). Author, critic, and film producer.

Gifted as a science fiction writer, film critic, cartoonist, glamour photographer, and director-editor-actor in erotic films, Rotsler was too intelligent to survive long in the porn world. His ambivalence is evident in his book *Contemporary Erotic Cinema* (1973), which analyzes the field in incisive and amused detail. Appreciation for the skill of performers such as MARILYN CHAMBERS is matched by scorn for beady-eyed hustlers such as RON JEREMY.

His own soft-core porn films as director, in some of which he also acts, are mediocre. They include *The Girl with the Hungry Eyes* (1967), *House of Pain and Pleasure* (1969), *Midnight Hard* (1970), and *Street of a Thousand Pleasures* (1972) (the latter two as Clay

McCord), and *Mantis in Lace* (1968), about a GO GO DANCER who commits a series of murders with kitchen implements and garden tools.

Out of place in the dog-eat-dog world of video porn, Rotsler returned to glamour photography, and to writing and illustrating science fiction, his first love. In increasingly poor health, he spent his last years odd-jobbing round the edges of the sex business, including ghosting autobiographies for phone-sex personalities. He also designed and executed the awards for the XRCO's annual HEART-ONS.

"When I started making films in 1965, I would cast personalities. Because when you're working at this level, you're not working with actors. You're lucky if you get someone who can act. But if you can get them in a certain state of mind, where it's just their personality, they love it. They're not working. They're just having fun."
—WILLIAM ROTSLER

ROUGH TRADE (U.S. gay slang, 1960s–present). Tough male prostitute, usually working-class, who offers an often violent sexual experience.

ROUND HEELS (U.S. slang, 1920s/1930s). Supposed sign of promiscuity—either because a woman whose heels were round would have a tendency to fall on her back, or, alternatively, because the heels of her shoes would become rounded down by such activity.

RUBBING UGLIES (Australian slang, 1990s–present). Sexual intercourse.

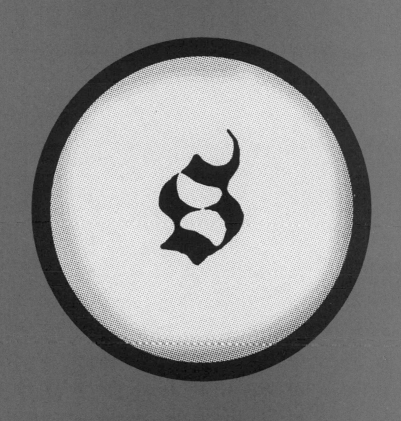

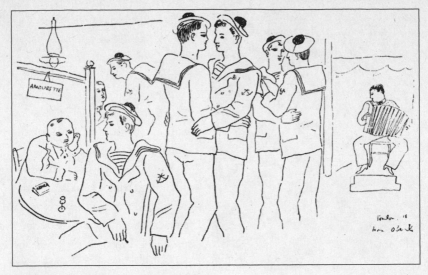

SAILORS DANCING TOGETHER IN FRENCH GAY BAR

SAILORS.

Conventionally, the sailor is shown as a horny heterosexual with a "girl in every port," whereas it's an open secret that many are gay or at least bisexual, particularly during long periods at sea. Even Winston Churchill, as First Lord of the Admiralty, acknowledged that "the traditions of the Navy" were "rum, sodomy and the lash." So well established was the practice that an informal regulation existed: homosexual acts became permissible once a ship had been out of port for thirty-nine days .The dichotomy was summarized in the truism "On land, it's wine, women, and song. At sea, it's rum, bum, and concertina."

Hetero sailors appear in U.S. musicals such as *Born to Dance*, *On the Town*, *The Fleet's In*, and in such dramas as *Since You Went Away* and *Cinderella Liberty*. Gay sailors in film are rarer but feature in Rainer Werner Fassbinder's film of JEAN GENET's *Querelle de Brest*, with Brad Davis as Fassbinder's sexual hero. More are found in literature. Celebrations range from George Melly's memoir of his gay life at sea in *Rum, Bum and Concertina*, and James Hanley's novel *Boy*, banned in Britain but published by the OBELISK PRESS in Paris, to the bawdy ballad "THE GOOD SHIP VENUS," where the cabin boy "lined his arse / with broken glass / and circumcised the skipper." In art, the muscled torsos and erect penises of sailors feature in JEAN COCTEAU's *Le Livre Blanche* and in the drawings of Gregorio Prieto and "TOM OF FINLAND."

ST. CYR, Lili (née Willis Marie Van Schaack) (1917–1999). U.S. dancer-actress-stripteaser.

Throughout the 1940s and 1950s, Lili St. Cyr was as famous as GYPSY ROSE LEE and SALLY RAND, even though, like them, she removed only a few clothes, and then only at the last minute. For one act, she lathered up in a solid silver bath, supposedly

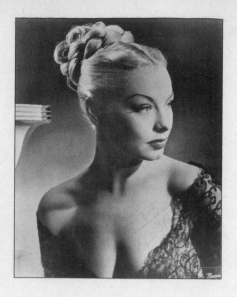

made for the Empress Josephine. Even with her covered in soap suds, her act was so inflammatory that a drunken Humphrey Bogart tried to barge into her dressing room. In another routine, the "Flying G," an invisible fishing line whipped off her G-STRING the instant the lights went out.

St. Cyr was often in court, accused on one occasion of "making the theater stink with the foul odour of sexual frenzy," though the charges seldom stuck. Less cautious in her private life, she had six husbands and many lovers of both sexes, one of whom could have been the young MARILYN MONROE. St. Cyr introduced her to the cameramen who photographed her first pinups, and Monroe did imitate St. Cyr's breathy voice and seductive body language, but it's unlikely they shared a bed.

Taken up by Howard Hughes, St. Cyr appeared in a number of his productions, including the 1955 *Son of Sinbad*, though she showed off more in two IRVING KLAW films, *Varietease* and *Teaserama*. In retirement, she opened a mail-order lingerie business, The Undie World of Lili St. Cyr, clients of which reputedly included MADONNA. In old age, she announced defiantly, "Only two things count in life—work and sex."

SALIVA PAJAMA (Italian slang, 1960s). To lick someone over the whole of their body.

JAMES BOND creator Ian Fleming told a friend "Sophia Loren had been on the set of one of her films in Italy, and the technicians had called down from their hoists that they'd like to give her a saliva pyjama." British performance artist Neil Hornick recalls, "For a one-man street theatre spectacle at the Glasgow Garden Festival, I stood at a corner, deliberately silent, gloomy, pale and haggard-looking, dressed in a shabby brown suit, tie and trilby, with a large notice hanging round my neck stating: 'LICK YOU ALL OVER—10P'. Most passersby reacted, as I anticipated, with surprise, revulsion and/or laughter. Little did I imagine that anyone would actually take me up on the offer. Unfortunately, one rugged Glaswegian matron insisted on doing just that, and I found myself duty-bound to oblige. I don't recommend the experience. She was no Sophia Loren. "

SALON KITTY. World War II Berlin brothel.

Ordered to set up a brothel to spy on foreign diplomats and the Nazi hierarchy, SS officer Walter Schellenberg took over the whorehouse of Kitty Schmidt at 11 Giesebrechtstrasse, and connected its rooms to recording equipment in the basement. Business

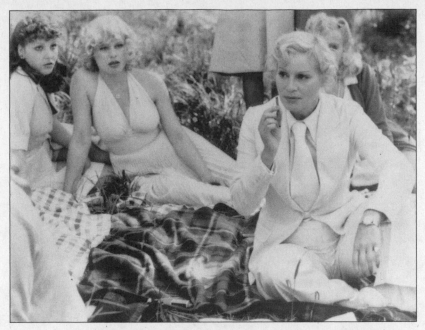

INGRID THULIN AS KITTY SCHMIDT WITH SOME OF HER GIRLS IN THE TINTO BRASS MOVIE *SALON KITTY*

continued as before, except when a client used the phrase "I come from Rothenburg," indicating he'd been sent there as a subject for surveillance. This alerted Schmidt to summon one of twenty prostitutes trained by Schellenberg in extracting information.

Except for some careless pillow talk from foreign diplomats, the scam never justified the effort. British intelligence quickly infiltrated it, and Salon Kitty mostly became a recreational facility for members of the SS and German high command, who used the girls, or spent hours giggling over tapes of their betters having sex. Allied bombing in July 1942 damaged the building and hastened its closing. Schmidt survived the war, but remained silent about Salon Kitty until her death in 1954.

ALSO

SALON KITTY (1976). Italian film. Directed by Tinto Brass.

Helmut Berger plays the Schellenberg character as a rogue officer who eavesdrops in order to blackmail his superiors. Ingrid Thulin is Kitty, and Theresa Anne Savoy is a prostitute who exposes the scheme. In Brass's version, the specialist whores, to test their "adaptability," are required to have sex with macabre and outlandish partners, including dwarves and a multiple amputee. Paradoxically, the effect of the film is to depict the Nazis as victims of the devious Schellenberg. The film is notable mainly as a warm-up by Brass for *CALIGULA*, in which Savoy, a protegée of BOB GUCCIONE, also starred.

SANCTUARY, THE. New York gay disco that occupied a deconsecrated church at the corner of Tenth Avenue and Forty-eighth Street. None of the furnishings had been removed; Bob Colacello, editor of Andy Warhol's *Interview* magazine, recalled leaning against a confessional and watching "a zonked-out dj spinning soul songs on the altar, the after-hours hustlers HEAVY PETTING in the side pews, the stiletto-heeled transvestites twirling under the strobe lights that flashed across the nave."

SANDSTONE RANCH.

From 1969 to 1976, the fifteen-acre Sandstone estate of John and Barbara Williamson in the Santa Monica Mountains of Southern California became, in the phrase of GAY TALESE, a "clothes-optional recreational center for adults." While its organizers always disavowed any intention to make it the center of SWINGER culture, its publicity did state that "open expressions of affection and sexuality are appropriate when mutual. While neither nudity nor sexual sharing are ever required, Sandstone does offer a serene setting where the real worth and dignity of human sexuality may be experienced." *JOY OF SEX* author ALEX COMFORT was a semi-permanent resident.

SATYRIASIS. See NYMPHOMANIA.

SCARIFICATION. Practice of cutting and scarring the skin so as to raise permanent ridges or bumps.

Employed by many African tribes to indicate manhood, it has been adopted by some Westerners as an erotic accessory. In one variation, beads are inserted under the skin of the penis, supposedly to heighten the pleasure of the person penetrated.

SCHWARZENEGGER, Arnold (Arnold Alois Schwarzenegger) (1947–). Actor and politician.

Austrian-born Schwarzenegger found fame in bodybuilding contests such as Mr. Europe, Mr. World, and Mr. Universe (which he won five times). Promoted by Joe Weider, publisher of *Muscle and Fitness* magazine, he won similar U.S. competitions during the late 1960s. However, as photographer George Butler noted, "Arnold was in a sport that no one liked, and he had a physique that people were repulsed by. In those days, the biggest problem we had was the homophobic attitude of the press. 'All of these bodybuilders are gay. We don't want anything to do with it.' " The fact that Schwarzenegger shared an apartment with Italian bodybuilder Franco Columbu ("The Sicilian Samson") didn't help. Nor did his assurances (and those of women friends) that he was heterosexual.

Yet within two decades of his arrival in the United States, and notwithstanding slurs such as critic Clive James's gibe that he resembled "a large brown condom stuffed with walnuts," Schwarzenegger was one of Hollywood's biggest stars.

Schwarzenegger, who had seen fellow bodybuilders Reg Park and Steve Reeves waste their best years heaving Styrofoam rocks around Rome's Cinecittà studios, knew sheer muscle wasn't in itself negotiable. But there had to be a way to make all that sweat saleable, and George Butler's book *Pumping Iron* suggested it. The 1977 documentary the book inspired gave Schwarzenegger a platform from which to articulate the pleasures of working out. As oxygenated blood raced through a muscle it created a "rush" comparable to orgasm. Every instant in which he gorged his tissues with blood, he experienced sexual ecstasy. "Get it?" his satisfied smile seemed to say.

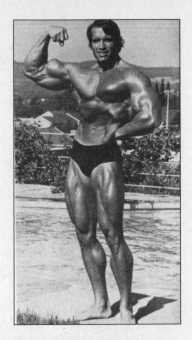

ARNOLD SCHWARZENEGGER

He underscored the lesson in a 1977 interview with *Oui* magazine, in which he went out of his way to establish his hetero credentials. "Bodybuilders party a lot," he said, "and once, in Gold's—the gym in Venice, California, where all the top guys train—there was a black girl who came out naked. Everybody jumped on her and took her upstairs, where we all got together. . . . Not everybody, just the guys who can fuck in front of other guys. Not everybody can do that. . . . Having chicks around is the kind of thing that breaks up the intense training. It gives you relief, and then afterward you go back to the serious stuff."

Once established as 100 percent male, Schwarzenegger was free to expose his softer side. He loosened up his lumbering gait with ballet lessons. ROBERT MAPPLETHORPE photographed him, and he was painted by Jamie Wyeth. A seminar on male sexuality at New York's Whitney Museum observed him in the flesh as a living work of art. As the pièce de résistance, he was fêted at a Manhattan cocktail party by publisher Viking. Guests included Jackie Onassis. After she and Arnold chatted for fifteen minutes, his future was assured.

SECOND SEX, THE (DEUXIEME SEXE, LE) (1949). Book by Simone de Beauvoir.

Pioneering work of sexual philosophy that articulated the contrasting attitudes of the sexes to one another. Taking its key from the existentialism developed by her companion Jean-Paul Sartre, de Beauvoir argues that women must redefine themselves in relation to men.

In her introduction, she writes, "humanity is male and man defines woman not in herself but as relative to him; she is not regarded as an autonomous being." In a quote from the philosopher Julien Benda, which many subsequently attributed to her alone, de Beauvoir says of Man, "He is the Subject, he is the Absolute—she is the Other."

SEMEN.

Difficult to depict in painting or drawing, semen acquired new erotic significance with the appearance of cinema. By the 1960s, the FETISH had a substantial contingent of admirers, who demanded to see it on-screen, making the MONEY SHOT an essential component of any porn picture. In Richard LaGravanese's script for Terry Gilliam's 1991 *The Fisher King*, video rental store proprietress Mercedes Ruehl quizzes a borrower, "Whatcha looking for? A story? What?" When he mumbles, "Something with semen," she thrusts a tape into his hand. "Here y'are," she says. "*Creamer vs. Creamer*." A further subgroup favors FACIALS, where semen spatters the woman's face. In 1989, the photographic artist Andreas Serrano excited controversy with his creations, which incorporated his own blood, urine, and semen. Works included *Frozen Semen* and *Ejaculation in Trajectory*. See BUKKAKE.

72. The same as a "69," but with three fingers inserted into the appropriate orifices.

SEWING CIRCLE, THE (U.S. slang, 1920s–1940s). Lesbian social group within the Hollywood film and literary community.

Originally denoting a sorority that gathered socially to sew, usually quilts, the term *sewing circle* was adapted to cover private parties of upper-class lesbians, and the informal power circles they created, particularly in the Hollywood film industry from the 1940s onward.

The LESBIANISM that flourished in Germany under the Weimar Republic migrated to British and U.S. film in the early 1930s with a number of actresses and technicians, including Leontine Sagan, director of *Maedchen in Uniform*, and dancer Valeska Gert. Sapphism flourished in Hollywood. So long as a woman married or indulged in occasional relationships with men, she could pursue a lesbian lifestyle undisturbed. Joan Didion cites director Otto Preminger saying approvingly, "A nice lesbian relationship, the most common thing in the world. Very easy to arrange. Does not threaten the marriage."

Greta Garbo was the *éminence grise* of the so-called Sewing Circle, abetted by sometime lover Mercedes d'Acosta. Other members, active or emeritus, included MARLENE DIETRICH, director Dorothy Arzner, Judy Garland, Tallulah Bankhead, Patsy Kelly, Joan Crawford, Katharine Hepburn, Katharine Cornell, Barbara Stanwyck, Marjorie Main, Nancy Kulp, and Agnes Moorehead.

Though some members frequented Santa Monica gay bars such as the Golden Bull and S.S. Friendship, they convened mostly at the homes of members such as Dolores Del Rio, then involved in a LAVENDER MARRIAGE to Cedric Gibbons, gay MGM art director, or Maria Huxley, who was both bisexual and a procurer of women for her writer husband. "Maria Huxley tamed women for Aldous," wrote novelist May Sarton. "The young tigress, you know; she broke them in." When the circle convened at the Huxley home, one of Maria's lovers, such as the artist Eva Hermann, or "another nubile girl would lie face-down on a mirrored coffee table, while onlookers photographed or stroked her."

"Confidentially, I've had them both, darling—and they were terrible."
—TALLULAH BANKHEAD, OF THE BRIDE AND GROOM AT A WEDDING

SEX (1926). U.S. play by MAE WEST.

West played Margy LaMont, a prostitute in a Canadian BROTHEL. The play ran for 375 continuous performances on Broadway before the police closed it down and sentenced West to ten days' imprisonment for corrupting the morals of youth.

SEX AND THE CITY. U.S. cable TV series and 2008 film. Highly successful HBO sitcom (94 episodes between 1998 and 2004) inspired by Candace Bushnell's book of the same name, which derived in turn from a series of columns in *The New York Observer*.

The series follows the sex lives of four independent professional New York women, including a publicist, a lawyer, and an art dealer (Kim Cattrall, Cynthia Nixon, and Kristin Davis), who profess to shun permanent relationships yet nevertheless define themselves in relation to the men they habitually pursue. Narrated by the articulate but chronically dissatisfied columnist Carrie Bradshaw, played by Sarah Jessica Parker, *Sex and the City* cut benchmarks for cable TV in the discussion of sexuality, and inspired a number of similar programs, including the lesbian-themed *THE L WORD*.

sex, lies and videotape (1989). U.S. film. Directed by Steven Soderbergh.

Soft-spoken James Spader travels the United States coaxing women into describing their sex lives on videotape, to which he later masturbates. A visit to old college friend Peter Gallagher and his subsequent involvement with Gallagher's unhappy wife (Andie MacDowell) and her sensual sister (Laura San Giacomo), who's also Gallagher's lover, shakes up the lives of all four, mostly for the better. Made for $1.6 million, the film won the Palme d'Or at Cannes and received an Oscar nomination for writer-director-editor Soderbergh. *sex, lies and videotape* helped launch the new independent U.S. cinema, and accelerated sales of portable VIDEO recorders.

SEX MACHINES (1920s–present). Mechanisms that duplicate the motion of copulation.

The twentieth century's first sex machine was imagined by the French writer Alfred Jarry. His 1902 novel *Le Surmale* (*The Supermale*) features an athlete who, after single-handedly beating a six-man team in a bicycle race, has sex with eighty-two women. When he shows no signs of exhaustion, an English inventor creates a sex machine something like an electric chair, which finally drains his erotic energy but kills him in the process. The "Excessive Machine" of BARBARELLA and the "Orgasmatron" of *Sleeper*, by WOODY ALLEN, were variations on the same idea, though less lethal.

Real sex machines were first built by amateur eroticists in the 1920s but subsequently turned into a minor industry. Most use an electric motor and cam to drive a shaft with a dildo attached. Simpler types combine a stool and dildo. The user straddles the stool and rocks back and forth, causing a dildo to rise and fall. The two were combined to create the SYBIAN. See also GYNOIDS.

SEX TAPES.

As sexual indiscretions go, the writing of effusive love letters is exceeded only by the recording of a sex video. That so many celebrities have succumbed to the temptation reveals tellingly their degree of intelligence.

Discounting STAG FILMS of the sort attributed to later stars such as JOAN CRAWFORD, gay porn films featuring future action star Chuck Connors, and the film, shot early in her career, of MARILYN MONROE giving a BLOW JOB, the first homemade porn to create headlines was that of aging "Brat Pack" actor Rob Lowe cavorting at the 1988 Democratic Convention with two girls, one of whom was later revealed to be underage. Lowe's career didn't suffer, and he went on to star in the hit series *The West Wing.*

In 1994, disgraced Olympic figure skater Tonya Harding featured in a graphic "wedding video" with her husband, Jeff Gillooly. (Harding subsequently embarked on a new show business career as a wrestler, for which, as the tape proved, she had a natural aptitude.) In 1996, a tape of *Baywatch* star Pamela Anderson performing oral sex on her then-husband, rock drummer Tommy Lee, was supposedly stolen by a construction worker remodeling their house. It quickly become public property, with—it must be said—some benefit to Anderson's flagging career, even though the couple made strenuous, though finally unsuccessful, attempts to retrieve the tape and sue those who had exploited it.

That the release of an apparently clandestine piece of porn could jump-start a career or jolt an ailing one was not lost on the world's has-beens and wannabes, so nobody was very surprised when a sex tape surfaced in 2004 that made an overnight celebrity of bubble-headed hotel heiress Paris Hilton. Shortly after, she began a brief and, so far, undistinguished career in movies and reality TV.

SEXUAL FREEDOM LEAGUE.

Formed in New York in 1963 by twenty-one-year-old Jefferson Poland, the SFL stated its aims as promoting sexual activity among members and agitating for reform of the abortion and censorship laws. The SFL tradition of ORGIES developed when Poland moved to the San Francisco area, relocating the League at the University of California, Berkeley. He first attracted national attention in August 1965 when he led a "Nude Wade-in" at Aquatic Park, a public beach in San Francisco.

In 1966, he relinquished the East Bay League to Richard Thorne, a charismatic African American. As the frequency of sex parties increased, members more interested in the League's political and social aims formed their own group. Leadership of the non-sex branch passed to Alida Reyenga, while UC Berkeley student Sam Sloan took over the pro-sex group. The latter hosted twenty-eight nude parties, the last of them on Christmas Eve 1967, usually regarded as the date at which the League expired.

SHEMALE (1990s–present). Shorthand term for transsexual in process of transition from male to female. Most have acquired some female characteristics through hormone treatment but still retain male genitalia.

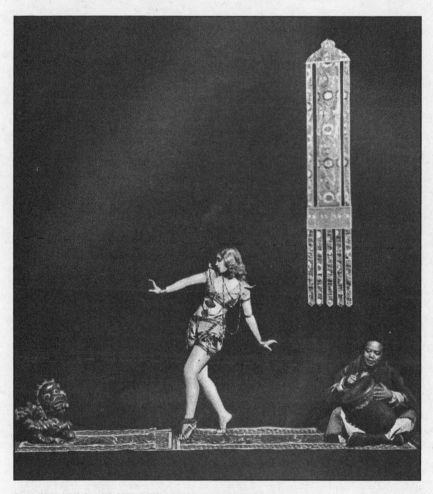

GILDA GRAY, WHO CLAIMS CREDIT FOR INVENTING THE SHIMMY

SHIMMY (Sometimes Shimmy and Shake, Shake and Quiver, Shimmy Sha-Wobble, Hooche-Cooche) (1893–1920s). Erotic female dance in which the feet remain stationary but the body moves provocatively. Probably from French *chemise*, a "shirt" or "shift."

Versions of the Shimmy can be found in Haitian voodoo and African tribal dances, and even in Russia, where an agitated dance, the *horon*, was supposedly inspired by the mating movements of the *hamsi*, a species of anchovy that, like the Californian grunion, stands on its tail in wet sand and quivers spasmodically to fertilize its eggs.

As a dance, it appeared late in the nineteenth century as the "Shake and Quiver." In 1893, various dancers using the name LITTLE EGYPT performed it as the "Hooche-Cooche" in New York and Chicago. The "Shimmy Sha-Wobble," is mentioned in a song called *The Bullfrog Hop*, in 1908. Gilda Gray popularized the word *shimmy* in 1918, when she described her dance as "shaking her chemise," though MAE WEST also claimed to have invented it, and sang "Everybody Shimmies Now," in the show *Sometime* (1919). In 1922, it gained international prominence with Armand Piron's song "I Wish I Could Shimmy Like My Sister Kate."

The Shimmy revived in the 1950s, once dancing couples were no longer required to touch, and gained impetus from the 1960s *BEACH PARTY* cycle of films. Dancers of the Freeze, the Swim, the Surf, or the Stomp simply struck a pose and undulated, quivered, or shook. During the 1960s, GO GO DANCERS popularized tasseled or fringed dresses, which such dances served to show off. In her 1975 piece *Sue's Leg*, to music of Fats Waller, choreographer Twyla Tharp cleverly toyed with the erotic possibilities of the Shimmy, showing one of her dancers standing in place and shrugging a loose shirt on and off her upper torso.

SILVER, Jean "Long Jean" (Aka Joan Beattie, Jean Fulda, Jeanne Silver, Long Jeanne Silver) (19??-). U.S. porn actress.

The left leg of Silver, a thalidomide victim, tapered to a stump just below the knee. In 1977, desperate for work, and knowing that the MITCHELL BROTHERS sought all physical types for their films, she volunteered her services, describing herself as "handicapped and horny." Seeing her potential, the Mitchells first featured her as a stage act at their Kopenhagen Lounge. Her small stature permitted her to use her truncated lower leg as an outsized penis. She did so with some skill, even doubling it back to insert it in her own vagina, as well as the vaginas and rectums of others—sometimes to such depth that audiences became alarmed.

Launched on the porn scene, Silver moved to New York, and found her niche in LEATHER, SPANKING, and ENEMA films, some of them for ALEX DE RENZY, and including the notorious 1977 *WATERPOWER*. She also came out as a lesbian, living initially with porn star Sharon Mitchell, then with ANNIE SPRINKLE, a relationship forged during the two days they were jailed for participating in a photoshoot for *Love* magazine in which Silver's stump played a major role.

"SILVER, Long Dong" (*né* Daniel Arthur Mead) (1960-). U.S. porn actor.

Bermuda-born Mead starred in a few porn films in the 1980s, on the strength of a penis so long he could tie a knot in it. Once the organ was exposed as a fake, he retired, and would have been forgotten had his name not surfaced during the 1991 U.S. Supreme Court confirmation hearings on the appointment of Clarence Thomas. Senator Orrin Hatch produced a former female associate of Thomas who testified that "he spoke about acts that he had seen in pornographic films" and also mentioned Silver. Despite this evidence, Thomas was appointed to the Court. (Paradoxically, a former page to Senator Hatch, Eliza Florez, enjoyed, as "Missy Manners," a brief X-rated career, notably in *BEHIND THE GREEN DOOR: THE SEQUEL*.)

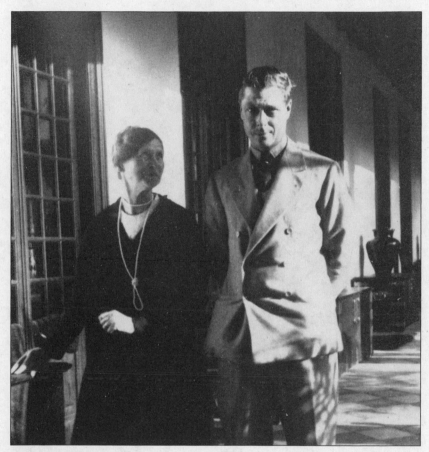

DUKE OF WINDSOR

SIMPSON, Wallis (later DUCHESS OF WINDSOR) (*née* Bessie Wallis Warfield) (1896–1986). Socialite.

Twice-divorced, U.S.-born Simpson married the future Edward VIII, heir to the English throne, precipitating his abdication in 1936. Rumors claimed that while living in China with her first husband, Simpson visited brothels to learn the technique of vaginal constriction known as the "Shanghai Squeeze," or CASANOVA CLIP. Reputed to "make a matchstick feel like a Havana cigar," these skills supposedly turned the sexually unsophisticated Edward into her abject slave.

Mrs. Simpson was also credited with mastery of *FANG CHUNG*, a Chinese form of oil massage in which the erogenous zones are stimulated one by one over a long period, leading to a spectacular climax that can be almost indefinitely delayed by finger pressure on the

"I have found it impossible to carry the heavy burden of responsibility and to discharge my duties as king as I would wish to do without the help and support of the woman I love."
—EDWARD VIII
. ABDICATION SPEECH

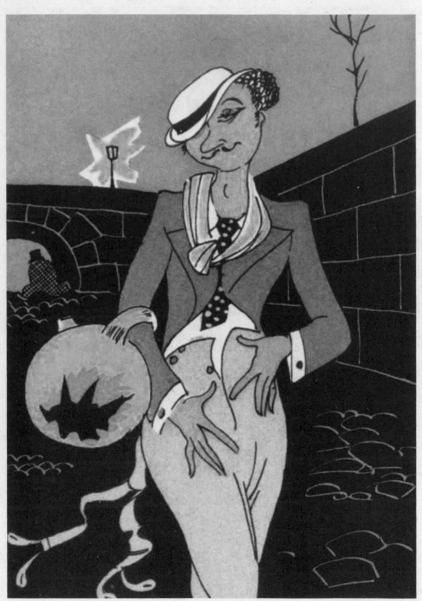

PARODY IMAGE OF A "SISSY MAN" AFTER A GAY ENCOUNTER ON THE BANKS OF THE SEINE, PARIS, 1930s.

area between the urethra and the anus. Even wilder claims were made for her sexual dominance of the complaisant prince. One courtier described glimpsing the duchess in nurse's uniform whipping the duke, who was dressed only in a diaper.

SISSY and SISSY MAN (U.S. slang, 1880s-1940s). Male displaying effeminate characteristics.

Though once widely used as a synonym for *homosexual*, *sissy* wasn't always uncomplimentary. African American women feared "sissy men" as serious competitors for the affections of their men. In Thomas Dorsey's *Sissy Blues* (1926), Ma Rainey sang:

> Some are young, some are old.
> My man says sissies got good JELLY ROLL.
> My man's got a sissy, his name is Miss Kate.
> He shook that thing like jelly on a plate.
> Now all the people ask me why I'm all alone.
> A sissy shook that thing and took my man from home.

Another blues lament runs,

> Woke up this morning with my troubles in my hand.
> Can't get me a woman, gonna get me a sissy man.

69. Mutual oral sex—so named because the Arabic numeral mimics the relative positions of those involved.

SIZE QUEEN (U.S. slang, 1980s-present).
Person of either sex preoccupied with penis dimensions in sexual partners.

SLASH FICTION (International, 1960s-present). Amateur pornography, mostly by and for women, which imagines gay relationships between the paired male stars of TV series conventionally separated by a solidus, or "slash," e.g., Batman/Robin, Starsky/Hutch.

Writers in *Star Trek* fanzines were the first to propose a gay relationship between two of its characters. In *Amok Time* (1967), scenarist Theodore Sturgeon shows Spock as a victim of "Pon Farr," a periodic frenzy to reproduce. In the episode, Spock and Capt. James Kirk fight, apparently to the death, but fans preferred a conclusion in which Kirk satisfied Spock's mating urge by becoming his lover.

Diane Marchant's 1974 *A Fragment Out of Time* is regarded as the first *Star Trek* slash novel, but the idea soon spread to other series with dual male stars (e.g., *Starsky and Hutch, Randall and Hopkirk, Deceased*), then to boy bands and to different-sex series such as *The X Files*. The cast of the British sci-fi TV series *Blake's 7*, disturbed by slash fiction inspired by their characters, tried to have it banned, without success.

SNOWDROPPING (Australian slang, 1960s). Stealing female underwear from outdoor clothes lines.

***SNUFF* (1976).** Argentine/U.S. film. Directed by Michael and Roberta Findlay and Horacio Fredriksson.

In January 1976, *Snuff* opened at a cinema off Times Square. Posters showed a woman's body chopped by giant scissors, under the slogan "The Bloodiest Thing That Ever Happened in Front of a Camera." In the film, members of a Manson-type cult in an unnamed Latin American country vow revenge on the rich. A man is castrated, another shot, and a pregnant woman butchered. At the conclusion of this scene, the director and film crew are seen walking into the shot. A pretty blond production assistant tells the director she found the scene sexually arousing, and he invites her to join him on the bed.

Feminist writer Beverly LaBelle, describing the film, went on, "They start fumbling around in bed until she realizes that the crew is still filming. She protests and tries to get up. The director picks up a dagger that is lying on the bed and says, 'Bitch, now you're going to get what you want.' What happens next goes beyond the realm of language. He butchers her slowly, deeply, and thoroughly. The observer's gut revulsion is overwhelming at the amount of blood, chopped-up fingers, flying arms, sawed-off legs, and yet more blood oozing like a river out of her mouth before she dies. But the climax is still at hand. In a moment of undiluted evil, he cuts open her abdomen and brandishes her very insides high above his head in a scream of orgasmic conquest. The End . . . Fade into blackness. There are no credits listed in the final moments of the film."

Indeed no credits were listed—perhaps out of embarrassment. *Snuff* was a fake. Originally called *Slaughter*, it had been shot in Argentina in the mid-1960s. Ten years on, producer Allan Shackleton resurrected it. The added "murder" of the production assistant was shot in New York. As the final touch, he arranged for protestors to picket the theater. "Pickets sell tickets," he told the press. New York district attorney Robert Morgenthau quickly uncovered the hoax and refused to prosecute. Feminist groups all over the United States, however, made it a cause célèbre.

SNUFF FILMS (1980s–present). Film in which a performer is actually murdered.

"There has been . . . a rumour that persisted for a long time during the years 1975–78 about 'snuff movies,'" wrote French critic Michael Caen in 1991, "that is to say films in which the actors, the actresses were really put to death. No specialist—I think of AL GOLDSTEIN—has seen them. Nor could the FBI or the police find them."

Few topics occupied so much energy in the porn debate during the 1970s as the existence or otherwise of snuff films. To some feminists, they were the inevitable next step in pornography. That men were capable of such things, radical campaigners such as Andrea Dworkin didn't doubt. "Men love death," she said. "In everything they make, they hollow out a central place for death, let its rancid smell contaminate every dimension of whatever still survives. Men especially love murder. In art they celebrate it, and in life they commit it. They embrace murder as if life without it would be devoid of passion, meaning, and action, as if murder were solace, stifling their sobs as they mourn the emptiness and alienation of their lives."

In 1979, the feminist lobby cited an anonymous ex-porn actress who claimed, "One agency in Los Angeles sent a woman out on an assignment with a man who killed her and took pictures of how he tortured her. The business just froze. Models went to work with their boyfriends, and some stopped coming in altogether. Everyone was terrified. That didn't last long though. People need money in order to live." The actress wasn't identified, nor the filmmaker, nor the agency.

Feminist ideologue Gloria Steinem was equally vague in 1983, claiming that snuff movies had been "driven underground (in part because the graves of many murdered women were discovered around the shack of just one filmmaker in California). . . . The last screening of a snuff movie showing a real murder was traced to the monthly pornographic film showings of a senior partner in a respected law firm; an event regularly held by him for a group of friends including other lawyers and judges." Which filmmaker? Which lawyer? Why was nobody prosecuted? In more than two decades since these statements, no hard evidence of snuff films has emerged.

The 1990 film *Henry: Portrait of a Serial Killer* shows the confederate of a serial murderer taping a rape-murder. Even though the killers on whom John McNaughton based his film made no such recordings, such videos undoubtedly exist. But fears that they will find their way into porn cinema are unfounded—not out of repugnance or fear of retribution on the part of pornographers, but because there's no audience. Neither blood nor death itself are sexually fetishized for most people, so only an infinitesimal number are interested in seeing someone killed on-screen.

Hollywood has fitfully addressed the possibility of snuff films. In *Videodrome* (1982), cable TV operator James Woods scorns the art porn offered to him by a Japanese dealer and goes looking for something "stronger." He finds it in a private channel on which a naked girl is tortured against an electrified wall of wet clay. The show is "just torture and murder. No plot. No characters. Very realistic." Otherwise, movies accept that snuff exists in the tiniest of niches. In *8mm* (Joel Schumacher, 1999), investigator Nicolas Cage tracks down the perpetrator of a snuff film, but Andrew Kevin Walker's script is honest enough to show him as someone who makes such things on order for private clients, not with any idea of their reaching an audience. A *CSI Las Vegas* episode also showed the investigators trapping a filmmaker who'd made snuff, but again as a one-off.

SNURGING (European and U.S. slang, 1920s-present). Sexual stimulation in sniffing girls' bicycle seats.

One of the most widely reported adolescent practices, snurging is celebrated in François Truffaut's 1958 short film *Les Mistons*, where the boys jostle to sniff the seat of Bernadette Lafont's bike.

SO (UK slang, 1900s). Euphemism for male homosexual—as in, "Is he 'so'?" (i.e., "that way"). (see also MUSICAL.)

SOFT-CORE. Erotic film or photography that doesn't show genitals, penetration, etc. Many films exist in both "soft" and "hard" versions. (See also HARD-CORE.)

SOHO. District of central London bounded by Oxford Street, Tottenham Court Road, Shaftesbury Avenue, and Lower Regent Street. (Not to be confused with Manhattan's SoHo, meaning "South of Houston Street.")

Soho is traditionally the RED LIGHT district of LONDON, and home to prostitution and pornography. For most of the twentieth century, both operated barely under cover, thanks to extensive corruption. Photographer-filmmaker GEORGE HARRISON MARKS recalled the milieu as it was around 1950. "There was an Obscene Publications Squad then. I was in Gerrard Street at the time. There were dozens of heavy porn bookshops and a very big porn [production] industry, which doesn't exist now, strangely enough. Proper hardcore stuff. The Old Bill [i.e., police] were paid off regularly. The stuff came from abroad, not home-grown. Soho was flooded with porn."

Crime novelist Robin Cook, alias Derek Raymond, whose novels of the London underworld, such as *The Devil Is Home on Leave* and *I Was Dora Suarez*, rest on firsthand observation, managed a Soho porn shop in the 1950s. He was taken aback when a group of policemen walked in and demanded "the films." After denying there were any on the premises, he called his boss—who explained that, far from wanting to bust the shop, the police were collecting entertainment for their Christmas party.

From the 1980s to the present, Soho became home to numerous sex shops, covert brothels, strip clubs, and the source of the prostitute cards that decorated the interiors of phone boxes throughout central London. Its narrow streets provided settings for a number of books and films, notably *Expresso Bongo*, *PEEPING TOM*, and *Absolute Beginners*.

SOPHISTIQUE SOFT. 1980s marketing term for the type of high-budget SOFT-CORE porn features typified by *EMMANUELLE*, with an emphasis on exotic locations and beautiful people.

SPELVIN, Georgina (Michelle Graham) (1936-). Also Chelle Grame, Merle Miller, Ruth Raymond, Georgette Spelvin, Claudia Clotoris, Ona Tural (pron. "Unnatural"). U.S. adult film actress.

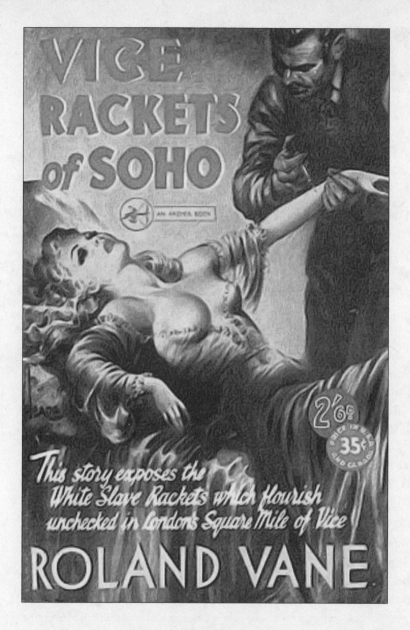

Shelly (sometimes Chelle) Graham ran away from home as a child to join the circus. Later she danced in USO shows, in the chorus of Broadway productions of *The Pajama Game*, *Guys and Dolls*, and *Cabaret*, acted Off-Broadway, worked as a dance director, appeared in TV commercials, and held a desk job in advertising, where she met GERARD DAMIANO. In 1962, she played a brief lesbian scene for RADLEY METZGER, to liven up the U.S. version of the French film *Les Collegiennes*. Thereafter, she appeared anonymously in several porn LOOPS, and played small roles in adult features.

In the summer of 1968, Graham, divorced three times and living in a lesbian relationship, was working as a captain of dancers on the Barbra Streisand musical *Hello,*

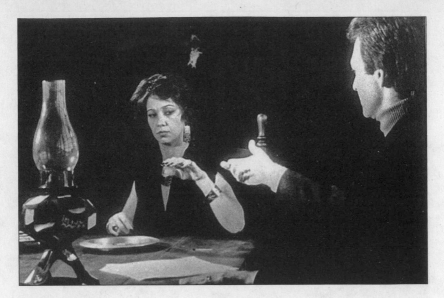

GEORGINA SPELVIN

Dolly! at Garrison, in upstate New York. About 10:00 p.m., she'd leave the set, get the train to Manhattan, shoot two porno LOOPS, catch the 5:00 a.m. train and be back ready to work when director Gene Kelly called, "Action." She got $1,500 for her work on the musical and only $100 for each porn film. Asked why she bothered for $200 a night, Graham said, "I did it because I was a star in those films, and in *Hello, Dolly!* I was just in the background."

Her break came when Damiano cast her in his first feature after *DEEP THROAT, THE DEVIL IN MISS JONES,* then shooting on a ranch owned by co-star HARRY REEMS. Graham claims she simply applied for a job as the unit caterer and cook. Damiano had already chosen a younger actress but decided Graham would be more credible as the middle-aged librarian of the story. His offer added another one-liner to the porn lexicon. Graham recalled, "They told me, 'We'll give you $100 a day and all the cock you can eat.'"

Unimpressed, she recruited her partner, Judith Hamilton, credited as "Clair Lumiere," to play opposite her in the lesbian scene. She also took a *nom de porn,* "Georgina Spelvin," a version of "George Spelvin," the pseudonym used by stage actors who don't wish to be identified.

As Spelvin, she appeared in more than seventy adult films. In addition, she had small roles in the low-budget horror film *I Spit on Your Corpse!,* for which she also served as costume designer, and the 1984 comedy *Police Academy,* as the prostitute who hides in a lectern to fellate Commandant George Gaynes, a role she repeated in *Police Academy 3: Back in Training.*

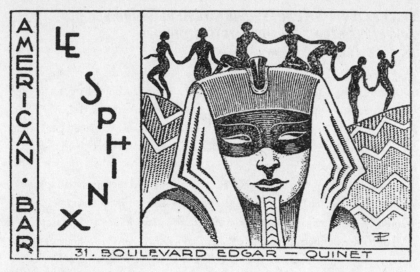

ADMISSION CARD TO LE SPHINX

SPHINX, LE (1926–1946). High-class Paris BROTHEL on Rue Edgar Quinet, opposite Montparnasse cemetery.

Famous for its Egyptian décor, mirrored rooms, and the beauty of its girls, the brothel was patronized by MARLENE DIETRICH, Duke Ellington, sculptor Alberto Giacometti (who claims to have contracted a sexually transmitted disease there), and HENRY MILLER, who wrote copy for its brochures and was paid in "trade."

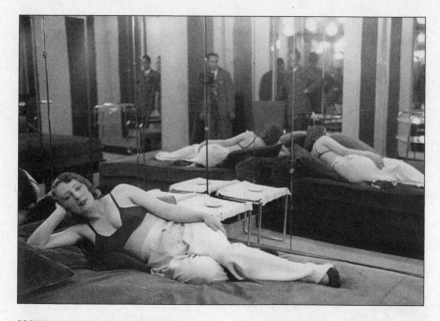

ROOM IN LE SPHINX, WITH PROSTITUTE AND CLIENT

SPICY DETECTIVE STORIES, SPICY WESTERN STORIES, SPICY ADVENTURE STORIES, SPICY MYSTERY STORIES (c. 1934–1940s). U.S. pulp magazines.

Published by the improbably named Culture Publications, the *Spicy* pulps were so popular that proprietors Harry Donnenfeld and Frank Armer could charge twenty-five cents a copy rather than the customary ten cents. Covers, usually by H. J. Ward, were lurid, featuring semi-naked young women being tortured, or terrorized by monsters, human or animal. Customarily, his illustrations appeared in two forms, with the uncensored version reserved for more sophisticated city buyers.

Culture paid top rates to writers, yet never copyrighted their material, assuming nobody would ever wish to reprint it. Most authors hid their identities rather than be identified with the magazines' S&M content. Hugh B. Cave, for instance, masqueraded as "Justin Case." Others, particularly Robert Leslie Bellem, used pseudonyms only to disguise the fact that they sometimes wrote entire issues. New York mayor Fiorello La-Guardia, who had already campaigned against BURLESQUE, put Culture Publications out of business when he took exception to Ward's cover for the April 1942 *Spicy Mystery*, which showed a semi-naked girl hanging from a hook in a meat locker while being menaced by a thug holding a very large knife.

Culture's and Bellem's most enduring invention was Dan Turner, a private eye always being stunned by a beautiful half-naked woman or by the butt of a forty-five. The cliché plots and terminology of the Turner stories were parodied, along with *Spicy Detective* itself, by S. J. Perelman in his essay "Somewhere a Roscoe," but a few years later the bestselling novels of MICKEY SPILLANE, an enthusiast for Bellem and Turner, demonstrated the longevity of the *Spicy* formula.

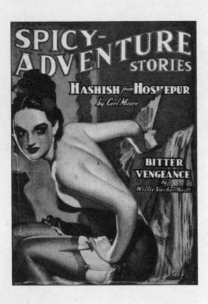
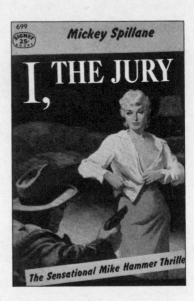

SPILLANE, Mickey (Frank Morrison Spillane) (1918–2006). American writer.

An ex-fighter pilot, Spillane began writing for comic books, contributing scripts to *Superman* and *Captain Marvel*. When publishers rejected his idea for a comic featuring hard-boiled private eye "Mike Danger," Spillane turned the character into "Mike Hammer," and wrote a novel instead. He claimed it took six days to finish *I, the Jury*, which was published in 1947, to instant success. It ends with Hammer shooting his nude but treacherous lover in the stomach with a forty-five, to revenge the death of a war buddy. When, in her last breath, she asks, "How could you?" he responds memorably, "It was easy." Terry Southern praised this climax as making "Malaparte, Céline and other high priests of the *roman noir* look like a bunch of pansies."

Though he lifted much from Dashiell Hammett's *The Maltese Falcon*, Spillane's work was closer to the pulp tradition of magazines such as *Black Mask* and particularly *Spicy Detective*. He acknowledged only one literary influence—John Carroll Daly, pulp writer-creator of the private eye Race Williams. His debt to the pulps was emphasized when Signet issued his novels in paperback with cover illustrations worthy of *SPICY DETECTIVE*.

Spillane's (and Signet's) run of bestsellers continued with *Vengeance Is Mine* and *My Gun Is Quick* (1950), *The Big Kill* (1951), and *Kiss Me Deadly* (1952), the last made into a film by Robert Aldrich. *Kiss Me Deadly* begins with Hammer encountering a woman on the highway, nude under a raincoat. She's subsequently tortured to death with a pair of pliers—by, as it turns out, Communist fifth columnists, who had became Spillane's primary villains. In *One Lonely Night*, Mike Hammer machine-guns forty of them—reduced by the publisher from eighty, which was thought "too gory."

Spillane was admired by artists as unlikely as filmmaker Stanley Kubrick and polemical novelist Ayn Rand. Rand praised his anticommunism, as did John Wayne, who expressed his patriotic appreciation by presenting Spillane with a Jaguar XK140. When it was stolen with the manuscript of a new novel inside, Spillane mourned the car; the book, he said, simply meant the loss of three days' work.

Identifying unashamedly with his characters, Spillane dressed as Hammer, even playing him in a movie, *The Girl Hunters* (1963), and marrying the blond model who posed nude for the cover of *The Erection Set*. He shrugged off the scorn of better authors. "Those big-shot writers," he sneered, "could never dig the fact that there are more salted peanuts consumed than caviar." His knowledge of his market was acute: "The first page sells your book," he said. "The last page sells your next book." Few people read him today, but he's survived by his image. As Raymond Chandler said of Sherlock Holmes, he was "an attitude, and a dozen lines of unforgettable dialogue." Of Spillane's unforgettable lines, the best may be his response to the news that Hemingway had attacked him in print. Spillane asked innocently, "Hemingway who?"

> *"I don't have fans. I have customers."*
> —MICKEY SPILLANE

SPLIT BEAVER. An image in which the vagina appears with the lips parted. See BEAVER.

SPORT FUCKING. Fornication exclusively for pleasure, without emotional commitment.

Sport fucking originally meant the promiscuity enjoyed by people emerging from a restrictive relationship, but was subsequently widened to include sex as a form of exercise. Traditionally, one vigorous sexual act gave the same aerobic benefit as running three times round London's Thurlow Square.

Opinion is divided among athletes about whether sex improves performance. According to British boxing champion Gary Stretch, "sex tires you greatly and you need to keep your energy. Six weeks before every fight, I wouldn't allow myself to look at a woman." In a variation of this rule, middleweight champion Jake LaMotta would invite his beautiful teenage wife to visit him in his dressing room before each fight, encourage her to excite him, then plunge his penis into ice water just before orgasm, so as to enter the ring aroused but unsatisfied.

All sports stars of either sex agree on the aphrodisiac effect of the sporting life. Basketball player Wilt "The Stilt" Chamberlain claimed twenty thousand sexual partners, each so desirable that "the average Joe would have proposed marriage on the first date." Magic Johnson, diagnosed as HIV-positive in 1991, said, "I can't pinpoint the time [of infection], the place or the woman. It's a matter of numbers." An anonymous British athlete confessed, "Athletics is a fuckfest; that's the only word for it." Of the Commonwealth Games, he continued, "I know of athletes who have no chance of making the finals in their event but just go for the party. You have people employed for the sole purpose of handing out free condoms. The village is so testosterone-filled that it goes on from the first day to the last."

SPORTING (U.S. slang, late 1800s and early 1900s). Relating to prostitutes or prostitution.

A SPORTING HOUSE or SPORTING PALACE was a BROTHEL; SPORTING WOMEN were prostitutes. "Sporting Life" is the PIMP character of DuBose Hayward's *Porgy* and, subsequently, of George Gershwin's opera *Porgy and Bess*.

> *I hope those sporting ladies don't get sunburned. I like 'em white as pastry.*
> —THOMAS MCGUANE, IN HIS SCREENPLAY
> FOR *THE MISSOURI BREAKS* (1976)

SPRINKLE, Annie (*née* Ellen Steinberg) (1954–) (Aka Annie Sprinkles). U.S. actress.

After a career as a prostitute, Sprinkle drifted into porn in the mid-1970s, and appeared in two hundred LOOPS, shorts, and feature films, some for longtime partner

GERARD DAMIANO. Even in the unbuttoned world of porn, Sprinkle's choice of roles was regarded as extreme, in particular her appearances in S&M films such as *Bizarre Styles* and *Kneel Before Me*, the latter cited by the MEESE COMMISSION as conspicuously violent. She also acted with, and for a time was the lover of, handicapped porn performer LONG JEAN SILVER.

Sprinkle relaunched herself in the 1980s as a performance artist and lecturer—a therapeutic process, she claimed, "to heal and transform my life." For a piece called "A Hundred Blow Jobs," she mimed fellatio with a dozen dildoes. "I played a tape of all the abusive remarks I'd heard, like, 'Suck it, you bitch!' and I sucked on all these different dildoes. I'd cry and gag and really get in touch with the pain each time. After a dozen times, I would no longer cry or gag—because I had transformed and exorcised that demon."

Slides prepared by Sprinkle quantified the total length of the penises sucked in her career (equivalent, she estimated, to the height of the Empire State Building) and summarized with a "pie chart" graphic her motives for entering porn. Money represented one-third of her reasons, followed by "Didn't Know What Else I Wanted to Do" and "Love and Attention." The wedge given to "Sex" was almost invisible.

Like ILONA STALLER in her live show, Sprinkle concluded her presentation by spreading her legs on the edge of the stage and inviting the audience to examine her, a way of "demystifying" the female body. The show, which received some federal funding, was denounced by reactionary senator Jesse Helms. Sprinkle continued to present it through the 1990s, though only to audiences of women or CROSS-DRESSING men.

STAG MOVIE (1920s–1980s). Pornographic short film, usually of one reel (i.e., nine minutes). So named because it was seen by uniquely male "stag" audiences.

In 1986, the report of the MEESE COMMISSION would frankly acknowledge that "stag films are a familiar and firmly established part of the American scene . . . shown privately, not only by individual citizens, but also by civic, social, fraternal and veterans' organizations." It decided that 44 percent of male adults had seen at least one stag film. (A 1986 *Time* survey revised that to 77 percent.)

While the commission branded professional porn as an encouragement to crime, it took a benign view of stag films, believing they "represent the preferences of the middle-class American male." It noted that in the stag world, "male homosexuality and bestiality are relatively rare, while lesbianism is rather common. In recent years, there has been an increased emphasis on group sex, usually three or four individuals, but as many as seven have been noted in a single film. Many stag films attack certain forbidden social and sexual themes; for example, taboos against miscegenation, cunnilingus, and fellatio are constantly assaulted in American stag films, while foreign countries with a strong religious base have a significant anti-clerical strain in their stag films. The taboo against pedophilia, however, has remained almost inviolate. The use of pre-pubescent children in stag films is almost nonexistent."

U.S. society and law traditionally tolerated nonprofit "stag" screenings. Films shown in private to consenting adults without payment of admission conveniently fell through the crack between the laws against pornography and those protecting free speech and the right to privacy. Pornographers also evaded the postal laws by sending their films on the road with a projectionist, who often, in imitation of the BURLESQUE tent shows, traveled the same route each year, presenting his program at anything from twenty-five to one hundred dollars a night to audiences as large as two hundred.

Such screenings often took place at the premises of fraternal groups such as unions and lodges, which generally owned the largest hall in town and whose members were not of the arrestable class. "Three shots of corn likker," wrote Nelson Algren of lodges in his novel *A Walk on the Wild Side*, "and the whole stuffed zoo—Moose, Elks, Woodmen, Lions, Thirty-Third Degree Owls and Forty-Fourth Degree Field Mice—begin to conspire against the very laws they themselves have written." In Bloomington, Indiana, the American Legion announced stag screenings in the local paper.

Equally honored as an institution was the private stag night (*Stag Party* was one of HUGH HEFNER's original titles for *PLAYBOY*). At this male equivalent of the bridal shower, men ritually mourned the end of a friend's bachelorhood with gorging, boozing, and whoring. Their milieu was exploited often by U.S. writers and filmmakers, e.g., Paddy Chayefsky's TV play and film *Bachelor Party*.

Purists argue that readily accessible video porn, in eradicating the communal experience of the stag screening, with its camaraderie and ribald commentary, robbed society of a valuable social institution, as slick modern pole dance shows superseded BURLESQUE with its bellowed exhortations to "Take it off!" However, as suggested by episodes of the U.S. TV series *Ally McBeal* and *The West Wing*, in which male characters shamefacedly confess to have gotten drunk at such parties, enjoyed watching strippers, and sometimes having sex with them, the stag night still flourishes.

STALLER, Ilona (née Ilena Anna Staller). Aka "La Cicciolina," Elena Mercuri) (1951–). Hungarian Italian actress and politician.

Sometime model Staller made her first erotic films in Italy in the mid-1970s and was soon a familiar face (and body), readily identified by her nickname "La Cicciolina," meaning "The Little Pinchable One," her pink teddy bear, and a trademark pink dress that revealed one bare breast.

A skilled self-publicist, Staller used her notoriety to launch a political career. To protest apathy toward the Chernobyl disaster, she was driven around Rome and Milan nude except for a radioactive carnation. In 1987, she won election to the Italian parliament as a Radical Party candidate, running on a platform of relaxed censorship, NATURISM, and sexual rights for prison inmates. To celebrate her victory, she paraded in Rome's Piazza Navona, hugging her bear and triumphantly pulling down her dress to show her breasts.

Breaking with the Radical Party, Staller launched the *Partito dell'Amore*, or Party of Love, recruiting fellow porn actresses such as Moana Pozzi as supporters. At the same time, she inaugurated a startling stage act, part sex, part politics. Stalking near-nude round a set featuring Gothic lighting effects and giant diabolic images, she alternated four-square songs in her little-girl voice—they sounded like Calvinist hymns fed through an electronic beat box—with political homilies. Men were invited onstage to examine her body, fondle her, even have sex with her—not for erotic effect, but to emphasize their shared humanity.

In 1989, flamboyant and handsome U.S. NeoPop artist Jeff Koons caught her show and went backstage to suggest a collaboration. The plan to make a film together metamorphosed into a sexual liaison. Koons shrugged off the fact that neither spoke the other's language. "Ilona and I were born for each other," he announced. "She's a media woman. I'm a media man. We are the contemporary Adam and Eve."

Koons documented their relationship in photographs of the couple naked and, in some cases, copulating. From these, he created giant plastic and wooden sculptures, installations and paintings—including one called *Ilona's Asshole*, which premiered at the Venice Biennale as *Made in Heaven*. They married shortly after.

Staller announced her retirement from politics and porn at the end of 1991, and also her pregnancy. A son, Ludwig, was born in 1992. But widespread hostility to *Made in Heaven* strained the marriage, as did the languishing of the *Partito dell'Amore*. Now under the presidency of Moana Pozzi, it failed to win a single seat at the 1992 elections. At the British premiere of *Made in Heaven* the same year, Staller and Koons announced their divorce, citing "differences between our cultural and social standing." When Staller defied a court order by spiriting Ludwig out of the United States, Koons spent millions of dollars on an unsuccessful ten-year struggle to regain custody. Meanwhile, Staller resumed her porn and political activities, even offering to have sex with Iraqi dictator Saddam Hussein if he would release foreign hostages. "You can't change somebody who was involved in the profession she was involved in," Koons said despairingly in 2007.

STANLEY V. GEORGIA. A landmark 1969 case in which the U.S. Supreme Court reversed the decision of the Supreme Court of Georgia that it was illegal to possess pornography, even when it was not being offered for sale.

"If the First Amendment means anything," decreed Justice Thurgood Marshall, "it means that a state has no business telling a man, sitting alone in his house, what books he may read, or what films he may watch." Reflecting a new climate of acceptance, the Court also decreed that to be classed as "obscene," a work must be "patently offensive" and have no "serious artistic, literary, political, or scientific value when taken as a whole." See *ROTH V. UNITED STATES*.

STANTON, Eric (1926–1999) (*né* **Ernest Stanzoni).** Erotic illustrator.

Stanton's Amazonian women, tall and massively breasted, with flowing manes of hair, set the tone for fetish art in the United States after World War II. He started drawing while in the navy, and worked as a dancing waiter and knife-thrower in vaudeville.

For a time, he shared a studio with Steve Ditko, and worked peripherally on Ditko's *Spiderman*, the influence of which is evident in his work.

In 1947 he won a job with IRVING KLAW, and illustrated numerous NUTRIX publications. He proved particularly expert in CAT FIGHTS and at depicting a dominatrix in command of a cringing male submissive. After the demise of Nutrix, Stanton's work, which included a comic strip, *Blunder Broad*, a parody of WONDER WOMAN, was sufficiently respected to command a large private market. As the acknowledged dean of fetish artists, he was consulted by ALFRED KINSEY during the latter's research.

STARK, Koo (*née* Kathleen Dee-Anne Stark) (1956–). Actress and photographer.

U.S.-born Stark, who starred in two British erotic films, *Emily* (1976) and *Cruel Passion* (1977), and had a small, albeit deleted, role in *Star Wars*, became the girlfriend of Prince Andrew, then second in line to the British throne, who smuggled her into Buckingham Palace on a number of occasions. Once her film career became public, the Royal Family terminated the romance. She later became a successful portrait photographer.

STEELY DAN. Strap-on penis or dildo invented by William Burroughs for his novel *Naked Lunch* (1959). Adopted as a stage name by rock musicians Donald Fagen and Walter Becker.

> *"Mary is strapping on a rubber penis. 'Steely Dan III from Yokohama,' she says, caressing the shaft."*
> —FROM *NAKED LUNCH*, BY WILLIAM BURROUGHS

STILETTOS. Women's spike-heeled shoes, typically black and in patent leather, a feature of FETISH and pedophile erotica.

STONEWALL RIOTS.

Early on the morning of Saturday, June 28, 1969, eight New York City police, only one in uniform, raided the Stonewall Inn, a Greenwich Village gay bar. They had ample justification. Stonewall lacked a liquor license, was a known pick-up spot for gays, lesbians, and CROSS-DRESSERS, and featured seminude male GO GO DANCERS. However, until then, police had been warned not to provoke the city's growing homosexual community.

The resentment felt by New York gays in general at this apparent harassment flared into a riot. Retreating into the bar, the police called for reinforcements as the mob tried to batter down the door with a parking meter, then set the building on fire. The battle fought between four hundred police and an estimated two thousand protestors ended with thirteen arrests, and injuries on both sides. Disturbances continued for another week, resisting even the efforts of tactical groups formed to battle Vietnam War protestors. As violence escalated, the crowd spontaneously chanted, "Gay Power!" the first public use of this later-iconic slogan. In July, the GAY LIBERATION FRONT was formed, largely as a result of the militancy engendered by Stonewall, and the following June, on the anniversary of the riots, ten thousand people marched from Greenwich Village to Central Park in a telling demonstration of gay power.

STORY OF O (See **HISTOIRE D'O**).

STORYVILLE. Brothel quarter of New Orleans.

Pianist and composer "Jelly Roll" Morton recalled "they had everything in the [Storyville] District from the highest class [brothel] to the lowest—creep joints where they'd put the feelees on a guy's clothes, cribs that rented for about five dollars a day and just had about enough room for a bed, small-time houses where the price was from fifty cents to a dollar and they put on naked dances, circuses and jive. Then, of course, we had the mansions where everything was of the highest class . . . Mirrors stood at the foot and head of all the beds. It was in those mansions that the best of the piano players worked." The U.S. Navy closed down Storyville in 1917 as a health risk to servicemen, but not before it had served as the cradle of jazz. See BELLOCQ, E. J.; JAZZ.

STREAKING (UK slang, 1970s). Running naked through a public place, usually before spectators, and often to achieve some satirical effect or for profit.

LADY GODIVA may constitute the first streaker, but the first examples of modern streaking occur around 1904. The practice reappeared spontaneously among U.S. college students in the late 1960s. In 1974, Michael O'Brien, an Australian, ran naked across the field at an England-vs.-France football match. The same year, Los Angeles sex shop owner Robert Opel, possibly with the connivance of Jack Haley, Jr., that year's telecast producer, streaked at the Oscar ceremony, cueing presenter David Niven to comment, "Probably the only laugh that man will ever get in his life is by stripping off and showing his shortcomings." Streaking dwindled in the 1990s, and survives mainly as an advertising stunt. Mark Roberts of Liverpool claims to hold the world record of four hundred streaking episodes, including one at the 2006 Winter Olympics, where he appeared at a curling match between Britain and the United States naked except for a rubber chicken, and with the name of an online gambling website printed on his back.

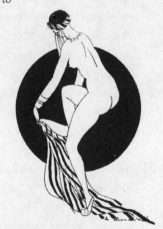

STRIP POKER. Variation of the card game in which players remove a piece of clothing for each hand lost.

STRIPTEASE. Theatrical performance involving the removal of clothing for erotic effect.

STRIPTEASE, PARIS, 1930s

No two authorities agree about the origin of striptease. Women and, less often, men for millennia have removed their clothing in a provocative manner for the benefit of sexual partners. Salome's Dance of the Seven Veils represents an early authenticated example of such a performance in public, The ritualized theatrical form, however, is an invention of the nineteenth century, documented in the 1896 film *LE COUCHER DE LA MARIEE.*

Burlesque popularized striptease as performance, creating the ritualized "bump and grind" style in which the dancer shook her breasts and made suggestive movements with her hips while removing her costume. Variations included tassels attached to the nipples, which the dancer could rotate. The predictability of these routines helped make stars of dancers such as GYPSY ROSE LEE and LILI ST. CYR, less because of their beauty than for the imagination with which they performed.The extinction of burlesque in the 1940s drove striptease into bars, where it was often presented in cabaret under theatrical conditions, with atmospheric lighting. Paris's CRAZY HORSE SALOON became the most famous of such clubs.

STRYKER, Jeff (*né* Charles Casper Peyton) (1962–). U.S. adult film actor.

Most of the 1980s generation of male X-rated stars that included Tom Byron, Randy West, Mark Wallice, and Jeff Stryker emerged from modeling, TV commercials, and male strip shows such as CHIPPENDALES. All of them, but especially Stryker, were not so much actors as movers, who communicated their sexuality in dance, not drama.

In *The Switch Is On* (1985), the first and most successful of the bisexual, or "switch," films, Stryker performed an extended nude dance in a shower room, which established his stardom overnight. Sex shops began selling neoprene facsimiles of his genitals, advertised as "Authentically Proportioned," and even though it was later revealed that they were exaggerated, there was a considerable demand. The Netherlands issued a stamp with his likeness, and he was invited to model for avant-garde Paris couturiers, but his career dwindled, though his CV continues to claim truculently, "I am the highest paid and most world-wide well-known male performer in the history of the adult industry. I have replicas of my body parts which are said to be the best selling ever. I have a 12 inch anatomically correct action figure made of myself. . . . I do not do auditions, the name and image alone will sell a movie. I do not do bit parts; if I do not star in it, I am not in it."

STUNT COCK (porn slang, 1960s–present). Porn performer able to achieve erection to order; frequently brought in to double for stars in close-ups.

A male of only average penile dimensions is wasting his time trying to get into porn unless he can "delay and deliver," ejaculate repeatedly, or is a WOODSMAN, able to remain erect for long periods. Such men become "stunt cocks." Marc Stevens, who appeared in films such as RADLEY METZGER's *Private Afternoons of Pamela Mann* and also in *THE DEVIL IN MISS JONES*, basked in the title, and in his ability to achieve erections at will. Directors hired him by the day as insurance, in case a performer couldn't perform. As "Jerry Butler," the conventionally hung Paul Siederman also built a career on his ability to come (he claims) fifteen times a day. In the film *BOOGIE NIGHTS*, new porn performer "Dirk Diggler" excites near-reverence in entrepreneur Jack Horner for a similar ability.

SUCK (1969–1973). Amsterdam-based sex periodical.

Advertised as "The First European Sex Paper," *Suck* was co-founded in 1969 by a group, including Jim Haynes, former co-publisher of the "underground" paper *International Times*, playwright Heathcote Williams, his girlfriend, the model Jean Shrimpton, and Germaine Greer, author of *The Female Eunuch*. Edited from Amsterdam to evade British obscenity laws, the paper printed the first gay guide to Europe and a collection of oral sex tips, and helped organize the two WET DREAM FESTIVALS.

Suck prospered in the libertarian climate following May 1968. To protest against censorship had become essential to one's liberal credentials. To be acquainted with erotica was stylish. To participate was chic. The paper's organizers fell out when it published a nude photograph of Greer; "face, pubes and anus framed by vast buttocks," she wrote self-deprecatingly later. Greer resigned, claiming the other editors had reneged on a promise also to appear naked. The paper limped along and, in 1973, expired.

SUITCASE PIMP (U.S. slang, 1960s–present).

Male companion of a porn actress who tries to insinuate himself into her career.

SULLIVAN, David (1949–). British entrepreneur.

The passing of Britain's 1967 Criminal Justice Act protected pornography against frivolous prosecutions, freeing publishers to circulate hard-core magazines to "subscribers," and exhibitors to screen in private clubs the sort of films already seen openly elsewhere in Europe. Among those to exploit this market was a young economics graduate from Leeds, David Sullivan. He built up a mail-order pornography business serving, he told the LONGFORD committee, twenty-five thousand "book club members."

Lord Longford baited Sullivan with some seductively wriggling generalizations about Unhealthy Cravings and Unnatural Acts, but secure in a buoyant market and an administration that encouraged free enterprise, the publisher retorted that he supplied only consenting adults, and did so as a simple businessman. "Anyone with any initiative would want to get on, make money, be a success, in any field," he pointed out. With Britain relishing its North Sea oil revenues and negotiating for a seat at the groaning table of the European Economic Community, Longford found it hard to argue.

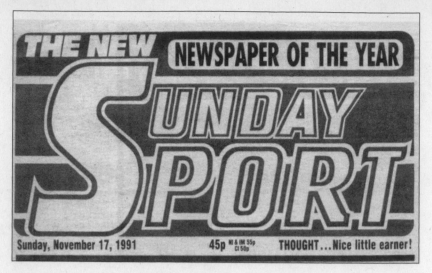

DAVID SULLIVAN'S HIGHLY SUCCESSFUL SEX TABLOID *THE SUNDAY SPORT*

Sullivan realized that a magazine or film arriving under plain wrapper appealed uniquely to the British taste for the furtive. To serve this market, he launched Conegate, which published magazines such as *Climax* and *Whitehouse*, the latter cheekily named after the most vocal of Britain's moralizers, MARY WHITEHOUSE. He also opened a chain of sex shops and produced soft-core feature films featuring his mistress MARY MILLINGTON. Even after he served a 1982 jail sentence for "living off immoral earnings," Sullivan's business acumen survived. Prohibited, as a convicted felon, from owning sex shops, he launched the erotic tabloids *Daily Sport* and *Sunday Sport*, the profits of which far exceeded anything he'd earned from earlier businesses.

SUMMER OF LOVE. The North American summer of 1967.

Like the student revolution of 1968, the Summer of Love was a spontaneous explosion of energy too long stifled by bureaucracy and repression. The spark was provided by such events as the "Human Be-In" at Golden Gate Park, San Francisco, on January 14, 1967; the "Nude Wade-In" at Aquatic Park, related to the SEXUAL FREEDOM LEAGUE; and the international radio broadcast in May of the Beatles's "One World," ending with a live debut performance of "All You Need Is Love." The same month, Scott McKenzie's song "San Francisco" became a hit. Written to publicize the Monterey Pop Festival, it pinpointed San Francisco as the center of pilgrimage for "people in motion," and promised "Summertime Will Be a Love-In there."

In June, two hundred thousand people converged on the festival. As the summer warmed up, college students on vacation, hippies, drop-outs, inquisitive tourists, and "Flower Children" gravitated to San Francisco and, specifically, the Haight-Ashbury area, a center for the production and distribution of hallucinating chemicals. Watching this wave of license head toward their city, local politicians feared the invaders might

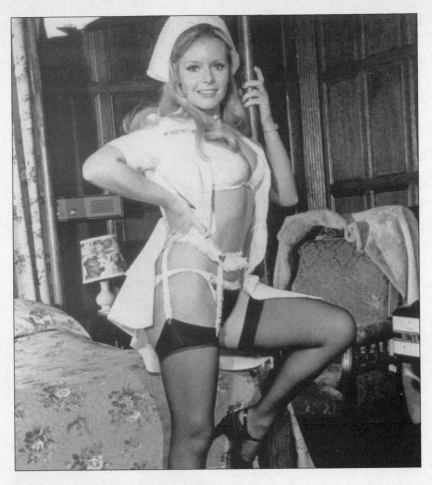

SULLIVAN'S MUSE MARY MILLINGTON IN *COME PLAY WITH ME*

take "love" literally and indulge in mass fornication. As early as January, one such administrator, scared of an influx of horny students for the "Human Be-In," demanded rhetorically, "Would you let thousands of whores waiting on the other side of the Bay Bridge into San Francisco?"

No such mass orgy took place. Most visitors were content to drift through the summer days in a fog of marijuana or LSD. Of those who stayed on, some found work in the sex industry that flourished in the liberated atmosphere and congenial legal climate of California. A few performed in porn LOOPS produced by the MITCHELL BROTHERS, while one migrant from the East Coast, MARILYN CHAMBERS, became the star of their first feature, *BEHIND THE GREEN DOOR*.

"SUPERMAN" (193?–198?). Cuban star of 1950s live sex shows.

Advertised as "a freak of nature . . . twelve inches—thirty centimeters—one foot of Superprick," "Superman" reigned supreme at Havana's Teatro Shanghai throughout the 1950s and 1960s. The Shanghai, built to house Chinese opera, offered what Graham Greene described as "a nude cabaret of extreme obscenity, with the bluest of BLUE FILMS in the intervals." Most people came to see Superman, who performed naked except for a blue-and-red velvet cloak, like that of the Man of Steel. Women in the front rows reputedly competed to be splashed by his semen.

Superman in his prime is mentioned by Mario Puzo in his novel *The Godfather* and in Francis Ford Coppola's film, where his performance so impresses Fredo Corleone that he lets slip the information that he's betrayed the family. Robert Redford seduces two thrill-seeking tourists by taking them to the show in the film *Havana* (1990). In Graham Greene's *Our Man in Havana*, local British agent Wormold also attends the Shanghai with visiting spymaster Hawthorne. Although Greene, in his memoirs, describes "watch(ing) without much interest Superman's performance with a mulatto girl (as uninspiring as a dutiful husband's)," he was sufficiently enthusiastic, during a visit to post-revolutionary Havana for the filming of *The Comedians*, to make an unsuccessful search for him. Superman's fate is unknown, though Pedro Juan Guitierrez's novel *Dirty Havana Trilogy* depicts him as an aging invalid, with legs and genitals amputated because of diabetes-related gangrene.

SURREALISM. Artistic movement that celebrated the primacy of the unconscious, the irrational, and the dream.

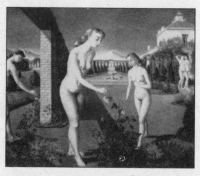

Surrealism grew out of the Dada movement and the experience of founder André Breton working in a psychiatric hospital during World War I. He became convinced that the greatest art sprang from the completely natural and spontaneous: dreams, random violence, and sex. (The only acceptable reason for not attending the daily séances at which Breton held court was that one had been making love.)

SURREALIST PAINTING BY ANDRÉ DELVAUX

Breton, the son of a policeman, disapproved of pornographic films, as he did of brothels and homosexuality, preferring instead to adulate the simple adventure serials of Louis Feuillade. Other surrealists disagreed. Paul Eluard, Luis Buñuel, Louis Aragon, René Crevel, and MAN RAY all participated in porn, and some regularly visited bordellos such as *LE CHABANAIS*.

Crevel, though homosexual, roughed out a brief treatment for a porn film called *The Geography Lesson*, in which a map of the world, particularly phallic Italy, comes to life and wreaks havoc in a girl's classroom. Eluard enjoyed a complex sex life with his wife, Gala, which included sharing his sexual adventures with her via letter and·in *PARTOUZES* with lovers such as Max Ernst.

In 1930, Eluard, Gala, and Ernst visited Cadaqués, in Spain, where Luis Buñuel and Salvador Dalí were shooting their film *L'Age d'Or*. Dalí fell in love with Gala, who remained with him for the rest of his life.

Although Breton embraced the concept of *l'amour fou*—a "mad love" that transcended all logic—he was nevertheless systematic in his attitude to sex within the surrealist group, and held a series of seminars on the subject, as part of which members were asked to complete questionnaires detailing their sexual tastes and preferences.

SWEATER GIRL (1930s-1950s).
Shorthand term for girl who looked good in a tight sweater.

Typified by the first appearance of Lana Turner as the teenage murder victim in *They Won't Forget*. In 1949, a U.S. competition to elect a Sweater Queen ended in an argument over the thinness of the sweater itself, so two queens were elected.

Obscene cinema, what a marvel! It's exhilarating; a discovery. The incredible life of enormous and magnificent organs on the screen. The sperm that leaps. And the life of loving flesh, all the contortions. It's glorious. And very well made, a tremendous eroticism. . . . It's a very pure show without theatrical effect. The actors don't move their lips, at least not to speak, it's a "silent" art, a "primitive" art; passion vs death and stupidity. They should show this in every theatre and in schools. It would result in workable marriages—the first; sacred unions, multi-faceted. Alas, poetry is not born yet.

—PAUL ELUARD, IN A LETTER
TO HIS WIFE, GALA, APRIL
1929

SWEATER QUEEN (gay slang, 1990s-present). Derogatory term used by macho gays to describe men who avoid overt identification as homosexuals, often working in professions that deal directly with the straight public, and for which they can wear attire that doesn't advertise their sexual preference.

SWEDEN.
In 1969, French president Georges Pompidou described his ideal for France as "Sweden, but with a bit more sun." Most of Europe shared his view of its northern neighbor as a beacon of rational humanism and enlightened social legislation. The Swedes had followed DENMARK in the 1970s in lifting most restrictions on pornography, and as early as 1968, in the film *Dom kallar oss mods* (*They Call Us Misfits*), permitted unsimulated sexual intercourse in a film on general release.

Tourists visiting Stockholm in the hope of unbridled vice, however, encountered something far chillier. Intensely private people, somber and introspective, the Swedes hungered not for the pleasures of the flesh but for forests, lakes, and a cleansing emptiness. They could be open about sex because it didn't interest them very much.

The film that most firmly established Sweden's credentials as a center of sexual experiment was Vilgot Sjoman's 1967 *Jag är nyfiken—en film i gult*, retitled in English *I Am Curious—Yellow*. In a quasi-documentary, Lena Nyman conducts a survey of the state of Sweden's liberal society, which included testing its degree of sexual permissiveness by having semi-public sex in a number of locations around Stockholm. In fantasy sequences, she also rounds up all twenty-three men with whom she has had sex before the film and, finding them guilty of having exploited her, ropes them to a tree and blows them up. Sjoman followed up in 1968 with the less successful *Jag är nyfiken—en film i blått*, known as *I Am Curious—Blue*, which recycled much of the first film's material, but from a different political perspective.

As long as it lasted, however, the image of Sweden as a haven of sexual liberalism made money for everyone. The Swedish AU PAIR became a stock figure of myth, portrayed as a sexual athlete, ready to romp for the price of a beer. The German producers of *Der Ostfriesen-Report* (1974), a compendium of jokes about the supposed stupidity of people from East Friesia, retitled it *Swedish Playgirls*, even though it was shot in Munich and had not one Swede in it.

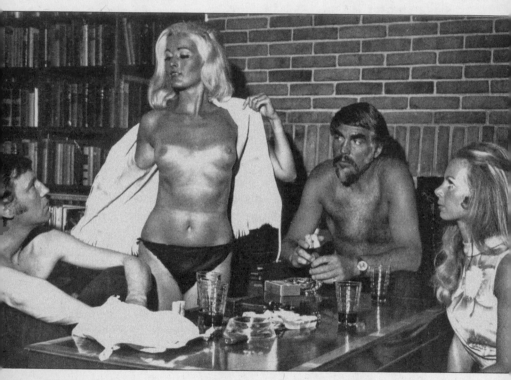

STILL FROM THE BRITISH FILM *THE WIFE SWAPPERS*

SWINGING (1950s–present). Couples trading partners for casual sexual encounters.

Although wife swapping and similar practices have a long pedigree, swinging is generally agreed to have begun on U.S. military bases during the 1950s. At Key Parties, couples tossed their car keys into a bowl and paired off randomly, depending on which key they chose. Rick Moody's novel *The Ice Storm* (filmed by Ang Lee in 1997) extracts humor from the unwillingness of the husband with a glamorous wife to accept a fat or ugly woman for the night.

The practice flourished to the extent that an association for swingers, the SEXUAL FREEDOM LEAGUE, was set up in Berkeley, California, early in the 1960s. Some organizations issued badges, indicating the wearer as a full paid-up member of the swinging culture, and magazines proliferated in which couples advertised their needs and desires. In France, known as *echangisme*, swinging was embraced with equal enthusiasm. Centers of swinging included PLATO'S RETREAT in New York and, in California, the SANDSTONE RANCH. A plate on the door of Hugh Hefner's original Chicago PLAYBOY mansion read in Latin SI NON OSCILLAS, NOLI TINTINNARE (IF YOU DON'T SWING, DON'T RING).

Cinema explored swinging in films such as *Bob and Carol and Ted and Alice* (1969), in which a couple who've swapped agonized over introducing their oldest and best friends to the practice, since it might ruin their friendship. It was deplored in the British quasi-documentary *The Wife Swappers* (Derek Ford, UK 1970), which exposed a so-called "wife-swapping cult," with overtones of organized crime and kidnapping. As a concession to the censors, the film includes a woman at a swapping party ranting at the participants, calling them "animals . . . you've taken the act of love and dirtied it . . . a woman isn't a sex machine; she's a childbearer!"

SYBIAN. A vibrator-based sex toy, in the form of a saddle, with two vibrators attached, designed to be ridden by a woman astride, one vibrator in her vagina, the other exciting her clitoris.

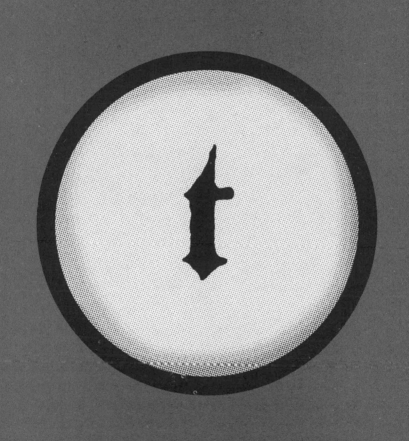

TABLE DANCING. (See LAP DANCING).

TAMPON. Plug, usually of compressed paper or fiber, for absorbing menstrual blood.

Used tampons figure in some twentieth-century erotic literature and in real life also. Hoki Tokuda, the twenty-eight-year-old wife of the septuagenarian

HENRY MILLER, recalled that her husband possessed a tampon with the blood and blond hair of MARILYN MONROE, sent to him by a maid who had souvenired it from a Philadelphia hotel. Prince Charles was memorably overheard discussing with his then-mistress Camilla Parker-Bowles that he might be reincarnated as a "tampon," so as to be even more intimately associated with her than ever.

TATTOO.

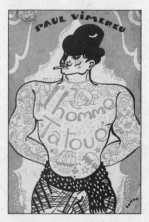

In 1796, Capt. James Cook wrote of the Polynesians, "both sexes paint their Bodys, *Tattow* as it is called in their language." Such tattoos, administered with wooden or bone spikes hammered into the skin, demanded endurance. As a consequence, tribal people and travelers who acquired tattoos displayed them as symbols of courage, voyages to exotic places, or membership of an exclusive brotherhood, e.g., military unit, street gang, or prison group.

Women, lacking such motives, were less often tattooed, the exception being prostitutes, who wore tattoos as far back as Pharaonic Egypt. Japanese *yakuza* gang members, supposedly to ensure that they were not infiltrated by informers, covered their bodies with elaborate *horimono* designs. The custom spilled over into their female companions, who sometimes submitted to erotic skin pictures. In *Shisei* (*The Tattooer*), a 1910 story by Junichiro Tanizaki, an obsessed artist drugs a woman and tattoos a spider on her back. Paradoxically, the tattoo, and the pain of acquiring it, don't disgust the woman but, rather, transform and elate her. She acquires the characteristics of the spider, and the power of life and death over the tattooist. In the 1981 film *Tattoo*, Bruce Dern, hired to BODY-PAINT tattoos on model Maud Adams, imprisons her and covers the finally acquiescent woman with the real thing.

Tattooing's male exclusivity disappeared with the development of the electric needle and more stable inks. Sideshow "tattooed ladies," usually the lovers or wives of tattoo artists, became a commonplace of carnival midways. They were celebrated in the song "Lydia, the Tattooed Lady," made popular by GROUCHO MARX.

In 1897, the *New York Herald* wrote that without a tattoo, "you cannot be *au courant* with society's very latest fad." Even then, a tattoo continued to mark the owner, male or female, as socially marginal. As late as 1920, a Boston judge dismissed a rape charge because the victim was tattooed. But in 1924, the U.S. heroine of Carl Van Vechten's novel *The Tattooed Countess* commemorated a punishing European romance by having the phrase *"Que Sais-Je?"* ("What do I know?") tattooed around her wrist.

From the 1960s, it became fashionable for women to sport "boutique" tattoos, usually of a small bird or a butterfly, on the buttocks or groin, or a more complex design at the base of the spine. "Giving a tattoo" to a lover indicated sexual submission. A 2006

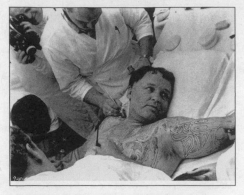

ROD STEIGER BEING MADE UP FOR HIS ROLE AS A TATTOOED MAN IN *THE ILLUSTRATED MAN*

study by the University of Chicago and Northwestern University found that nearly 50 percent of Americans between twenty-one and thirty-two have at least one tattoo or a PIERCING other than in an ear. Men and women alike say their tattoos make them feel sexy and rebellious, a 2003 Harris poll found. (See ARSE-ANTLERS.)

TAXI DANCER (U.S., 1920s–1930s). Dance hall "hostess," hired by the dance.

In taxi dance halls, customers bought a ticket, customarily for ten cents, entitling them to one dance, as immortalized by Lorenz Hart in the lyrics to "Ten Cents a Dance" (1930). Various subterfuges existed to cheat the client, e.g., tickets might apply to the number of songs played by the band, whether the buyer danced to them or not. Many taxi dancers doubled as prostitutes. In *Blonde Venus* (1932), Marlene Dietrich, introduced to showgirl "Taxi Belle" Hooper (Rita La Roy), sarcastically asks if she "charges for the first mile."

TEA.

The Chinese habit of drinking aromatic teas or infusions to scent the sexual juices gained favor in the West during the twentieth century. In Diane Johnson's *Le Divorce*, the American heroine, anxious to please her French lover, finds that an entire pot is needed to achieve a noticeable effect. Help arrived in 2006 in the form of Sweet Release Oral Sex Enhancement pills. Herb-based, they promised lemon-flavored vaginas and semen tasting of apples.

***TEA AND SYMPATHY* (1953).** U.S. play, by Robert Anderson.

The wife of an overbearing "jock" academic befriends a sexually confused male student, to whom she dispenses more than the traditional "tea and sympathy" expected of university wives. Leading him to bed, she delivers the play's most famous line: "Years from now, when you talk about this—and you will—be kind." Elia Kazan directed the play on Broadway, with Deborah Kerr and John Kerr. Vincente Minnelli filmed it in

1956 with the same cast but a framing flashback, censor-imposed, in which the hero, now married with children, revisits his college to hear that his lover regretted her lapse, and suffered for it.

TEA-BAGGING (U.S. slang, 1990s). Sex act in which a lover takes the entire scrotum into his or her mouth.

TEA ROOMS. See COTTAGING.

TELEPHONE SEX, TELEPHONE DATE. See PHONE SEX.

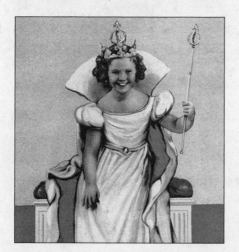

TEMPLE, Shirley (1928–). U.S. film star and, as Shirley Temple Black, ambassador and diplomat.

The most popular child actress of all time, Temple had a devoted PAEDOPHILE following. According to legend, a movie executive once FLASHED her in his office. Unfazed, she responded, "I thought you were a producer, not an exhibitor." Only Graham Greene was courageous enough, in a 1937 review of John Ford's *Wee Willie Winkie*, to discuss Temple's covert eroticism. "Infancy with her is a disguise," he wrote. "Her appeal is more secret and more adult. . . . Watch the way she measures a man with agile studio eyes, with dimpled depravity. Adult emotions of love and grief glissade across the mask of childhood, a childhood skin deep. . . . Her admirers, middle-aged men and clergymen, respond to her dubious coquetry, to the sight of her well-shaped and desirable little body, packed with enormous vitality, only because the safety curtain of story and dialogue drops between their intelligence and their desire." Furious at this slur on their nine-year-old star, 20th Century Fox sued for libel on Temple's behalf. They bankrupted the magazine that published the review, and forced Greene, then a penniless novelist, to pay £1,500 of the damages.

"10" (1979). U.S. film. Directed by Blake Edwards.

On a scale of one to ten, the perfect woman would be a ten. In the film, songwriter Dudley Moore becomes infatuated with the putatively peerless Bo Derek and pursues her recklessly, only to be stricken by scruples at the last moment. The film's use of *Bolero* by Ravel gave new popularity to the piece, already a standard of the erotic repertoire. ANNETTE HAVEN has a small role as a porn actress.

TICKLER (or FRENCH TICKLER). See CONDOMS.

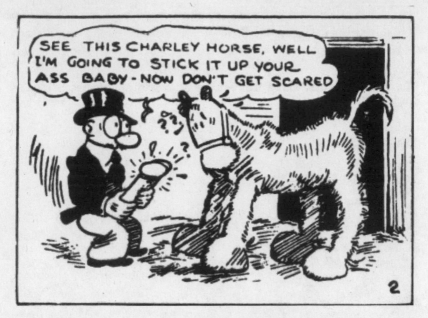

PANEL FROM TIJUANA BIBLE BASED ON THE COMIC STRIP *BARNEY GOOGLE*

TIJUANA BIBLE (U.S., 1920s–present). Pocket-size pornographic comic booklet, so called because tourists often brought examples back from holiday trips to Mexico, where the booklets were supposedly printed.

The crudely drawn "bibles" depicted the imaginary sexual exploits of movie stars (e.g., MAE WEST, Clara Bow, JEAN HARLOW), comic-strip characters (Dagwood and Blondie, Popeye), and sometimes public figures (Edward VIII, WALLIS SIMPSON, and even Gandhi). Enthusiasts for comic-book history continued to produce them into the 1990s, with "bibles" devoted to writer Salman Rushdie and/or President Ronald Reagan. Ironically, the same horizontal pocket-size format was adopted for the Armed Services Editions paperbacks issued during World War II for distribution to servicemen abroad.

***TO BEG I AM ASHAMED* (1938).** UK novel by "Sheila Cousins" (pseudonym for Ronald Mathews).

Supposedly the memoirs of a London prostitute, the tepid *To Beg I Am Ashamed* takes its title from the story of the Righteous Steward in the Bible: "Then the steward said within himself, What shall I do? for my lord taketh away from me the stewardship: I cannot dig; to beg I am ashamed." First published in Paris by the OBELISK PRESS, it appeared in England in 1953, when it was furiously attacked by the press, and banned. For a time, Graham Greene, who frequently patronized prostitutes, was rumored to be the author, but at most he may have supplied "local color" to Mathews, who was a colleague.

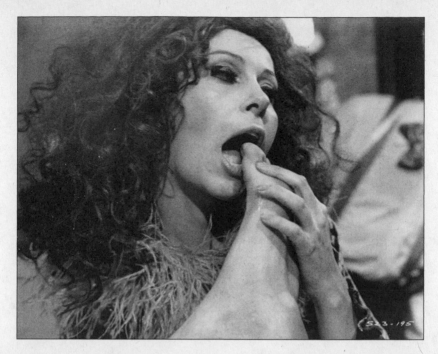

TOES.

An area of anatomy overdue for erogenous reexamination, though not entirely ignored by eroticists. In *THE JOY OF SEX*, ALEX COMFORT (who had lost the fingers on his left hand) explained that flexible or elongated toes can substitute for fingers or a penis. Sarah Ferguson, estranged Duchess of York, made the front pages in August 1992 when paparazzi snapped her, bare-breasted, having her toes sucked, poolside, by a lover. In the film *Flashdance*, Jennifer Beals uses her bare foot to fondle Michael Khouri under a restaurant table, while in his memoir *A Little Learning*, Evelyn Waugh recalls a fellow schoolteacher rhapsodizing over the pleasure of introducing a young boy's foot into his trousers.

Toenails, too, are not without appeal. For the title sequence of Stanley Kubrick's film of *LOLITA* (1962), the London company Chambers and Partners shot male hands carefully lacquering the nails of a female foot. British playwright Alan Bennett mentions an actress who claimed she seduced Japanese men with the invitation "Would you like me to cut your toenails in the warmth of my own home," but no reliable evidence has emerged of this particular fetish.

"TOM OF FINLAND" (*né* Touko Laaksonen) (1920–1991). Artist.

A gay counterpart of ERIC STANTON, Finnish-born Laaksonen discovered the homoerotic attraction of military men as a lieutenant in the Finnish army during World War II. In peacetime, while working in advertising, he drew husky men, almost invariably in uniform—occasionally, controversially, Nazi—with bulging muscles and even more engorged genitals, barely concealed in overtight trousers or jeans.

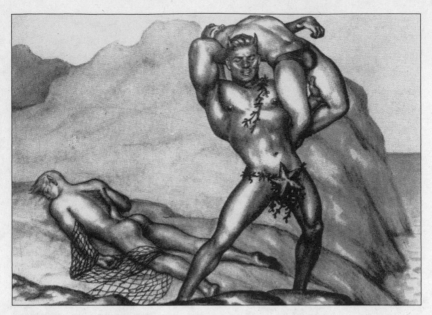

GAY PORN BY "TOM OF FINLAND"

In 1957, his picture of a Finnish lumberjack featured on the cover of U.S. magazine *Physique Pictorial*. As "Tom of Finland," he became synonymous with "cruising cycle cops in straining black leathers, doughboys in uniform, lumberjacks and longshoremen, together with a brooding anonymous cast of sexual outlaws, all roaming a crepuscular erotic realm in search of orgiastic, often sadomasochistic ritual copulation" (Neil McKenna). Laaksonen left advertising in 1973 to concentrate on his fetish drawing, and the production of "Tom of Finland" leather gear. "I am not ashamed that I draw men having sex," he said. "I work hard to make sure they are proud men having happy sex."

TONGUE BATH (U.S. slang, 1920s). Cunnilingus.

TOPLESS. Bare-breasted. Also BOTTOMLESS.

TOP SHELF. By law, British erotic magazines must be sealed in plastic and placed on the top shelf of the shop, out of reach of minors. See *BINIBONG*.

TOSSING SALAD (U.S. slang, 1990s–present). Vigorous licking of the testicles.

TRAINS.

The body of erotic mythology inspired by trains falls into two categories: one, the train as phallic symbol; the second, the effect of the motion on passengers. The train is often represented as a penis, particularly when plunging into a tunnel, e.g., the express bearing Cary Grant and Eva Marie Saint in *North by Northwest*. Jean Renoir traded on the coitus-like motion of the pistons and driving rods of the locomotive in his *La Bête Humaine*. The supposedly aphrodisiac effect of its swaying motion is expounded in *Silver Streak* (1976), by Ned Beatty, only to see Gene Wilder put it into practice with Jill Clayburgh; while Cary Grant in *Notorious*—Hitchcock again—finds his embrace of Ingrid Bergman disturbed and intensified when the motion of the train sends them rolling across the compartment wall. Of memorable erotic scenes in sleeping compartments, Jack Lemmon in *Some Like It Hot*, sharing a couchette with MARILYN MONROE, stands out. Metro trains present an entirely different attraction. In Michel Houellebecq's novel *Platforme*, middle-aged men take the last Metro of the night in order to expose themselves or masturbate to a captive audience of young women heading home. See *CHIKAN DENSHA*.

TRAIN, TO PUT ON . . . or PULL A (Australian/U.S. slang, 1960s). To submit to serial group sex. Also "to put on an onion."

TRAMP (U.S. slang, 1910–1980s). A prostitute, though sometimes simply an amoral woman with a taste for slumming, cf., Rodgers and Hart's song "The Lady Is a Tramp," from *Pal Joey*.

TRANNY (slang). Shorthand for *transvestite*. See CROSS-DRESSING.

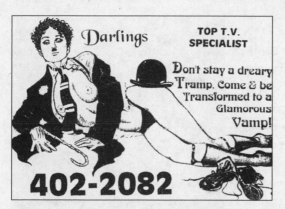

LONDON PROSTITUTE CARD OFFERING "T.V.", I.E., TRANSVESTITE SERVICES

TRANSSEXUAL. A person who undergoes surgery and hormone treatment in order to change his or her sex. See WEGENER, Gerda.

TRANSVESTISM. See CROSS-DRESSING; DRAG.

TRAYNOR, Chuck (*né* Charles Everett Traynor) (Aka Howard Dale, Howard Muniz) (1937–2002). U.S. producer and actor.

Married to both LINDA LOVELACE and MARILYN CHAMBERS, and responsible for the career of the former, Traynor, a gun-toting ex-bar owner, drug dealer, and PIMP, accumulated a rich history of violence, and influenced the world of pornographic film out of all proportion to any creative contribution.

According to rumor, Traynor was to have acted in *Deep Throat*, but was unable to maintain WOOD. Instead, he's credited as "Production Manager." Lovelace later made Traynor the scapegoat for all her transgressions, claiming that he forced her to become a prostitute, to undergo silicone breast implants, to marry him, and, finally, to appear in porn films, even standing over her with a pistol to force her to fornicate with a dog in the 1972 *DOG FUCK*—an absurd claim to anyone who has seen the film, since she plainly participates with enthusiasm. This is borne out by HARRY REEMS. While labeling Traynor "an asshole," he denies he was even present for most of *DEEP THROAT*. "Damiano sent him away because he would get jealous of how much [Lovelace] was enjoying the sex. She was really into it." Lovelace's most telling revenge on the aggressively straight Traynor is her accusation that during a sex party with SAMMY DAVIS, JR., she persuaded him to join her in fellating the star.

TRICK, TRICKING. Prostitute slang for a paid sex act.

TROMBONE. Sexual act in which a male crouches on all fours while a partner applies lips to the anus and simultaneously masturbates him, the combined actions being thought to imitate those of a trombone player. See RIMMING.

TURNER, Lana (*née* Julia Jean Mildred Frances Turner) (1921-1995). U.S. film actress.

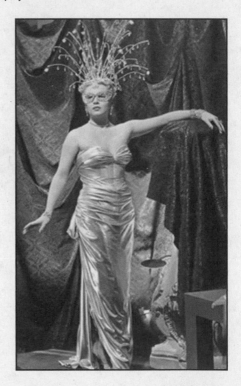

Eight times married, a chronic alcoholic, the central figure in several sensational affairs and one murder, Lana Turner was the archetypal Hollywood bad girl, with a man-eater reputation. "She was amoral," said one producer. "If she saw a stagehand with tight pants and a muscular build, she'd invite him into her dressing room." In 1958, her lover at the time, gangster Johnny Stompanato, former bodyguard of gang boss Mickey Cohen, was stabbed to death in her home. Turner's thirteen-year-old daughter, Cheryl Crane, admitted to the crime, but after hearing testimony of Stompanato's mob connections and brutality toward Turner, the jury deliberated for only twenty minutes before returning a verdict of justifiable homicide.

Vindictively, the Stompanato family leaked Turner's hysterical letters to her lover, and claimed that she, not her daughter, had murdered him when he threatened to leave her: Crane, they asserted, was persuaded to confess to the crime in the knowledge that no jury would convict her. Turner's relationship with Stompanato is referenced in Curtis Hanson's film *L.A. Confidential*, while the rumors about Stompanato's murder and Turner's alleged involvement clearly inspired WOODY ALLEN's *September*. See ALLEN, Woody; SWEATER GIRL.

TWINK (1960s-present). Pedophile slang for an attractive young boy. See also CHICKEN HAWK.

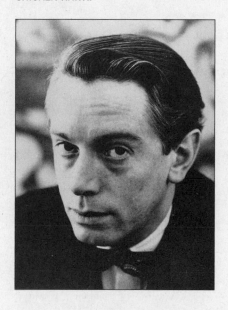

TYNAN, Kenneth (1927-1980). UK theater critic, journalist, and entrepreneur.

A suave mouthpiece for that generation of British intellectuals—painter David Hockney, film director John Schlesinger, playwright John Osborne—who took their reclusive, dusty pursuits and dragged them into the limelight, Kenneth Tynan was, as Tom Stoppard said at his memorial service, "part of the luck we had." However, Britain's artistic establishment never forgave him his lurid private life, including a highly public "open marriage" to novelist Elaine Dundy. In Schlesinger's 1971 *Sunday, Bloody Sunday*, a couple at a London party noisily debate their tormented relationship. As the wife histrionically pulls open her dress, an exasperated guest mutters, "Not those tired old tits again." Everyone recognized the models for these characters as Tynan and Dundy.

Once he gave up criticism, Tynan's career faltered. He abandoned a biography of sex theorist WILHELM REICH, and never found money for the one movie he tried to direct, a celebration of his sexual enthusiasm, spanking. *OH! CALCUTTA!*, his erotic stage anthology, made money, but a follow-up, *Carte Blanche*, flopped. His diaries document visits to Paris and Berlin sex clubs, an agonizing account of a vodka ENEMA, and some chewy celebrity anecdotes: JOHN F. KENNEDY screwing MARLENE DIETRICH in the White House, and Tynan refusing to sleep with Vivien Leigh under Olivier's roof, only to watch her climb into bed with Dundy.

In the last decade of his life, he started an affair with an unsuccessful actress who cooperated in his enthusiasm for caning and CROSS-DRESSING, Tynan's favorite role being as silent movie actress Louise Brooks. Of this relationship, he wrote with enormous satisfaction "I have achieved sexual fullfilment."

Inevitably, Tynan is remembered less as the witty critic than, in the words of fellow critic Michael Billington, "the spanker, the star-fucker, the sexual obsessive, the suave and ultimately ailing hedonist" and the first person to use the word *fuck* on British TV. But though he deserved better, he expected no less. Life ended for him when the sex died. Made impotent by his illness, he quoted Voltaire's despairing verse on encountering the same tragedy.

> One dies twice, I see that well.
> Unable to love or be loved—
> That's unbearable.
> By comparison, death is nothing.

"A good epitaph," he commented in his diary. Within eighteen months, he was dead.

"UGLY GEORGE." See URBAN, George Peter.

UP SKIRT (slang, 1960s-present).

From the early days of the century when, as Cole Porter remarked, "a glimpse of stocking was looked on as something shocking," men have lusted to see up women's skirts, even when there was no more on show than underwear. In the 1930s and 1940s, the common knowledge in show business that certain stars, notably Carmen Miranda and JEAN HARLOW, were naked under their costumes, fed a popular fetish, manifested at its most extreme by nuns warning their Catholic charges to avoid shiny shoes, for fear of offering a glance up their skirts. See CROTCH SHOT.

URANIAN. Omnibus term for pedophile literature and art.

URBAN, George Peter (aka "Ugly George") (1942-). Filmmaker.

As "Ugly George," Urban roamed Manhattan throughout the 1970s and early 1980s with a video camera, accosting women in the street, and persuading them—often with surprising ease—to remove some or all of their clothing while he taped them, transmitting the recordings on his cable access show *Truth, Sex, and Violence*. Urban's anticensorship, pro—free speech stance was sufficiently popular for celebrities such as John Lennon and Yoko Ono to appear as guests.

UROLAGNIA. Sexual pleasure derived from urine, from either being urinated on or urinating in public.

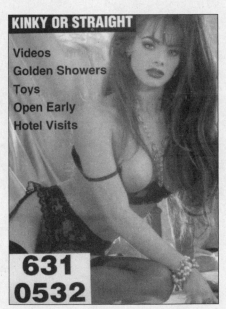

LONDON PROSTITUTE CARD OFFERING "GOLDEN SHOWERS"

Urinating has always had an element of sexuality, which twentieth-century eroticists have explored, particularly in New York. Jackson Pollock famously urinated in the fireplace of Peggy Guggenheim, with whom he was having an affair. In the course of gay orgies involving ROBERT MAPPLETHORPE, ANDY WARHOL created a series of "Chemical Paintings" by persuading his partners to urinate on prepared canvases, changing the tones by having them ingest various substances.

S&M clubs such as New York's MINE SHAFT featured steel tubs where enthusiasts could lie while being pissed on—"the real thing," noted one report righteously, "as distinct from the warm ammonia squeezed from a rag onto dupes as they lie back, eyes obediently closed, at some of the city's more expensive brothels." Among street prostitutes, the conventional code for urolagnia, aka a "golden shower" or "golden stream," is a six-pack of beer rattled out a car window.

Dominatrices specializing in WATERSPORTS typically offer to urinate in the client's mouth, or on his chest or genitals. One London expert offered a choice of locations: Clients could elect to be pissed on in her Watersports Chamber, on a rubber mat in her Dungeon, or in her Medical Chamber, where she could also administer an ENEMA and make them hold it in. If preferred, she could perform the services while wearing a rubber nurse's uniform.

In RADLEY METZGER's film *L'Image*, a beautiful sex slave is forced to crouch and urinate within sight of diners at a fashionable Paris restaurant. In urophagia, fetishists derive pleasure from drinking urine. Devotees recommend eating grapefruit to give flavor to the urine, and soda or beer to dilute it. To be avoided are asparagus, which adds pungency, and beet, which colors it red. Followers of the Japanese fetish *omorashi* ("to wet oneself") are aroused by the discomfort of a full bladder or by the sight of someone in the same state, ideally a woman, who exhibits visible discomfort, e.g., crossed legs. See TEA; WARHOL, Andy; MINE SHAFT, THE.

VADIM, Roger (Roger Vladimir Igorevich Plemyannikov) (1928–2000).
French film director, writer, and actor.

Although an indifferent director, Roger Vadim had the same instinct as Hugh Hefner for judging the sexual tastes of the male audience. His melodramas were as chintzily overdecorated as the settings for *PLAYBOY* centerfold photo shoots, and just as effective in tweaking latent male lust, as were the actresses he favored—BRIGITTE BARDOT, Annette Stroyberg, Catherine Deneuve, Jane Fonda—and made his stars, mistresses, or, frequently, wives.

Both the title of his first film, and its advertising ("And God . . . Created Woman . . . But the Devil Created Brigitte Bardot") caused problems in Anglo-Saxon countries, by taking the name of the deity in vain.. In most countries, it was retitled *And Woman Was Created.* Despite this, it was an enormous hit. Jeanne Moreau credits Vadim with launching the New Wave, since his film's frank eroticism and youthful cast drew to the movies a new audience bored with the *cinema de papa*—Daddy's cinema.

But after his initial success, Vadim's penchant for flowing robes, plunging horses, and hot-eyed stares, and his improbable heroines—space girls, incestuous lovers, women who believe themselves the reincarnation of Don Juan or who want to die of an orgasm—deterred American audiences. Subsequent films, such as *La Ronde* (1964), *La Curée (The Game Is Over)* (1966), and *BARBARELLA* (1968), all with his then-companion Jane Fonda, mostly failed.

To the end, Vadim remained a uniquely European purveyor of a specialized erotic vision. Aside from *Et Dieu . . . Crea la Femme,* his most enduring film is the 1960 *Et Mourir de Plaisir (To Die of Pleasure),* a sensuous adaptation, with lesbian and necrophilic overtones, of Sheridan LeFanu's vampire story "Carmilla." Shot around the ruins of Hadrian's villa, outside Rome, it starred his then-wife Annette Stroyberg, and boasted a faux-baroque score by avant-garde composer Jean Prodromides. However, despite the international cast, English dubbing, and a new title, *Blood and Roses* also flopped.

VALENTINO, Rudolph (*né* Rodolfo Alfonzo Raffaelo Pierre Filibert Guglielmi di Valentina d'Antonguolla) (1895–1926). Italian American actor.

When Rudolph Valentino entered movies, the hero of fiction, theater, or film was either a tight-lipped man of action or a cringing wimp in thrall to a dominating woman. Valentino was neither. As worn by him in *The Sheik* and *The Son of the Sheik,* the robes of an Arab chieftain didn't look like fancy dress, and he could tango in *The Four Horsemen of the Apocalypse* as if it were just one step from taking his partner to bed.

Never mind that he'd arrived as a penniless emigrant from Italy, and worked as a busboy, movie extra, dance partner, and GIGOLO. He was made for the movies. On his lips, the intertitles of silent film came to life. In *The Sheik,* he carries off blond bubblehead Agnes Ayres to his tent. "Why have you brought me here?" she quavers. Valentino raises one incredulous eyebrow. "*Mon dieu,*" he says, "are you not woman enough to know?"

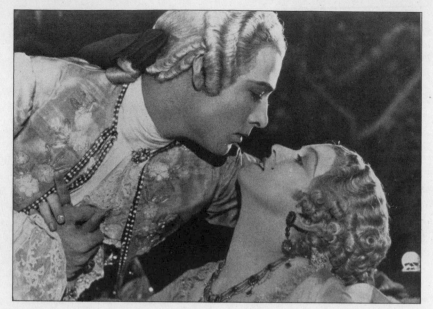

VALENTINO "SISSIFIED" AS MONSIEUR BEAUCAIRE

Agnes blushes and averts her eyes. She knows very well, as does every woman in the audience.

In real life, Valentino was no sheik. Somewhere between homosexual and asexual, he was happiest in his clifftop mansion Falcon's Lair, dabbling in poetry and consorting with gay friends such as Norman Kerry and Ramon Navarro, whom he presented with a gold-plated life-size dildo, presumably modeled from his own penis. In 1968, Navarro would be murdered by two gay hustlers he'd invited to his home. According to legend, they choked him to death with the Valentino dildo.

Since his career demanded it, Valentino married—twice, both times to lesbians. The second, Natacha Rambova, alias cosmetics heiress Winifred Hudnut, bullied him into effete roles for which he was draped in ropes of pearls as *The Young Rajah* and powdered and bewigged as *Monsieur Beaucaire*. Alarmed at Valentino's dwindling popularity, producer Joseph Schenck cooked up a romance with his most incendiary star, Polish import Pola Negri, whose career also needed a jolt, and cast him in *The Son of the Sheik*. It became his greatest hit, but posthumously, since he died before its release. Negri gave the performance of her life at his funeral, bewailing a nonexistent love, while the funeral director, distressed by the emaciated look of Valentino's corpse, substituted a wax effigy for the lying-in-state.

VAMP (U.S. slang, 1910–1930). Verb: To exercise sexual attraction flagrantly as a means of seduction. Noun: A woman who does so.

Rudyard Kipling was the first to christen the predatory female a "vampire" in his 1897 poem "The Vampire," which included the notorious dismissal of women as no more than "a rag, a bone and a hank of hair." The corruption *vamp* first appears in Katharine Kaelred's 1910 Broadway play *A Fool There Was*—a phrase also extracted from Kipling's poem—but was popularized in the 1915 film version, the star of which, THEDA BARA, is identified simply as "The Vampire." She bewitches wealthy men with her smoldering look, orders "Kiss me, my fool!," only to discard them when their fortunes and vitality are drained.

VENUS, V (19??-). U.S. porn actress.

The prototype of other grossly overweight performers in CHUBBY CHASER films such as *Tons of Love*, this five-hundred-pound lady with a prominent tattoo, whose flesh hangs round her in valances of white blubber, figured under the *nom du film* V. Venus in a number of MITCHELL BROTHERS productions, including *Behind the Green Door: The Sequel*. WILLIAM ROTSLER, encountering her on the set of an orgy scene, remarked, "You look like you're having a good time," to which she replied, "Hell, yes! If it wasn't for movies like this, I'd *never* get laid!"

VIAGRA. Proprietary name for the anti-impotence drug Sildenafil citrate.

VIBRATOR. For the last half of the nineteenth century, the recreational value of the vibrator was one of the best kept secrets of the medical profession. Doctors reserved the machine for the treatment of "female hysteria" and "congestion of the genitalia" and to encourage the circulation of the blood in injured muscles. Some ran by clockwork, like wind-up toys, or were driven by compressed air. The British Macauras Blood Circulator from about 1902 required the user to turn a handle, rather like that of an egg beater.

An electrical vibrator was patented by Kelsey Stinner in the 1880s. Hamilton Beach patented a simpler version for home use in 1902, the fifth domestic appliance to be electrified, after the sewing machine, fan, teakettle, and toaster, and about a decade before the vacuum cleaner and electric iron. Advertised as muscle-relaxers and aids to home massage, early vibrators followed the design of the pistol-grip hair drier. Interchangeable attachments included a disc studded with flexible plastic spikes for scalp massage and a mushroom-shaped bulb supposedly for use on muscle cramps. A knob regulated the intensity of the vibration.

GERSHON LEGMAN claimed to have conceived a vibrator in the 1920s and worked with an inventor to perfect it. It's likely that he was one of many researchers working to streamline the machine. Some clockwork vibrators of the 1930s had adopted the phallic shape, but it wasn't until the appearance in the 1970s of the first battery-operated vibrators that the now-familiar electrical torpedo became standard.

Militant feminism and the appearance of shops such as San Francisco's Good Vibrations accelerated the sale of vibrators. Feedback from enthusiastic users encour-

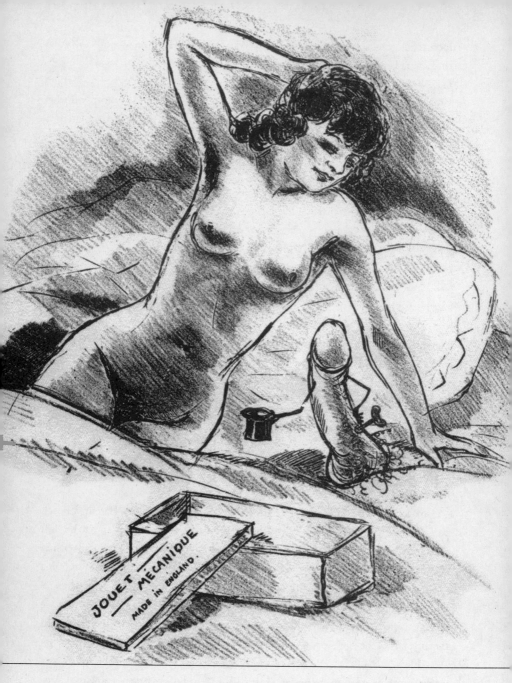

CLOCKWORK VIBRATOR, FRENCH, 1920s, BUT DESCRIBED AS "MADE IN ENGLAND" ON THE BOX (HENCE THE TOP HAT, DOFFED POLITELY)

aged the development of new models designed for specific needs: the two-pronged Rabbit, which stimulated both the vaginal entrance and the clitoris; the double-penetration model, serving both vagina and anus; the slim, cranked variety with a bulbous end, more effective for exciting the G-SPOT. Slimmer models were produced for anal use, often in metal, since some users enjoyed the coldness and even keep theirs in the refrigerator.

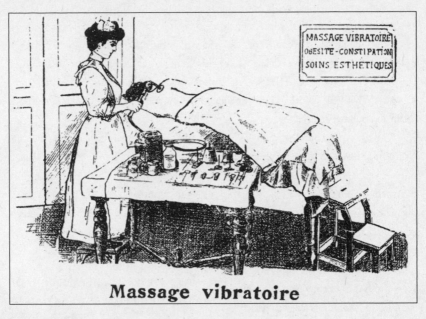

"MEDICAL" VIBRATOR TREATMENT, PARIS, 1909

MOTHER (*looking at erotic photos taken by her daughter and boyfriend*): *This is your room. You did these things right here? In my house?*
DAUGHTER: *Well, I thought someone in this house ought to be having sex—I mean with something that doesn't require batteries.*
—SCRIPT FOR *PARENTHOOD* (1989),
BY LOWELL GANZ AND BABALOO MANDEL

VICTIM (1961). UK film. Directed by Basil Dearden.

Pioneering drama exposing the plight of gays in Britain, where homosexuality remained a crime until the Sexual Offences Act of 1967. A bisexual barrister, played by gay actor Dirk Bogarde, attracts the attention of both the police and blackmailers when a young lover is targeted by the police. The film reiterates the point made by the German film *ANDERS ALS DIE ANDERN*, in 1919, that gays often prey on their own; the blackmailer in both films is very pointedly identified as homosexual.

VIDEO.

The arrival of the video recorder and player in the mid-1970s transformed the market for all films, but especially for porn, which played an important role in the industry-wide change. (Some even attribute the failure of the Betamax format to the greater availability of porn on Sony's technically inferior VHS system.)

Video was cheaper to make and distribute than film, so production costs plunged, accelerating output. Video also removed many of its problems with censorship and the law. Reformers who'd felt confident at picketing an X-rated theater were powerless to enter the living rooms of Middle America.

Since video was easily copied, the larger porn producers could produce cassettes in bulk, and flood the market. Casualties of this change included pioneers BILL OSCO and the MITCHELL BROTHERS. Asked in 1987 about production plans, Artie Mitchell said, "What's the point? You make a video movie and the Koreans take it in the back room and dub ten copies."

With almost no porn being made on film, adult cinemas everywhere were closing. (In the film *BOOGIE NIGHTS*, producer Jack Horner's loyalty to film over video, and his refusal to abandon professional performers for amateurs, signals his downfall.) Most filmgoers were not sorry to see the demise of X-rated movie houses. "If there was a legitimate grievance against [sex movies]," wrote Gay Talese, "it was that the box office's admission fee of $5 per customer was too high a cost to pay for the inferior quality of the films, the sophomoric scenarios, the unconvincing acting even in the bedroom scenes in which the actors were constantly losing their erections and futilely trying to simulate intercourse."

> *The day of going into a sleazy theater and having a rat crawl up your leg is over.*
> —ANN MYERS PERRY, PRESIDENT OF THE ADULT FILM ASSOCIATION OF AMERICA, 1977

Video not only hugely increased the porn audience but also changed its nature. Almost all patrons of X-rated cinemas had been men, but within a few years, 33 percent of adult videos were being rented by male-female couples, only then followed by men alone (26 percent), women alone (21 percent), male couples (12 percent), and female couples (8 percent).

Some adult-film personalities initially welcomed the shift to video and home viewing. ANNETTE HAVEN said in 1982, "The ladies watch the films while the men are away at work, and the men get together and watch the films after the ladies have gone to bed. . . . They'll watch them together maybe next year. Then a couple of years after that, they'll be watching them with their neighbors, and a couple of years after that, it'll be, 'Come on, Mabel, why don't we go down to the local theater and watch this adult movie on the big screen?' " Nobody anticipated that Hollywood would meet this new competition by increasing the amount of sexuality in mainstream films, and put such high-budget porn out of business.

By the early 1990s, about three hundred video porn cassettes were being issued every year in the United States, and 70 percent of all adult programming had shifted to Los Angeles, where technicians and equipment were cheaper and more readily available. Distribution ranged from ten thousand to fifty thousand copies for a hit. (Today, the number of titles has risen to fourteen thousand. The industry earns an estimated

$57 billion worldwide annually, $20 billion in the United States alone, where some eight hundred million titles are rented each year.)

Even more influential was the introduction in the mid-1980s of the home video recorder, allowing amateurs to create their own pornography, a possibility explored in the 1989 film *sex, lies and videotape*. The porn industry began buying it up for commercial resale, turning some talented enthusiasts into stars in their own sex lives.

The INTERNET gave added impetus to the spread of video porn. As well as the possibilities of purchasing erotic DVDs online without the necessity of visiting the rental store, services such as X-Tube acted as showcases of both amateur and professional porn, with the option of downloading the material directly to your computer.

VORONOFF, Serge Abrahamovitch (1866–1951). Surgeon, biologist, and medical experimenter.

As director of the Laboratoire de Chirurgie Expérimentale at the Collège de France, Russian-born Voronoff became famous for transplanting the organs of primates into human beings as an aid to rejuvenation. In his Villa Molière clinic in suburban Paris, he treated five hundred men between 1920 and 1929, either by implanting monkey organs, particularly testicles, or injecting the men with extracts from monkey glands. In his 1924 book *Forty-Three Grafts from Monkey to Man*, Voronoff claimed an 88 percent improvement in the patients' physical and mental state. Many men also claimed to be sexually rejuvenated by the surgery, but clinical trials never substantiated this.

Inspired, Voronoff transplanted simian ovaries into women as a "cure" for menopause, then implanted a human ovary in Nora, a monkey, which he tried to inseminate with human sperm. Not surprisingly, no child resulted, but the same year, Félicien Champsaur, whose sensational novels celebrated sexual depravity from ancient Rome to bohemian Montparnasse, wrote *Nora, Le Guenon Devenue Femme* (*Nora, The She-Monkey Turned Woman*). Nora evolves into a woman after being implanted with the ovaries of a Russian princess and a man's pineal gland. She becomes a star of the Paris stage with "her fantastic *ballet nègre*." Illustrations to the first printing show Nora dancing near-naked wearing a skirt of bananas identical to that worn by JOSEPHINE BAKER.

Even when the medical world largely rejected Voronoff's theories, doctors continued to apply them. Maurice Girodias credited a course of monkey gland injections with his decision to found the erotic OLYMPIA PRESS. Voronoff himself died from syphilis, supposedly contracted from one of his own transplants. During the 1990s there was speculation that his experiments might have been instrumental in importing the AIDS virus from primates into humans. See AIDS; BAKER, Josephine; OLYMPIA PRESS.

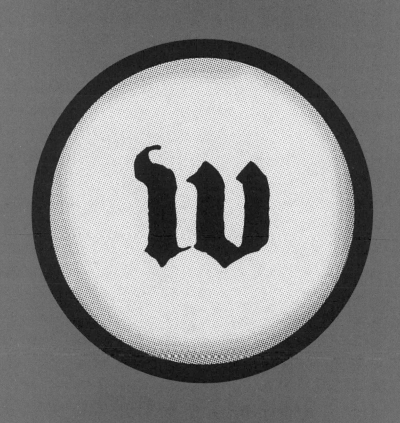

WARHOL, Andy (*né* Andrew Warhola) (1928–1987). American artist.

"Art will be remembered with distaste," Warhol decreed. "Westerns, pornography, science fiction, rock 'n' roll, Pop Art paintings are the supernatural truth, the unreal place where you really are, the place where your vision is." None of Warhol's work was outright pornography, but the films shot in his East Forty-seventh Street Factory shared porn's seedy settings and minimal technique. *Blow Job* (1963) tweaked the staid straight establishment by showing a forty-minute act of fellatio, but recording only the handsome face of the young man being fellated. *FUCK* (aka *BLUE MOVIE*) included thirty-three minutes of his stars Viva and Louis Waldon copulating—but in a film two hours long.

Though his graphic work was seldom erotic, Warhol, who was preoccupied with Hollywood and the evanescent nature of stardom, used sex extensively in his films. Many featured a roster of synthetic stars whom he had created, including Viva, Ultra Violet, Holly Woodlawn, and Candy Darling. In 1968, Valerie Solanas, mentally unstable founder of the Society for Cutting Up Men (SCUM), shot and almost killed Warhol. Ironically, her intended victim had been MAURICE GIRODIAS, whose OLYMPIA PRESS had published her *SCUM Manifesto*.

In the late 1970s, after visiting S&M clubs such as THE MINE SHAFT, Warhol became preoccupied with their imagery, and began his series of *Chemical* or *Piss Paintings*. After treating canvases with copper paint, he paid men to urinate on them, sometimes feeding them vitamin pills to change the chemistry of the urine. For the *Torso* pictures, Victor Hugo, a protégé of the designer Halston, arranged photo sessions for Warhol in his Nineteenth Street loft, paying young gay hustlers to perform in orgies. Warhol hovered around the edges, snapping POLAROIDS, then hurrying into the toilet for a private "organza." See PHONE SEX.

WATERPOWER (1977). U.S. film. Written and directed by Shaun Costello.

Porn film inspired by the activities of Richard Kenyon, THE ENEMA BANDIT. Costello cast JAMIE GILLIS, well known for his involvement in violent porn, and based the film on Martin Scorsese's *Taxi Driver*, even to using some of Bernard Herrmann's score. The result was an eerily accurate picture of the underside of the increasingly respectable adult erotica industry.

The twitching Gillis is excited to orgasm watching an enema being administered to a woman at the GARDEN OF EDEN, a club for bondage devotees, sadomasochists, and cross-dressers. As his first victim, he chooses that most seductive of uniformed women, an airline stewardess. Having spied on her through a telescope making love, he feels justified. "She's dirty," he reflects. "Just a toilet. If I cleaned her out she would be clean again. She'd thank me. She'd be glad I cleaned her out." He's finally tracked down by a cop played by C. J. Laing, noted in the porn world for her propensity for S&M roles.

But *Waterpower* was too raw for U.S. audiences. Its mafia financiers even reissued it, unsuccessfully, with GERARD DAMIANO's name on it, hoping people would be attracted by an association with *DEEP THROAT*. Finally they sold it to producer-distributor Reuben Sturman, who retitled it *Schpritz* and released it in continental Europe, where it was a huge success. French critic Pierre Gras hailed it as a "sulphurously Gothic masterpiece . . . joyously murky, *Waterpower* is a metaphor for the fantasy world of American hard-core which would like to rid, by sexual violence, Hollywood of its prudery. Jamie Gillis, a barbarous and Dionysiac brute, officiates genially over this Satanic Hollywood." See AVIATION; BONDAGE; CROSS-DRESSING.

In the fall of 1976, I was [rung by] Sid Levine, the front man for the porno unit of the Gambino crime family. I was their largest supplier of feature product. . . . He didn't waste any time. "Look, I'm a grandfather and I'm ashamed to have to ask you this, but they need an enema movie." Sid has been given an audio cassette recording of something called The Enema Bandit, *which has a scene where an effete Doctor, assisted by an evil nurse, is giving an enema to a bound and gagged young girl.*

—SHAUN COSTELLO

WATER SPORTS (1980s–present). Slang for all sex acts involving enemas or urine. See UROLAGNIA.

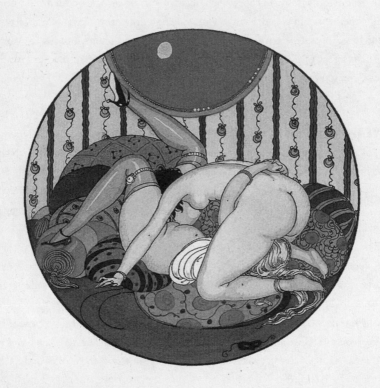

GERDA WEGENER LESBIAN IMAGE, 1920S

WEGENER, Gerda (1889-1940). Danish-born illustrator.

Wegener was among the most distinctive and flamboyant of the foreign artists who flocked to Paris before World War I. Her bisexual husband, Einar, posed for both her male and female characters. Wegener coolly introduced him as her sister-in-law, "Lily Elbe," a persona he assumed after becoming the first surgical transsexual. The couple amicably divorced, and Elbe married one of their male friends. Elbe hoped a further operation would allow her to bear children, but she died in 1931, probably from a failed ovarian transplant. Wegener subsequently became famous for her colorful erotic illustrations, often with lesbian themes.

WELL OF LONELINESS, THE (1928). UK novel, by RADCLYFFE HALL.

The Well of Loneliness describes the romantic relationship between Stephen Gordon, an upper-class Englishwoman who owes her male name to the fact that her parents hoped for a son, and Mary Llewellyn, whom she meets while serving as an ambulance driver in World War I. Unlike male homosexuality, lesbianism was not illegal in Britain, but Sapphic tendencies were regarded, in the words of one character, as the "unnatural cravings of [an] unbalanced mind and undisciplined body." Ostracized by their families, Stephen and Mary move to Paris, where they become members of the flourishing gay culture.

Hall meant the book as a tract in support of lesbian acceptance, and overloaded it with psychological and sexological references. It is reticent about sex—"and that night, they were not divided" is as close as it comes to an erotic description—but a British judge ruled it obscene for defending "unnatural practices between women," and the editor of London's *Sunday Express* fulminated, "I would rather give a healthy boy or a healthy girl a phial of prussic acid than this novel." The book's British publishers, Jonathan Cape, resourcefully backed a bootleg printing in Paris that sold even better than the British edition, and the book has never been out of print since.

The CROSS-DRESSING style of Hall's characters and their habit of addressing each other by surnames, like British clubmen, resonated with the GARÇONNE fad to create a style that soon became the dominant one for lesbians, leading to the aggressively male butch, or bull dyke, stereotype. A reaction to a more feminine style led to the emergence of the LIPSTICK LESBIAN.

WEST, Mae (*née* Mary Jane West) (1893-1980). American actress and playwright.

During the 1930s, few Hollywood personalities were as vulnerable to "impressionists" as Mae West. All it took was a hand on one hip, a sly sideways look, and the drawled "Come up and see me sometime." No matter that West never used this line, any more than Bogart said, "Play it again, Sam." What made the line work was its frank offer of sexual favors. With West, the come-on of the street whore infiltrated the drawing rooms of America.

Mary Jane West was born in Brooklyn into a vaudeville family. She started her career at five, and by fourteen was billed as "The Baby Vamp." A large bust and her six-inch platform shoes made walking difficult, so she developed a trademark hip-swinging stroll, and a variation on the provocative SHIMMY. Impatient with the feeble theatrical material on offer, she began writing plays, but it wasn't until 1926 that one of them, *SEX*, got onstage. Subsequent dramas such as *The Drag* and *Pleasure Man*, involving male homosexuality, cross-dressing, and even castration, did less well, but in 1928 *Diamond Lil* became a ma-

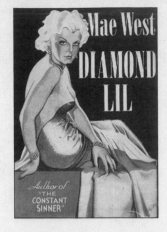

jor Broadway success, on the strength of which West won a small movie role opposite George Raft in *Night After Night* (1932). She rewrote her lines, starting with the first scene. A hatcheck girl exclaims, "Goodness, what lovely diamonds," and West responds, deadpan, "Goodness had nothing to do with it, dearie." Raft said resentfully, "She stole everything but the cameras."

Critics such as Graham Greene praised West. "The big-busted carnivorous creature in tight white sequins sits as firmly and inscrutably for inspection as the tattooed women in the pleasure arcades. The husky voice drones, the plump jewelled fingers pluck, the eyes slant . . ." But her films and others like them jolted Hollywood into establishing the self-censoring PRODUCTION CODE, forcing West into innuendo. "I've been places and seen things," boasts one lover. "That's funny," purrs West. "I've been things and seen places." Even more famously, she enquired, "Is that a gun in your pocket, or are you just happy to see me?"

West's films saved Paramount during the Depression, and by 1936 she was the United States' highest-paid woman. However, tightening censorship, as well as her age, forced her screen retirement. She wrote a bestselling autobiography, appeared on radio, and in stage shows where she could surround herself with bodybuilders and husky men in uniform. She attributed her apparent agelessness to a daily ENEMA and to repeated massages with cold cream. Salvador Dalí designed a couch that imitated her lips, and World War II air-men, after one look at their puffy flotation vests, called them "Mae Wests."

WET DREAM FESTIVAL (1970–1971). Short-lived Amsterdam event.

Two Wet Dream Festivals were held in Amsterdam, in 1970 and 1971, under the auspices of the magazine *SUCK*, and directed by one of its editors, James Haynes. A jury watched what Haynes called a "four-days-long orgy of smut films" and awarded first prize to *A Summer Day*, a documentary about BODIL JOENSEN, Danish star of ZOO-PHILIA porn. A retrospective award went to JEAN GENET'S *CHANT D'AMOUR*. Also honored was *The New Adventures of Snow White*, an erotic animated version in the series *Grimms Marchen von Lusternen Parchen*.

A second festival took place in October 1971. Though films were shown, the focus had shifted. Haynes told *Variety*, "We are not concerned with pornographic aspects primarily, but with the libertarian concept. It is an attack on paternalism because it asks why people can't see any image they want." To this end, "Love Rooms" were provided, and performance artist Otto Muehl invited to appear. Following a lesbian exhibition by two women, Muehl displayed a live goose, and announced that he would decapitate the bird, cover the severed neck with a condom, and use it to penetrate one of them. When animal-loving members of the audience prevented this from taking place, Muehl expressed his contempt by defecating onstage.

No third festival was held, although co-organizer William Levy did discuss a theater event to take place on a boat, during which all participants, either singly or in groups, would be required to achieve orgasm.

WHAT THE BUTLER SAW. Generic title for the mildly erotic short films shown on the earliest form of cinema, the arcade Mutoscope or Kinetoscope machines, where a penny bought a one-minute story on a continuous loop of film or, in cheaper versions, a succession of flip cards. So many of these films showed servants spying on their betters that Kinetoscopes became known as "What The Butler Saw" machines.

WHITEHOUSE, Mary (*née* Constance Mary Hutcheson) (1910-2000). British social reformer.

Whitehouse, a Catholic ex-teacher, became convinced of "a conspiracy to remove the myth of God from the mind of man." In 1965, she formed the National Viewers' and Listeners' Association, and launched a "Clean Up TV" campaign, harrying the government and in particular the BBC, as well as sex shops and events or publications that she saw as outrages against public decency. Where the law refused to act, she brought private prosecutions. Targets included the magazine *Gay News*, over a poem by James Kirkup, and the National Theatre's production of Howard Brenton's *Romans in Britain*, in which two actors, playing Roman soldiers, mimed the anal rape of a Briton. The latter suit failed because the witness sent by the NVLA had sat too far back in the theater to be sure whether the actor used his penis and not, as the performer insisted, a thumb. Her opponents parodied Whitehouse vigorously. DAVID SULLIVAN named one of his porn magazines *WHITE-HOUSE*, and the BBC a radio comedy program *The Mary Whitehouse Experience*. Though she won widespread notoriety, there's little sign that her efforts were successful.

WHORE. Prostitute, or, as a verb, to act as a prostitute, or, in a larger sense, to exploit your skills exclusively for gain. From the old German *horon*, a "female adulterer." Also HO or HOE.

A particularly damaging epithet, the term *whore* doesn't lose its power even as the German *hure* or the French *putain*, which has become an all-purpose curse, the Gallic equivalent of *fuck*.

Corrupted to *ho*, the word, like *nigger*, became common currency in U.S. street slang and rap lyrics, to the extent that both words lost their power as insults so long as they were used within the African American or gang community. A failure to realize this cost New York "shock jock" Don Imus his job in 2007, when he referred to members of the Rutgers University women's basketball team as "nappy-headed hos." During the ensuing uproar, rap star Snoop Dogg precisely defined the variant meanings of *ho* as used by him and by Imus. "We are not talking about no collegiate basketball girls," he told *MTV News*. "We're talking about hos that's in the 'hood that ain't doing shit, that's trying to get a nigga for his money. These are two separate things." See PROSTITUTE.

WHOREHOUSE. Antique term for a BROTHEL, or BORDELLO.

Whorehouse returned to general use in the 1970s and 1980s, beginning in 1969 with William Bowers's screenplay for the comedy Western *Support Your Local Sheriff*, which slyly named the town "hostess" Madame Orr and had Jack Elam explain he was "a horse-holder at Madame Orr's house." Ironically, the reemergence of the word occurred just as brothels were falling out of favor, supplanted by the MASSAGE PARLOR and the CALL GIRL. See *THE BEST LITTLE WHOREHOUSE IN TEXAS*.

WIFE-SWAPPING. See SWINGING.

WINDMILL THEATRE (1932–1966). London BURLESQUE theater.

In 1932, after failing as a venue for drama and foreign films, the Windmill Theatre in London's SOHO, owned by Laura Henderson, widow of a wealthy grower of jute in India, and managed by Vivian Van Damm, launched *Revuedeville*, a Paris-style program of continuous comedy, dancing, and music, enlivened by nude showgirls. Restrictions imposed by the LORD CHAMBERLAIN required that the girls remain immobile. All the same, audiences crowded the theater, even during the Blitz. The theater was bombed by the Luftwaffe, and an electrician killed, but shows continued, with the management proudly advertising "We Never Closed." Mrs. Henderson died in 1944, but Van Damm carried on until the 1960s, when the theater became a strip club.

Windmill shows gave many young Englishmen their first look at a nude woman— ostensibly Mrs. Henderson's motive, since her own son had died in World War I as a sexual innocent. A version of the Windmill was depicted in the 1942 musical *Tonight and Every Night*, with Rita Hayworth; in *Murder at the Windmill* (1949); and in Stephen Frears's *Mrs. Henderson Presents* (2005).

WOLF MAN, THE (*Der Wolfsmann*) (*né* Sergei Konstantinovitch Pankejeff or Pankeyev (1886–1979).

Pseudonym given by SIGMUND FREUD to his patient Sergei Pankeyev, who dreamed persistently of a tree full of white wolves. "It was night and I was lying in my bed.

Suddenly the window opened of its own accord, and I was terrified to see that some white wolves were sitting on the big walnut tree in front of the window. There were six or seven of them. The wolves were quite white, and looked more like foxes or sheep-dogs, for they had big tails like foxes and they had their ears pricked like dogs when they pay attention to something. In great terror, evidently of being eaten up by the wolves, I screamed and woke up." Freud deduced that Pankeyev had witnessed the PRIMAL SCENE of his parents having sex, probably "doggie fashion," or, alternatively, had witnessed dogs copulating. The case was central to Freud's 1914 paper *"Aus der Geschichte einer infantilen Neurose"* ("From the History of an Infantile Neurosis"). Even though Freud eventually declared his treatment over, Pankeyev, whose father and sister both committed suicide, was troubled by psychoses for the rest of his life. See FREUD, Sigmund.

WONDER WOMAN (1941–present). American comic book character.

Created, improbably, by William Moulton Marston, an academic best known as the inventor of the polygraph, or lie detector, *Wonder Woman* first appeared in *All Star Comics* #8, in December 1941. Ostensibly, she was based on the Greek goddess Artemis. Marston claimed that each element of her costume—skimpy bustier and skirt, knee-high red boots with spiked heels, and wrist bands—derived from some Greek deity, while her "Lasso of Truth" was created from the golden girdle of Gaea. Neither DC Comics nor the public seemed aware that character, costume, and stories of *Wonder Woman* celebrated classic FETISH tastes, or that Marston, an enthusiast for sexual BONDAGE, lived openly in a ménage-à-trois with his wife and a young student.

In addition to comic books, the character was featured in a 1975–1979 TV series starring Lynda Carter (ironically a born-again Christian), and in the *Super Friends* and *Justice League* animated series. Bondage enthusiasts, for obvious reasons, enjoyed *Wonder Woman*, and fetish artist ERIC STANTON parodied her in his own strip *Blunder Broad*. Through the early 2000s, Hollywood producer Joel Silver was engaged in trying to film a *Wonder Woman* feature.

WOOD. Porn film term for a hard penis. Hence "waiting for wood"—a delay in filming caused by a performer's inability to achieve an erection.

WORKING GIRL (U.S. slang, 1920s–present). Prostitute. Term invented to distinguish whores from "business girls," who had legitimate office jobs.

> *"'I don't like that man,' said the young stenographer. 'I said something about getting up early every morning and going down town. He raised his eyebrows, sort of surprised and interested, and asked me: "Oh, do you work?" . . . "I go to business," I told him. The very idea—him trying to make me out a working girl.'"*
>
> —*New York Herald*, February 1924

WORLD MODELING. Los Angeles agency founded in 1976 by Jim South in the suburb of Van Nuys, in the San Fernando Valley, much used by adult-film producers and photographers.

For decades, World Modeling has been one of the main companies channeling new talent into the world of magazine and video erotica. Its ubiquitous ads—GIRLS! EARN $250 A DAY AS A FIGURE MODEL! NO EXP. NEEDED!—made it the point of first contact for many later-prominent porn stars, e.g., GINGER LYNN and COLLEEN APPLEGATE.

WORMS. Prisoners in Russian jails are said to volunteer for garden duty not out of a love for nature and fresh air, but to gather earthworms, which, confined in a small jar, act as a surrogate vagina.

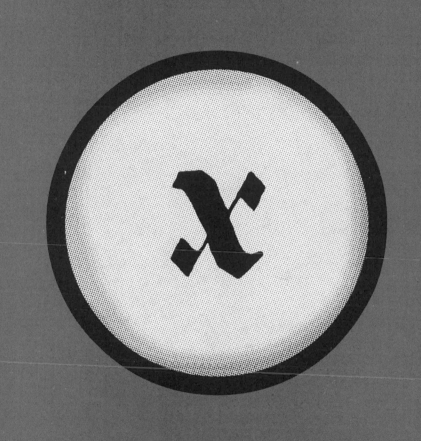

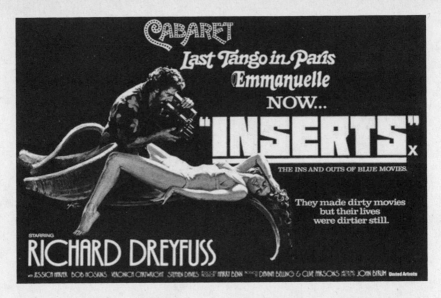

MAKING THE MOST OF AN X. EXTRAVAGANT PROMOTION BY A LONDON CINEMA FOR THE RELATIVELY MODEST FILM *INSERTS*

X-RATED.

Traditionally, the letter *X* signifies the forbidden, while its repetition, as in XXX, indicates conspicuously high quality or strength, as in alcohol. In science or mathematics, *X* can also designate an undiscovered or unknown element, as in the TV series *The X Files*, about supposedly hidden evidence of extraterrestrial and paranormal phenomena.

All these senses converge in the use of *X* to indicate images or texts too erotic or terrifying for general audiences. In 1951, the British Board of Film Censors introduced the first "X" certificate, signifying a film that could be seen only by people over sixteen. The American film industry's self-censorship body adopted a similar rating in 1968, effectively barring any X-rated film from general exhibition, except in "adult" cinemas. Producers and exhibitors saddled with an X rating had two alternatives: Some butchered the films until they met censorship guidelines. Others made a virtue of necessity and exploited the catchpenny connotations of "X," either by designating their product in multiples—"XXXXX"—or incorporating the letter into slogans, e.g., "X Was Never Like This," used to promote *EMMANUELLE*.

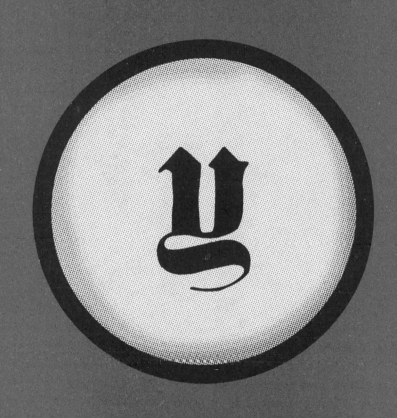

YEAGER, Bunny (*née* Linnea Eleanor Yeager) (1930–). U.S. glamour photographer.

Best known for having imported BETTIE PAGE into the glamour mainstream from the world of fetishist bondage and S&M. After early success as a blond beauty queen but failure as merchandiser of her own line of swimwear, Yeager moved into photography, where she enjoyed the considerable advantage of being sufficiently beautiful to act as her own model. In 1954 a friend introduced her to Page, who spent her holidays in Florida. They worked together on a number of photo series, including some famous shots with cheetahs at Africa USA, a local petting zoo. Initially Page was the benefactor in this relationship, since Yeager had little money to pay her. However, her shots were accepted by *PLAYBOY*, boosting Page to an entirely new level of public awareness. Yeager subsequently shot a number of centerfolds for *PLAYBOY*, and remained the preeminent female glamour photographer of her generation.

YIFF (slang, 1990s–present). Shorthand term for the branch of ZOOPHILIA involving sex with dogs. Said to be imitative of the yelp of a fox. See FURVERT.

YODEL IN THE VALLEY (U.S. slang, 1970s). Synonym for cunnilingus.

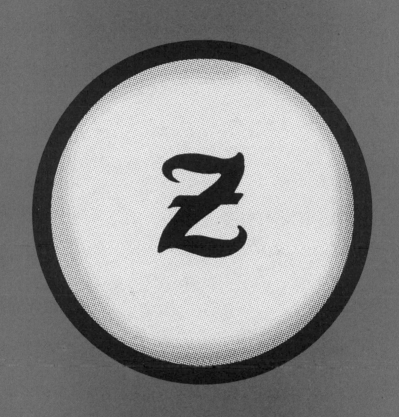

ZIPLESS FUCK. See *FEAR OF FLYING.*

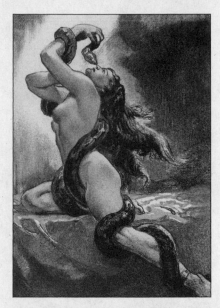

IMAGE FROM FRENCH EDITION OF GUSTAVE FLAU-
BERT'S *SALAMMBO*, SHOWING CARTHAGINIAN
PRIESTESS OF SNAKE CULT

ZOOPHILIA. Sexual intercourse with animals.

Zoophilia, sometimes called bestiality, appears in the erotic art and literature of all centuries. Dogs, goats, and chickens feature most commonly, though in *Gamiani, or Two Nights of Excess* (1833), Alfred de Musset describes his heroine enjoying sex with a donkey, a large dog, and an orangutan. In modern times, Port Said in Egypt was often mentioned as the site of exhibitions featuring women and donkeys.

Nevertheless, zoophilia mostly belongs with CONCEPTUAL SEX ACTS, more written about than performed.

Apes, as the closest creature to man, featured often in fantasies of animal sex. Experiments in Paris in the 1920s by SERGE VORONOFF in transplanting simian sex organs into humans triggered a rash of books about monkeys mating with women, including Felicien Champsaur's *Nora: La Guenon Devenue Femme*, and *Ouha: Roi des Singes* (*Ouha, King of the Monkeys*), about a lost white girl in the jungle and her rescue by a giant monkey. The book is dedicated to Voronoff.

Books about apes as sexual predators inspired Edgar Wallace's screenplay "The Beast," which became *King Kong* (1933). Howard Schulman's 1974 play *Censored Scenes from King Kong* even suggested that the original *Kong* showed sex between the ape and Fay Wray—in fact impossible, for no other reason than the giant ape was created from models and a few body parts—notably a face and a hand. In a very real sense, King Kong didn't exist.

The worldwide explosion of pornographic film in the 1960s and 1970s encouraged filmmakers and photographers to realize zoophilic fantasies. GEORGINA SPELVIN played with a python in *THE DEVIL IN MISS JONES*. For the 1978 porn feature *Different Strokes*, the director persuaded a dog to perform cunnilingus by having the actress's vagina stuffed with candy. (The scene, if indeed shot, never appeared in the film.) LINDA LOVELACE experienced no such problems with her appearance in *DOG FUCK*. Canine zoophilia subsequently became sufficiently popular to engender its own sexual sub-speciality, generally referred to as YIFF. Enthusiasts for zoophilia covered a wide range. In 1990, DEA agents raided the Berry Park estate of rock star Chuck Berry in Wentzville,

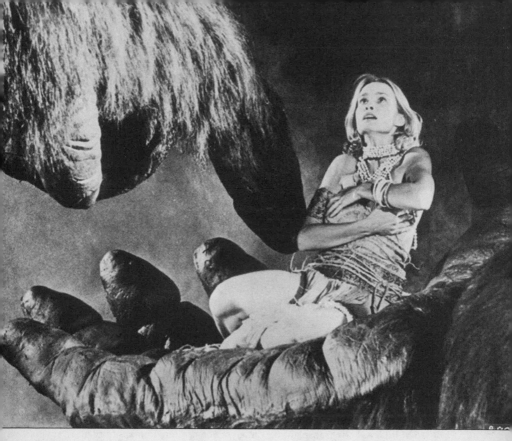

JESSICA LANGE IN THE HANDS OF A NONEXISTENT GIANT APE IN THE 1976 REMAKE OF *KING KONG*

Mississippi, and seized drugs, cash, sex videos, and eight-millimeter amateur zoophilia films.

During the 1970s, DENMARK and SWEDEN emerged as the major sources of animal porn, much of it starring Danish performer BODIL JOENSON and featuring not only dogs and pigs but also horses. Despite the horses being strongly fetishized, sex involving them has usually ended with nude riding and, very occasionally, the ritual mutilations described in Peter Schaffer's play *Equus*. Actual sex with horses beyond the fellatio demonstrated by Bodil Joenson is hazardous, as proved in 2005, when forty-five-year-old Kenneth Pinyan died of a perforated colon, near Seattle, Washington, after being penetrated by an Arab stallion.

Acknowledgments

An exhaustive list of the people who contributed to *Carnal Knowledge* would include the schoolmate who whispered that first incomprehensible anecdote about a traveling salesman and the farmer's daughter; the visitor from Europe who, after a visit to my childhood home, left behind an album of discreetly airbrushed female nudes; and the movie projectionist who invited an impressionable adolescent to view his collection of blue movies.

However, since the specific impulse to compile this book began about twenty years ago, during a two-year stay in Los Angeles, I owe the greatest debt of gratitude to those Angelenos who introduced me in the luxuriant garden of erotica that flourishes under California's sun.

Chief among these is the late William Rotsler, my witty and perceptive guide through that world of the flesh to which he devoted most of his life. Curtis Harrington, also sadly lost to us, shared with me his memories of working with Marlene Dietrich and Sylvia Kristel, while Kelvin Jones lent his photographic expertise to encounters with Ginger Lynn Allen, Hyapatia Lee, George "Big Mac" McDonald, and the members of the X-Rated Critics' Organization.

Otherwise, I can do no better than follow X-rated star Randy West who, in accepting the "Heart-On" for Best Sizzling Support (Male) at the 1989 X-Rated Critics' Organization Awards, thanked "all the women who made it hard for me, and all the men who made it easy for me."

Among the latter, I'm particularly grateful to the bibliographers, collectors, critics, and academics who were unstinting with their advice and assistance. These include the late John Brosnan and Bernardino Zapponi, and the happily living David Burke, Dr. Kristin Duncombe, Roger Faligot, Joel Finler, Terrance Gelenter, Anton Gill, David Hamilton, Charles Higham, Neil Hornick and Image Diggers, Patrick Kearney, Wolfgang Kuhlmey, Robert Lichtman, Patrick McGilligan, Michael Neal, Neil Pearson, Nicholas Pounder, Dr. Martin Simpson, Martin Stone, David Thompson, James Tindley, and Bill Warren. I am no less grateful to Anne Billson, Heather Hartley, Toni Johnson-Woods, Minor Knight, Anne LeChartier, Philippa Joy Thornton, and Carolyn See.

Specifically, however, and for reasons she least of all will understand,
this book is for Vickie Lynch, aka Hyapatia Lee.

"Thou wast not born for death, immortal Bird!"

PHOTOGRAPHIC CREDITS

A Bigger Splash. Copyright 1974 New Line Cinema.

Amarcord. Copyright 1974 New World Pictures.

Barbarella. Copyright 1968 Paramount Pictures Corporation.

Blonde Venus. Copyright 1932 Paramount Pictures Corporation.

Blue Movie (aka *Fuck*). Copyright 1972 Andy Warhol Films.

Caligula. Copyright 1982 Analysis Film Releasing Organization.

Candy. Copyright 1968 Buena Vista Pictures.

Come Play with Me. Copyright 1979 Tigon Pictures.

Confessions from the David Galaxy Affair. Copyright 1979 Tigon Pictures.

Diamonds Are Forever. Copyright 1971 United Artists.

Emmanuelle. Copyright 1974 Columbia Pictures Corporation.

Everything You Always Wanted to Know About Sex* *But Were Afraid to Ask. Copyright 1972 United
    Artists.

Fando and Lis. Copyright 1968 Cannon Film Distributors.

Gypsy. Copyright 1962 Warner Brothers Pictures.

Hardcore. Copyright 1979 Columbia Pictures Corporation.

Histoire D'O. Copyright 1975 Allied Artists.

The Illustrated Man. Copyright 1969 Warner Brothers/Seven Arts.

Inserts. Copyright 1974 United Artists.

King Kong. Copyright 1976 Paramount Pictures.

Lady Chatterley's Lover. Copyright 1981 Cannon Film Distributors.

A Life of Her Own. Copyright 1950 Metro-Goldwyn-Mayer.

Love and Death. Copyright 1975 United Artists.

Love Happy. Copyright 1949 United Artists.

Maitresse. Copyright 1976 Tinc Films.

Marilyn Monroe. Courtesy of New York World-Telegram and the Sun Newspaper Photograph
    Collection

9 $\frac{1}{2}$ Weeks. Copyright 1986 Metro-Goldwyn-Mayer.

Orphee. Copyright 1950 DisCina International.

The Wife Swappers. Copyright 1970 TransAmerican Films.

Women in Love. Copyright 1969 United Artists.

COVER GRAPHICS

Crash. Cover design by Bill Botten. Copyright Jonathan Cape 1973.

TEXTS

Christopher and His Kind by Christopher Isherwood (Farrar, Strauss and Giroux, 1976).

Memoirs of Hecate County by Edmund Wilson (Doubleday, 1946).

Sex in Australia by Gael Knepper. (J & G Publishing, Sydney, 1984).

"Echoes of the Jazz Age" from *The Crack-Up* by F. Scott Fitzgerald. (Norton, 1964).

Justine by Lawrence Durrell. (Dutton, 1988).

Wlt: A Radio Romance by Garrison Keillor. (Viking Penguin, 1991).

Poème by Louis Aragon, translated by "Zoltan Lizot-Picon" i.e., Christopher Sawyer-Laucanno and Mark Polizotti. (Alyscamps Press, Paris, 1996) .